THE
COLUMBIA
ENCYCLOPEDIA
OF
NUTRITION

THE
COLUMBIA
ENCYCLOPEDIA
OF
N U T R I T I O N

THE INSTITUTE OF HUMAN NUTRITION, COLUMBIA UNIVERSITY
COLLEGE OF PHYSICIANS AND SURGEONS

COMPILED AND EDITED BY

MYRON WINICK, M.D., BRIAN L. G. MORGAN, PH.D.,

JAIME ROZOVSKI, PH.D., AND ROBIN MARKS-KAUFMAN, PH.D.

G. P. Putnam's Sons
New York

G. P. Putnam's Sons
Publishers Since 1838
200 Madison Avenue
New York, NY 10016

Library of Congress Cataloging-in-Publication Data

The Columbia encyclopedia of nutrition.
Includes index.
1. Nutrition—Dictionaries. I. Winick, Myron.
II. Columbia University. Institute of Human Nutrition.
[DNLM: 1. Nutrition—encyclopedias—popular works.
QU 13 E56]
QP141.C69   1987   613.2′03′21   87-10782
ISBN 0-399-13298-8

Printed in the United States of America
1   2   3   4   5   6   7   8   9   10

Acknowledgments

We would like to thank the following past and present members of the faculty of the Institute of Human Nutrition, Columbia University College of Physicians and Surgeons, and the School of Dentistry and Oral Surgery for their help in compiling this encyclopedia: Drs. Pedro Rosso, Xavier Pi-Sunyer, Irwin Mandel, Louis Steinberg, Stephen ·Atwood, and Henry Sebrell, and Ms. Maudene Nelson. In addition, we would also like to express our appreciation for all the work put in by our staff, and in particular Faye Seltzer, for their help in typing and preparing the manuscript. Finally, thanks go to our editors, Adrienne Ingrum and Anton Mueller, for their help and advice at every stage of the manuscript and to Bill Adler, our agent, for his support during the project.

Introduction

In the last twenty years there has been a gradual heightening of interest in the prevention of chronic disease and the promotion of health among the millions of people who are not overtly ill. With this interest in disease prevention and wellness promotion has come a new interest in nutrition. Perhaps the oldest medical science, long neglected since it has been displaced by specific drug therapy, nutrition has become a major concern of the public at large and more and more it is becoming a major concern of the medical profession.

Evidence has become irrefutable that the right diet can lower certain people's risk for developing some of the most serious diseases afflicting our society. Conversely, the wrong diet can decrease longevity and increase the risk for these same diseases. Heart disease, cancer, osteoporosis, high blood pressure, obesity, anemia, and many other diseases are related to the food we eat.

In addition to preventing disease, there is some evidence that the quality of our lives can be affected by our diets. Our performance at work or school, our ability to participate in athletics, even the time it takes to fall asleep at night may depend to some extent on the food we eat and on the time we eat it. Finally, we are becoming more and more aware that proper nutrition varies among different individuals. Requirements for various nutrients differ for women and men; for children and adults; for the middle aged and elderly; for those pregnant and lactating, and even among different racial and ethnic groups.

This new awareness by the public and by health professionals has not been ignored by commercial interests anxious to promote a product or a nutritional scheme which brings financial gain. Nutrition has become big business. Hundreds of millions of dollars are spent on weight reduction schemes which are scientifically unsound and which do not work. In addition huge sums are being spent on nutritional supplements touted to do everything from curing baldness to preventing enlargement of the prostate gland. Often these substances are innocuous compounds for which people use their hard earned money in the hope of avoiding difficulty later on or even worse curing some disease for which no nutritional treatment is known. Sometimes, and especially when taken in large amounts, the substances advocated may be dangerous.

"Nutrition education" comes from radio and television commercials, from an assortment of magazine articles, from government documents, from supermarket promotions, even from word of mouth.

Perhaps at no time has there been a greater need for an authoritative book on the subject of nutrition to document what is known and what is not known; what dietary changes are appropriate and what are not; when supplements should be taken and when they are unnecessary; which supplements may be dangerous and at what levels. For this reason the authors of this volume decided to undertake the task of writing an encyclopedia of nutrition. This book is not, nor does it seek to be, totally comprehensive, covering in depth all aspects of nutrition. Rather, it has focused on those issues in nutrition and diet which most concern us in our desire to lower our risk for certain diseases and to promote good health and well being.

The editorial board is composed of professionals who have specialized in nutrition and who are currently or were recently on the faculty of Columbia University's College of Physicians and Surgeons. They have tried to evaluate all available evidence before reaching a conclusion or recommending dietary modification.

The approach taken in the major entries has been not only to discuss what should be done but also to discuss why it is important. Thus the intent has been, not to simply prescribe a diet or nutritional plan, but to present the evidence as it exists and from that evidence decide on the best practical measures.

The topics covered are extremely varied. From anemia and atherosclerosis to women's nutrition and zinc deficiency. Some topics are covered in much more depth than others, depending on the importance to human health. The book is not an attempt to offer "home remedies" but rather to increase knowledge. For we believe that only with increased knowledge can informed decisions be made. It is only by being informed that people can evaluate the mass of nutrition information, some of it subtly disguised, coming out every day, and make the kind of dietary modifications, if any, which will offer the best chance of lowering their risk for certain chronic diseases and improving the quality of their lives.

Myron Winick, R. R. Williams, Professor of Nutrition and Professor of Pediatrics, Columbia University College of Physicians and Surgeons

THE
COLUMBIA
ENCYCLOPEDIA
OF
NUTRITION

ADDITIVES

The main functions of food additives are to preserve foods in a way that will prevent spoilage and contamination, to improve the taste of foods, and to make foods appear more appetizing. We are totally dependent on food additives to ensure a safe and adequate food supply for our city dwellers. Food is moved thousands of miles from the point of production to the cities, and even with the availability of improved methods of refrigeration the potential for spoilage and contamination with disease-causing bacteria during transit is great. The need for additives to minimize these dangers is obvious. Less clear is the need to add substances merely to improve taste or to restore color, although some would maintain that such substances increase the consumption of nutritious foods.

Recently, people have become disturbed by the increasing use of additives because of proven health risks associated with some of them. Saccharin, the artificial sweetener, is one such substance that has been implicated as a risk factor for bladder cancer. A number of coloring dyes have also been associated with increased cancer risk. Salt, perhaps the oldest food preservative, has been linked to high blood pressure. During the last few years, food additives have also been blamed for hyperactivity in children.

Clearly, this is a difficult area in which to make generalizations. Each additive must be considered individually. The benefits obtained by using a particular additive must be balanced against the risks involved with its use. A good illustration of this would be an additive essential to prevent spoilage. Here we might accept a health risk associated with the additive if it was considerably smaller than the risk of consuming the contaminated food. By comparison, any substance added to food strictly to enhance its appearance (i.e., to improve its color), should not be added to food if it brings with it any significant health risk at all.

Although this may seem simple and logical enough, it has been the center of a great deal of controversy, because any two experts in the field may make different judgments when faced with the same facts. Let us consider the case of saccharin. It improves taste, yes, but are there any other benefits to be derived from its use? Some say yes, because it reduces calories and helps prevent obesity. However, no study has ever shown that saccharin has any significant part to play in a weight-loss program, or that it has any long-term effect on the incidence of obesity. But does saccharin present any significant health hazard in the amounts added to foods? Saccharin given in huge doses to animals does cause cancer. But these doses are never reached by even the most devoted saccharin users. Hence, is the health hazard of any real significance? The law says yes. In 1958, Congress passed the Delaney Clause, which states that any substance added to our food supply causing cancer in even one laboratory animal when administered in any dose must be removed. Saccharin qualified and was ordered off the market. The public outcry was so great that Congress was pressured into passing a special law extending its use. Because of its imprecise nature, the concept of benefit versus risk had moved from the scientific to the political arena.

Because a judgment is involved, the Delaney Clause is at once both too restrictive and not restrictive enough. It is too restrictive because it defines cancer risk in a way which may not be appropriate. It is not restrictive enough because it does not deal with other health risks which may be equally as dangerous as cancer.

The question of food additives and hyperactivity in children is another complicated issue. In 1973, Dr. Benjamin Feingold reported that children diagnosed as hyperactive markedly improved when placed on a diet free of all food additives. This report aroused a great deal of interest because of the large number of children suffering from this disorder. Studies were carried out comparing the additive-free "Feingold Diet" with an equally restricted diet containing food additives. Neither the parents nor the children knew which diet they were following. The results of most of these studies confirmed Dr. Feingold's claim; about half of the children did improve. However, it was not due to the removal of food additives—the same degree of improvement was shown on both diets. The results of one study confused the issue more by showing that there was slightly more improvement in a group of under-three-year-olds on the additive-free diet.

Clearly, these results do not justify the removal of all additives from the food of all hyperactive children. Rather, they show that a change in dietary pattern, with or without the removal of food additives, may be of benefit. There may also be a small number of hyperactive children under three years of age who could benefit from specifically removing food additives from their food. This is not to say that some food additives are not capable of producing hyperactivity in children who are sensitive to them. Red dye II, which is commonly added to foods, has been shown to increase hyperactivity for a short period of time in some already hyperactive children, when administered in large amounts. However, at present there is little evidence to show that food additives, as they are currently used, contribute significantly to the problem of hyperactivity in children.

In this modern society, it is not possible to produce enough food to feed everybody without the use of chemical fertilizers and food preservatives. These substances have, in fact, become a necessary adjunct to life. However, the use of antibiotics in food production has associated with it such major health hazards that the risks clearly outweigh any advantage it may have. Such practices should be banned in the US, as they have been in other western countries.

The decision as to whether or not any additive is used in our food supply should be based on a number of questions. First, why is the additive being used? Second, what are the health risks when a particular additive is used in the amounts added to foods? These risks must be assessed based on the highest cumulative amounts an individual is likely to consume. Obviously, there should be different standards for a preservative as opposed to flavors and colors. Third, if there is a health benefit to be derived from using a particular additive, is there a safer way of achieving the same benefit?

Although the present system of regulating the addition of chemicals to food is far from perfect, our food supply is still one of the safest in the world. (See also ANTIOXIDANTS; ASPARTAME; FOOD PROCESSING.)

ADOLESCENT

During adolescence our food requirements are higher than at any other time in our lives. Failure to meet those needs may delay growth and sexual maturity. Even before adolescence our food intake has a profound effect on sexual maturation. Taller and heavier children tend to reach puberty before thinner and lighter ones. Thus, nutrition has a great impact on the timing and successful completion of the tremendous changes that go on in our bodies as we go through puberty.

NORMAL GROWTH

Boys usually reach puberty somewhere between the ages of twelve and fourteen years, and girls a little earlier, between nine and thirteen years. Boys and girls really grow up at this time in what is termed the "adolescent growth spurt." Usually they gain as much as 15 percent of their adult height. Boys tend to gain more weight at a more rapid rate than girls do during adolescence, which accounts for their higher energy and protein requirements. As one would expect, they lay down much more muscle and less body fat than do girls. It is worth noting that although we attain almost our full height by about twenty years of age, girls can grow approximately another centimeter after that time and boys can grow twice that much. Actually, human muscle mass and skeletal mass are not at a maximum until about forty years of age.

ENERGY AND PROTEIN

Energy and protein needs are high in adolescents because of their rapid growth rate. However, adolescents do tend to eat even more than the usual recommended allowances. Provided that the energy they consume is balanced by their energy expenditure, there is a lot to be said for allowing adolescents to eat according to the dictates of their appetites. However, if this equation does not balance, there will be a tendency to become overweight. Obesity is prevalent among adolescents, and can destroy the child's self-image and impair normal social and psychological development. Fat adolescents are definitely discriminated against by their peers as well as by adults. As a result they can become socially isolated, depressed, and bored, which can cause further overeating, only serving to promote the condition of the obesity.

A reducing diet for obese adolescents must be selected with great care. Severe energy restrictions divert dietary protein to be used for energy instead of for tissue production, which can, in turn, lead to stunted growth. Weight reduction is best achieved by restricting those foods rich in calories, like high fat and high carbohydrate foods. Treating the obesity in a group setting sometimes helps obese children, as the group support they receive improves their self-image and makes giving up those well-loved cookies, cakes, and candies easier to bear. Regular physical exercise can also be useful.

VITAMINS AND MINERALS

Vitamin requirements are increased for all adolescents due to the demands of growth. To meet the increased energy demands, higher than adult levels of thiamine (B_1), riboflavin (B_2), and niacin (B_3) are necessary. They enable a person to break down large quantities of carbohydrates in order to provide energy. Folacin (folic acid) and vitamin B_{12} are both required for tissue growth, so the requirement for these also increases. In addition, skeletal growth necessitates adequate vitamin D intake. Vitamins A, C, and E are all essential to keep this new tissue in working order.

American adolescents tend to fall short of what we consider to be the optimal intake of several vitamins. Some young people take as little as 50 percent of their folacin requirements, which could lead to anemia and stunted growth. Vitamin B_6 deficiency is also prevalent, impairing the body's ability to use dietary protein. There are also signs of less serious deficiencies of vitamins C and A.

As far as minerals go, calcium, iron, and zinc are most likely to be in short supply. All are needed in increased amounts during the growth spurt—calcium for normal skeletal growth; zinc and iron for skeletal and muscle growth. In addition, iron is essential for the increased volume of blood which is now being made by the body to supply the extra growing tissue with nutrients.

The faster a person is growing, the more calcium is needed. The body does its part by retaining more dietary calcium than at other times in the life cycle. However, modern teenagers are doing their best to make calcium deficiency a problem! They drink less milk and eat fewer dairy products—which are practically the only excellent sources of calcium in the American diet. To absorb calcium most efficiently, the diet should have a calcium to phosphorus ratio of 1:1. The more phosphorus, the less calcium absorbed. Our average diet has a ratio of 1:3, because many processed foods, sodas, and meats have such a high phosphorus content.

Between 5 and 15 percent of American adolescents are anemic. Boys increase their muscle mass and blood volume faster than do girls, accounting for their higher dietary need for iron. On the other hand, girls lose about .5 milligrams of iron per day as a result of menstruation. While iron is most easily absorbed from meat, absorption from plant sources, such as beans and green vegetables, can be enhanced if a person consumes a food high in vitamin C, like orange juice, along with the iron-containing food.

Zinc is necessary for growth and sexual maturation. Four hundred milligrams of this mineral are retained per day by the male and a little less by the female. It has been shown that many adolescents consume far less than needed—especially girls, who often consume less than half of the recommended allowance. The richest sources of zinc are meat, seafood, eggs, and milk. Any food containing protein also contains zinc (about 1.5 milligrams of zinc for every 10 grams of animal protein). Vegetable sources like legumes and cereals contain less zinc. Hence, adolescents who are strict vegetarians must pay particular attention to this nutrient. (See VEGETARIAN DIETS.)

As you can see, good nutrition at the time of adolescence is essential for normal growth and development. You might even say that this is the time of your life when you are sowing the seeds of future health. (See entries for specific vitamins and minerals.)

NUTRITIONAL PROBLEMS OF THE PREGNANT ADOLESCENT

Although the actual number of births to mothers under the age of nineteen years is now on the decline, teenagers gave birth to over 17 percent of all babies born in America in 1977 (according to the latest figures) as opposed to 13.9 percent in 1960. This means that 570,000 babies were born to teenage mothers—of which 42,000 were born to girls under the age of sixteen. While the social implications of this situation have created a great deal of concern, the medical aspects of the problem are no less important.

Pregnant teenagers have an increased number of spontaneous abortions, premature deliveries, and complications during pregnancy. These include preeclampsia and eclampsia, diseases characterized by high blood pressure, edema (abnormal accumulation of body fluids), and abnormal kidney function. Juvenile mothers also have a greater number of abnormal deliveries, such as prolonged labor, and require a larger number of cesarean sections. The latter is usually due to a disproportion between the diameter of the pelvis and the infant's head. Obviously, the abnormal deliveries lead to a higher risk of serious complications for both the mother and the infant.

Teenage mothers also have a tendency to have smaller babies than do more mature women. For example, the number of infants weighing less than 5 pounds 8 ounces is two to three times more common in mothers under twenty years of age. These smaller infants are more sensitive to the consequences of a difficult labor and can have more complications during the first days of life than larger infants.

The great majority of full term infants born weighing 5 pounds 8 ounces or less have suffered growth retardation. This means that the mother has not been able to provide the unborn baby with proper nutrition or the other elements necessary for adequate prenatal growth. Fetal growth retardation is a serious problem, especially when it is severe. One of the organs affected by retarded growth is the brain and studies have shown that small babies (who are not premature) are more prone to have learning disabilities, behavioral problems, and lower IQ scores later in life. All these problems are manifestations of a still indeterminate type of brain damage.

The most important factors believed to be responsible for some of the pregnancy complications and fetal growth retardation that afflict the juvenile mother and her baby are immaturity of body functions, in-

adequate prenatal care, and poor nutrition.

The immaturity factor is not necessarily an age-related problem. The onset of puberty is different in every person and although the average age of menarche (the first menstrual period) is around thirteen years of age, it may occur as early as nine years of age (and in a few cases, even earlier) and as late as seventeen years of age. Physical growth usually continues for another four to five years after menarche, after which time a girl reaches full physical maturity. At this point, the immaturity factor should not influence the outcome of pregnancy in the young mother and, for all practical purposes, a teenage pregnancy can be considered comparable to an adult one. Most girls over seventeen are likely to fall into this category. Thus, the young pregnant teenager is the focus of most concern since not only is she more immature in terms of body function, but she is also less likely to have regular medical care and an adequate diet. Dietary surveys of pregnant adolescents have found inadequate protein and caloric intake, while low intakes of iron, calcium, and vitamin A are also common.

The nutritional requirements of a pregnant teenager are much higher than that of a mature woman since the teenager is still growing herself. Her needs, therefore, will parallel her rate of body growth at the time when pregnancy begins. Thus, dietary recommendations should be carefully adjusted to each individual need and to the nutritional status of the adolescent at the start of pregnancy. An extremely young teenage mother with an adequate nutritional status should be encouraged to gain her estimated growth increments in weight in addition to the expected weight gain of pregnancy. Thus, an adequate weight gain for a pregnant teenage mother could range from 27 to 35 pounds. If she was underweight at the start of pregnancy, the estimated weight deficit should be added to the recommended weight gain.

In addition to an adequate caloric and protein intake to achieve these body weight goals, a teenage mother should receive generous supplements of iron and calcium in addition to the vitamin and mineral supplements routinely prescribed to pregnant women. The guide given below will provide each of the es-

sential nutrients and approximately 2000 calories per day. (See PREGNANCY.)

ALCOHOL ABUSE

More and more high school children are becoming chronic alcohol users. Boys have traditionally indulged in alcoholic beverages before the legal age, but now girls are beginning to do the same in alarming numbers. At the present time, 39 percent of all school adolescents are moderate drinkers and 28 percent are considered to be problem drinkers.

While it is true that this represents smaller numbers than among the adult population, these children very often have other drug problems which makes the situation worse. Younger and younger children are using marijuana, cocaine, PCP (known as "angel dust"), and other dangerous narcotics. While we are just beginning to understand the ad-

---

DAILY DIET GUIDE FOR PREGNANT ADOLESCENTS

Food	Minimum Number of Daily Servings
Whole or low-fat milk	4
Fruit (fresh & juices)	6
Vegetables (raw & cooked; yellow/orange & green)	3–4
Whole grain and enriched breads & cereals	6–8
Meat, fish, poultry, beans, & peanut butter	6 oz
Eggs	1

verse effects of these drugs on the brain, we are well aware of the negative effects of alcohol on the mind and body. First, if children are intoxicated during school hours they are less able to learn and this affects their school performance and ultimate career goals. Second, alcohol and its degradation products destroy brain cells. Finally, alcohol causes secondary nutrient deficiencies.

Alcohol compromises a person's nutritional status in several ways. Every gram of alcohol is equivalent to seven calories. Alcohol contains no nutrients and hence it could be termed "empty calories" in the same manner as "junk food." By taking in a good deal of energy in this nonnutritious fashion, other more nutritious foods will be displaced from a child's diet. This will cause a reduction in the protein, vitamin, and mineral intake—nutrients needed for optimum growth and development. Alcohol also irritates the lining of the stomach and intestines, which reduces the appetite and thus prevents a child from getting the nutrients needed to sustain the adolescent growth spurt.

Certain specific nutrients critical to growth are particularly affected. In a chronic alcohol user, dietary zinc is poorly retained in the body and an abnormally high percentage of this mineral is excreted in the urine. The absorption of certain vitamins, such as folacin, is also greatly impaired. As mentioned earlier, both zinc and folacin are essential for growth. Adolescents, like any type of chronic alcohol user, are also very likely to sustain liver damage and as a result the liver's retention of vitamins A and B_{12} will be reduced, which can lead to deficiencies in these nutrients.

As you can see, this problem of alcoholism in the younger generation is extremely serious. Not only does it impair nutritional status and decrease growth, but by affecting a person's ability to learn, it prevents the adolescent from realizing his or her potential and so reduces the quality of life in the future. (See AL-COHOL.)

VEGETARIANISM

A meatless diet can be more than adequate in protein, calories, and all other nutrients needed by a teenager. A diet eliminating all foods derived from animal sources, including milk, milk products, and eggs, will be dangerously low in vitamin B_{12} unless the diet includes *tempeh* (a fermented soy product), brewer's yeast, or B_{12} supplements.

An adolescent should be cautious when a meatless diet is adopted without a thorough familiarity with planning the proper nutritional balance. Unlike meat-containing diets where the protein is completely usable, vegetarian diets require matching grain foods with beans, peas, and nuts. The result of this process, called *protein complementing,* makes just as beneficial a pool of dietary proteins as those found in meats. There is also need for caution when former food habits are abruptly altered to accommodate new eating habits like vegetarianism. (See VEGETARIAN DIETS.)

ATHLETICS

A teenage athlete takes his or her diet very seriously. But, misconceptions often obscure the correct advice. Calories are critical to provide the energy needed for growth, training, and performance. An intake exceeding 3000 calories per day is needed for someone involved in daily workouts. More than half the calories should be from carbohydrates—preferably from starchy foods rather than from sweet ones. Protein need not be a central focus, since the additional amount required is usually eaten in the array of foods which comprise an average teen's diet.

Supplements should not be necessary when most foods eaten are whole grain, fresh, or unprocessed. Fluid intake is frequently underplayed. Water and other beverages should be plentiful—one to two quarts per day is fine. At the starting line and during competition it is best to take in only plain water or very dilute beverages.

AGING

For years we have had nutrient requirements for young adults, both male and female, for pregnancy, infancy, and adolescence—but there is not a single nutrient for which there is a recommended daily allowance for men and women sixty-five and older. Even worse, there is no data base on which to formulate such recommendations. For the present, any recommendations we make must be based on a combination of experimental results, clinical experience, and logical deduction, and so must be considered tentative.

Perhaps we should begin by asking the question: Why should older individuals have different requirements for certain nutrients? The answer lies in understanding some of the changes that occur with aging. First, older people produce less saliva and often have poor dentures. This can cause difficulty with very dry foods. By simply consuming moister and softer foods, or in some cases by dividing food into smaller pieces, the problem can be solved.

Aging also brings about a decrease in the amount of acids secreted by the stomach. This may seem surprising, since so many older people complain about heartburn. The truth of the matter is that although there are indeed food items which produce "heartburn," often the "heartburn" is not caused by increased acidity but by other factors, such as gas production. Certain spicy foods, as well as other foods such as peas, beans, cabbage, and carbonated beverages, which have been proven to produce gas, are most often the culprits.

Reduced mobility and enzyme activity in the gastrointestinal tract, known to be associated with aging, often results in digestive difficulties in dealing with certain foods. For example, after eating dairy products, cramps and diarrhea may occur because of a reduction in the activity of lactase, an intestinal enzyme which breaks down lactose, the principal sugar in dairy foods. The solution here is not to stop consuming all dairy products, but instead to eat them in smaller amounts, and at many times throughout the day. Remember, dairy products contain large amounts of calcium, a very necessary nutrient—particularly for older women who are prone to osteoporosis (brittle bones) because of a loss of calcium from their bones, which is accelerated after menopause. (See OSTEOPOROSIS)

The motility of the intestine decreases with age. Motility is the involuntary folding and unfolding of the intestine which "moves" the food

through it. A decrease in this movement causes food to remain in the
intestine for a longer period of time,
producing harder stools and resulting in constipation. Some investigators blame the lack of fiber in our
diets for this problem. Indeed, fiber
will shorten the transit time of foods
(the length of time necessary for foods
to go through the intestine). In addition, a lack of fiber has been blamed
for the higher incidence of colon cancer and diverticulosis in the United
States, compared with other populations. The obvious solution to this
problem is to increase the consumption of foods high in fiber. However,
many of these foods may be hard to
chew and digest, which is a major
problem for older people. We recommend consuming foods which are
softer but still have a high fiber content, for example, cooked carrots,
cooked cereals such as oatmeal, and
cooked cabbage.

Aging affects certain senses:
taste, smell, vision, and hearing. Obviously, this then affects the types of
foods chosen by an older person. Salty
and sweet taste sensations can decline markedly with age, and so older
people often prefer foods which are
richly seasoned. The noise from
chewing carrots also adds to their
eating enjoyment. Some investigators claim that two-thirds of the sensation of taste depends on the ability
to smell. How a food looks is extremely important to its psychological appeal. Older people often have
problems with their vision and hence
should eat in well-lit rooms, with
enough color (both in the food and
in the surroundings) to stimulate their
senses.

These changes indicate that the
very process of aging requires some
alterations in the kinds of foods ingested.

There is a second aspect to the
problem of nutrition and aging which
could, in the long run, prove of more
fundamental importance—our lifelong pattern of eating habits. The in-
triguing suggestion has been made
that we can in some way delay or
change the aging process by changing our eating patterns early in life.
Certain diseases which are much more
common in the elderly, such as atherosclerosis and cancer of the colon,
are associated with long-term eating
patterns. Recent evidence suggests
that other diseases, such as osteoporosis and periodontal disease
(causing loose teeth), may in part be
caused by a faulty calcium and phosphorus balance which begins in the
early thirties for women and in the
forties for men. In these diseases, as
well as certain others, one cannot expect dramatic cures by correcting dietary abnormalities in the older
individual. It has taken decades for
the damage to be done, and it cannot
be reversed in a relatively short time.
However, even in later life dietary
alterations may prevent further pro-

gression of abnormalities and in some cases may even improve the situation.

CALORIES

There is good evidence (as well as good theoretical grounds) for recommending the intake of fewer calories by older individuals. First, older people are less active and hence expend less energy. This is particularly so when an individual leaves a relatively active job for the more sedentary life of retirement. This caloric restriction may be lessened somewhat by keeping active in later life. For this reason, regular forms of moderate exercise, such as walking and swimming, are strongly recommended. Second, there are changes in the body's metabolism which cause it to require less energy. Third, older individuals tend to lose lean body mass, mostly due to some wasting of muscle. This results in an increase in the ratio of fat tissue to lean tissue, or a relative obesity—another good reason for consuming fewer calories.

Since there are other nutrients which should not be reduced and some which should actually be increased, the number of calories consumed requires a certain amount of discretion in the kinds of foods chosen.

PROTEIN

The few direct measurements of protein and amino acid metabolism in older people which have been made indicate that requirements are essentially the same as for younger adults. Thus, we would recommend, at present, an intake of no more than the recommended dietary allowance for protein for young adults (.8 grams of protein per kilogram of body weight daily). The protein should be of high quality so that all the required amino acids are provided. As we shall see, however, in order to limit the amount of saturated fat in the diet, some reduction of the ingestion of red meats and unskimmed dairy products is advisable.

FATS

The best way for an older individual to reduce the intake of calories is to reduce the total quantity of fat in his or her diet. This will have the added benefit of helping to lower serum lipid levels, thereby reducing the risk of coronary artery disease. Less fat in the diet may perhaps even reduce the incidence of colon cancer, a major killer in older people. Thus, we recommend that older people ingest no more than 30 percent of their calories as fat, and for those with high levels of serum cholesterol, we recommend even greater reduction. In addition, dietary cholesterol intake should be kept to less than 300 milligrams per day. (See ARTERIOSCLEROSIS.)

CARBOHYDRATES

Carbohydrates are consumed in two forms, as simple sugars and as complex carbohydrates. The complex carbohydrates can be further divided into those which can be broken down and assimilated by the body, such as starch, and hence are a source of calories, and those which are not broken down and hence pass through the gastrointestinal tract, to be excreted in the stool. This latter group falls into the category we call fiber.

Simple sugars are a pleasant source of low-bulk calories and must therefore be taken with caution and in moderation on any low-calorie diet. The starches found in potatoes or grains such as wheat, corn, or rice, if unrefined or enriched, contain other essential nutrients. While these foods add calories they also help to provide essential vitamins, minerals, and fiber—hence, complex carbohydrates. Fiber acts as a bulking agent and promotes rapid movement of the stool through the lower intestines, thereby preventing or reducing the severity of constipation.

Based on these considerations, we recommend that 55 percent of all calories consumed come from carbohydrates, mostly in the form of tubers, unrefined starches, and whole grain or enriched flours, and that the diet be high in fiber in the form of cellulose and bran. (See CARBOHYDRATE; FIBER.)

CALCIUM AND PHOSPHORUS

The amount of calcium absorbed by the body is governed to some extent by the body's needs and to some extent by the amount and form of calcium in our diet. Most older individuals are in negative balance; meaning they lose more calcium than they absorb. This results in a slow but progressive loss of calcium from the bones, its main storage site. Reversing this process is not simply a matter of consuming more calcium. To be effective, calcium must be increased, but phosphorus and protein intake (if very high) must be decreased.

The American diet is high in both phosphorus and protein. The typical protein intake, in the form of meat, poultry, fish, and dairy products, is twice the amount recommended by the National Academy of Sciences in the recommended dietary allowances. Therefore, a slight reduction would still be within the range of adequate protein consumption. The major sources of phosphorus are meats and carbonated soft drinks (containing phosphoric acid).

To promote optimal calcium absorption we recommend, particularly for older individuals, around 1 gram of calcium per day, combined with the elimination of phosphate-containing beverages and the previously mentioned slight reduction in protein intake. (See CALCIUM; OS-TEOPOROSIS; PHOSPHORUS.)

IRON

Iron is converted from its nonabsorbable form to its absorbable form by the action of hydrochloric acid in the stomach. Many older individuals secrete less hydrochloric acid than normal and hence may be absorbing iron poorly. We recommend the ingestion of 18 milligrams of iron daily in the ferrous (absorbable) form. The best way to ensure such an intake without consuming too much red meat or organ meat is to use fortified foods, particularly cereals (avoid sugared cereals, however). If this cannot be done, then iron should be supplemented in the form of tablets or drops.

VITAMINS

We know almost nothing about the actual vitamin requirements of older people. There are certain theoretical arguments for an overall reduction in B vitamins since caloric needs are reduced and the requirements of the B vitamins are dependent on the amount of calories consumed. On the other hand, there are arguments which make a good case for an increase of these vitamins since certain organs, such as the nervous system, may not be functioning optimally and most of the B vitamins exert their major biochemical effects on the nervous system. Thus, at the present time, we would recommend a balanced diet rich in whole grains and low-fat dairy products and would not recommend direct supplementation.

There is one vitamin, B_{12}, which must be combined in the stomach with a substance known as the intrinsic factor in order to be properly absorbed in the intestine. Older people may be deficient in the intrinsic factor and vitamin B_{12} absorption may therefore be poor. Vitamin B_{12} is present in all meats (and all foods of animal origin) and hence on a varied diet no problems should develop. For the elderly individual subsisting mainly on a vegetarian diet, however, supplementation is recommended.

DIETARY RECOMMENDATIONS FOR THE ELDERLY

Nutrient	Men	Women
Calories	2300/day	2000/day
Protein	56 gr/day	45 gr/day
Fat	25–30% of total daily calories (63–76 gr/ day)	25–30% of total daily calories (55–66 gr/ day)

DIETARY RECOMMENDATIONS

The preceding table summarizes our tentative dietary recommendations for the elderly. These recommendations are based on the considerations mentioned above and may need to be changed as new information is gathered.

(See also ARTERIOSCLEROSIS; CANCER; DRUG-NUTRIENT INTERACTION; OSTEOPOROSIS.)

ALCOHOL

The word alcohol as it is commonly used refers to the intoxicating substance in such beverages as wine, beer, and distilled spirits (that is, hard liquor—scotch, gin, vodka, etc.). The chemical name of this substance is ethanol.

While it is true to say that an occasional drink is not harmful to you, any form of *regular* drinking is a health hazard. The liver is the most susceptible organ to the noxious effects of alcohol; the end result of prolonged alcoholism could be *cirrhosis*. However, even from the time you take your first drink, alcohol impairs liver function and puts you in a high-risk group for high blood pressure, heart disease, and cancer.

There is a linear relationship between the amount of alcohol consumed and the risk of contracting cirrhosis of the liver. If you were to consume a pint of liquor a day for twenty-five years you would have a one in two chance of developing cirrhosis. This disease results partly from the direct effects of alcohol on the liver and partly as the result of malnutrition, common to heavy drinkers.

One gram of alcohol is equivalent to 7.1 kilocalories, one ounce to 71 kilocalories, one drink to 100–150 kilocalories. Hence, you can see that it is very easy to consume a large quantity of energy in this form. Unfortunately, alcohol has little nutritional value outside of its energy content and is simply another form of "empty calories." A person is satisfying his or her appetite with alcohol—taking, for example, 1000 kilocalories in this form—is unlikely to be able to obtain the needed nutrients from the rest of his or her diet. The following table shows the caloric content of some alcoholic beverages.

Alcohol consumption leads to gastric irritation and to a loss of part of the lining of the intestines. This loss impairs the processes of absorption of lactose (the sugar found in milk) and leads to an intolerance to milk and other dairy products, as well as decreasing the absorption of folacin (folic acid) and thiamine. Thiamine is essential for the metabolism of carbohydrate in the diet. Folacin is required for all forms of cellular division, including the production of red blood cells. Too little folacin leads to anemia and a reduced capacity to replace worn out tissues, such as those lining the digestive system, which are usually replaced every two or three days.

Alcohol also causes pancreatitis, which leads to impaired produc-

CALORIC CONTENT OF ALCOHOLIC BEVERAGES

	Approx. Amount	Calories	Alcohol (gr)
Liqueurs (cordials)	8½ tsp	65–75	6–7
Brandy, cognac	6 tsp	73	10.5
Gin, rum, vodka, whisky, 80 proof	9 tsp	104	15
100 proof	9 tsp	133	19.1
Champagne	4 oz	85	11
Dry sherry	2 oz	85	9
Muscatel, port	3½ oz	158	15
Red and sauterne (California)	3½ oz	85	10
Ale	12 oz	148	13.1
Beer	12 oz	150–160	18
Beer, light	12 oz	96–100	12–14.4
Cider, hard	6 oz	71	9.4
Daiquiri	3½ oz	125	15.1
Manhattan	3½ oz	165	19.2
Martini	3½ oz	140	18.5
Tom Collins	10 oz	180	21.5

tion of digestive enzymes and malabsorption of nutrients. Even beer, with a 5 percent alcohol content, will cause gastric irritation if consumed regularly. On the other hand, pancreatitis is more usually found in drinkers of hard liquor.

If it were the malnutrition arising from the consumption of alcohol that caused the liver disease, you would expect that a good diet to counteract the effects of the alcohol would eradicate the problem. Unfortunately, this is not the case. Although a good diet will be beneficial in limiting the damage, all the evidence shows that the alcohol itself has a direct toxic effect. Alcoholics consuming a good diet would simply be expected to take longer to develop cirrhosis. It should be mentioned that not all alcoholics contract cirrhosis. There seems to be a genetic predisposition to the disease, and at least 50 percent of all drinkers have been shown to have such a tendency.

As mentioned before, alcohol simply contains calories, and excessive indulgence can lead to high calorie intake. Unlike most sources of energy, alcohol cannot be broken down anywhere but in the liver. Neither can it be stored in the body. Hence, it must all be disposed of as quickly as it enters the body. This means that the liver must divert most of its activity to this process. As a result, other nutrients, especially protein and fat, will not be metabolized to any extent—which will lead to them being stored in the liver. This stored protein absorbs water ten times its own volume and so causes swelling of the liver—which impairs its function—and eventually leads to *ascites* (the liberation of fluid from the liver into the digestive cavity). Eventually, inactive fibrous tissue replaces the metabolically-active liver tissue. This condition is known as cirrhosis.

The protein that is digested is often only broken down to substances called amines and ammonia. These substances, which are harmful to the brain, build up to quite high concentrations in the blood if the alcoholic eats a mixed diet. An inability to break down the nucleic acids (RNA and DNA) found in all cells leads to high levels of uric acid in the blood. This is deposited as small crystals in the joints, causing pain. This condition is known as *gout,* which has been associated with "high living." Gout often leads to erosion of the joints and to arthritis.

The liver in the heavy alcohol consumer is unable to metabolize fat. Hence, fat deposition in the liver occurs, and produces a fatty liver—which further impairs its function. It also means that high levels of lipids occur in the blood, with an accompanying high risk of cardiovascular disease.

Alcohol is broken down in the liver to produce acetaldehyde, which in turn is broken down to nontoxic substances. Acetaldehyde is toxic to both the heart and the brain. It is broken down by a group of enzymes—microsomal enzymes—responsible for degrading just about every kind of drug and toxic substance that enters the body during your lifetime. When you consume alcohol, the microsomal enzymes increase their activity. This means that not only will a chronic alcohol user be able to get rid of alcohol from his system more quickly than a nondrinker but that he will also remove drugs faster. Hence, any drug that the doctor prescribes will have a less profound effect and will last a shorter period of time. This is why physicians should always know if their patients drink.

If an individual is intoxicated (drunk) at the time a drug is taken there can be extremely serious consequences. For instance, sleeping pills, which are relatively safe when the user is sober, can be lethal in the same dose when the person is drunk. This is because there is so much alcohol in the body that it successfully competes with other toxic substances present for degradation by the microsomal enzymes and overwhelms this cleansing mechanism. As a result, the other substances remain relatively unchanged in the body.

The chronic drinker's increased

ability to break down toxic substances can often lead to more serious problems. Drinkers can place
themselves in a higher risk group for
cancer. Many substances in our food
and the environment have the potential to cause cancer if they are
partially degraded. This degradation
takes place in the liver as a function
of the same microsomal enzymes that
degrade alcohol. Tobacco pyrolyzate is one such substance, dimethyl
nitrosamine (found in some beers) is
another, and tryptophan pyrolyzate
(formed when you cook meat) is yet
another. Alcohol has also been shown
to be toxic in pregnancy. (See PREG-
NANCY.)

Under normal circumstances,
the ability to degrade these substances is minimal and so they are
relatively harmless. However, with
heavy drinking, significant levels of
them are produced by the stimulating effect of alcohol. For instance, a
person who takes four or five drinks
a day and smokes ten cigarettes a day
has five times the chance of getting
lung cancer as compared with a nondrinker smoking the same number of
cigarettes a day.

Hormones are also broken down
more quickly in a heavy drinker. In
a man, testosterone (the male sex
hormone) is broken down more rapidly than normal in a heavy drinker.
Furthermore, the alcohol decreases
the production of this hormone by
the testes. Hence, you could say that

alcohol impairs a male's sexual performance.

No matter how you look at it,
moderation is the key word when it
comes to alcohol. A little alcohol (one
or two drinks a night) is perhaps not
a problem, but if your consumption
rises above this, health can be seriously compromised.

MODERATE ALCOHOL CONSUMPTION AND HEALTH

Consumption of fermented beverages is common in cultures all over
the world. In the United States and
other western cultures a cocktail or
a glass of wine with a meal has become a standard in many homes.
Does alcohol consumed in these
quantities pose a threat to health?

Except for pregnant women, the
answer seems to be no. Quite to the
contrary, moderate daily consumption of alcohol, for example, one glass
of wine with each major meal, could
be beneficial. The basis for this conclusion is derived from various
sources. Several studies have indicated that moderate consumption of
alcohol not only does not reduce life
expectancy, but it may, indeed, prolong life.

Moderate alcohol consumption
(five to ten grams per day) has been
shown to defer the effects of atherosclerosis. This effect is believed to
be mediated by its influence on the
metabolism of certain lipid-carrying

proteins in the blood (lipoproteins). People who consume moderate quantities of alcohol daily tend to have higher plasma levels of high-density lipoprotein or HDL and lower levels of low-density lipoprotein or LDL. This pattern of high HDL and low LDL levels has been found in people who do not develop serious atherosclerosis.

The possibility of a protective effect against atherosclerosis is probably the single most important beneficial influence of alcohol on health. Unfortunately, if atherosclerosis has already developed, the consumption of alcohol does not appear to improve the outcome of the disease. A few years ago, there were indications that ingestion of small quantities of alcohol could help patients with *angina pectoris* (chest pain due to coronary atherosclerosis). In this respect, alcohol ingestion compared favorably with *nitroglycerin* (a drug commonly prescribed for this complaint) in alleviating the pain, but it was later shown that the effect was purely due to the pain-killing effects of alcohol and not due to dilation of the coronary arteries as with nitroglycerin, and therefore was not protective against heart attack.

Alcohol has a favorable effect on food intake and digestion, especially in elderly or debilitated people. Alcohol can stimulate the appetite, while enhancing digestion by increasing both the secretion of gastric juices and the rate at which food passes down the digestive tract. This increase in gastric secretion is due to the increased output of hydrochloric acid in the stomach. The increased gastric secretion and increased motility help to shorten the time taken for food to move down the digestive tract, thus contributing to the reduction of the feeling of fullness after a meal, especially if the meal was a particularly heavy one.

Intake of small quantities of alcohol has also been shown to increase a person's ability to work hard physically. This may be due to the fact that alcohol increases blood flow to the muscles and that alcohol itself provides extra energy, which can be used for muscle work. However, most scientists believe that the effect is due to a reduction in the feeling of fatigue.

After alcohol ingestion, there is a small transient rise in body temperature with increased perspiration. This change can have a protective effect for a short exposure to extremely cold temperatures. However, since in the long run the effect of alcohol is to cool the body because of heat loss through the skin, alcohol use may become detrimental if the exposure to cold is prolonged.

Due to mechanisms not entirely understood, the ingestion of small quantities of alcohol has been found to alleviate *dysmenorrhea* symptoms (painful menstrual periods) in many women. The effect probably involves the relaxation of muscles in the uterine wall. This property of alcohol has been used as well to stop premature uterine contractions, therefore preventing premature birth by allowing the woman to carry through the pregnancy until the normal time for delivery. This treatment is effective at a time in pregnancy when the fetus cannot be affected. Unfortunately, the treatment is not always successful.

Alcohol can stimulate or inhibit the release of various hormones. One of the hormones whose release is inhibited is the antidiuretic hormone, which limits the amount of fluid lost from the body as urine. This explains the typical increased urinary output that follows alcohol ingestion, independent of the volume of alcoholic beverage ingested. Some people believe the increased urinary output may have a beneficial "cleansing" effect since body "impurities" are eliminated; this belief does not have any scientific basis.

The evidence demonstrates that alcohol consumption in moderation, immediately preceding or during meals, not only enhances the pleasure of eating a nice meal, but it has some effects which are beneficial to health. The only circumstance in which alcohol is totally contraindicated, even in small amounts, is when a person is regularly taking drugs that affect brain function, such as sedatives, antidepressants, tranquilizers, anticonvulsants, and hypnotics (barbiturates). Alcohol potentiates the effects of these drugs, resulting in marked sleepiness, impairment of motor coordination, and impaired judgment. (See also ARTERIOSCLEROSIS; PROTEIN-CALORIE MALNUTRITION.)

ALLERGY

An allergic response is defined as the production by the body of specific substances *(antibodies)* that react with foreign proteins *(antigens)* in a manner which usually renders the antigen inactive. This response is a major part of the body's immune system: It is called an *allergic response* only when it induces symptoms.

Certain food proteins, that somehow leak across the barrier of the gastrointestinal tract in minute amounts, can induce antibody formation and an antibody-antigen response. This response may take one of several forms, producing a specific set of symptoms. These symptoms may be respiratory, such as sneezing, running nose or ears, or wheezing; gastrointestinal, such as sores in or around the mouth, abdominal pain, vomiting, or diarrhea; dermal, such as wheals, itching, and rashes of all types; or neurological, such as dizziness or headache.

Foods that are often involved in an allergic response are milk, wheat, chocolate, corn, eggs, seafood, and nuts. Foods likely to cause an *immediate* response are fish, seafood, berries, and nuts. This response usually takes the form of a skin wheal that is raised, pale in the middle but surrounded by a bright red area, and extremely itchy. Sneezing, running nose and eyes, and sometimes wheezing and difficulty in breathing are other immediate reactions. Acute allergic symptoms, if severe, may require rapid treatment with drugs such as antihistamines and even Adrenalin.

A delayed response is more often observed when the allergen is in cereal, beef, eggs, pork, chocolate, certain legumes, or chicken. The actual antigen in this case is often a breakdown product formed by the digestion of the food. Delayed reactions may occur in the skin or respiratory tract, but often will produce gastrointestinal symptoms, such as diarrhea; or neurological symptoms, such as a headache.

As food usage changes, the prevalence of allergic symptoms caused by certain foods changes. Originally, for example, soya bean formula was introduced for babies allergic to cows' milk protein. However, more and more infants are now becoming allergic to soya bean protein. Corn is used far more frequently in manufactured foods than previously and allergy to corn protein is now being seen more and more.

In most cases, however, the solution is not that obvious and detective work must be done. The standard way to uncover the offending food is by what is called an *elimination diet.*

The principle is to feed the person a diet made up of foods that are rarely allergenic and then to introduce other foods one at a time. If nothing happens, the new food can be added to the diet. If an allergic response occurs, then the offending food is removed. After a short period it is introduced again. A second response confirms the initial impression and the food is then removed from the diet. Unfortunately, many allergic people are affected by more than one food and hence the diet must be continued until a wide variety of foods has been tested.

Once a food has been identified as allergenic it should be omitted from the diet for at least six months. After that it can be carefully tried again. If no allergic response follows, it can be carefully reincorporated in the diet. Although this procedure may sound simple, it is really quite time-consuming if you wish to avoid all suspected allergens. Hence it should not be undertaken if you only occasionally have an allergic reaction. The following table shows the array of foods that must be omitted if milk, egg, or wheat is suspected of being the offending food.

Some people think that this bothersome procedure can be avoided by skin testing. This is done by injecting a series of suspected allergens under the skin and seeing if a wheal appears in twenty-four hours. Although this procedure works well in detecting air-borne allergens (pollen, dust, etc.), it has very limited usefulness in detecting food-borne allergens. (See also CYTOTOXIC TESTING; INTOLERANCE.)

FOODS CONTAINING EGGS, WHEAT, AND MILK

Food	Products	Examples of Foods Containing These Products
Egg	Fresh or powdered eggs	Egg substitutes, baked goods, custard (flan), ice cream, hollandaise, mayonnaise, cutlets and breaded items, meringue, puddings, cream pie, pastas, fondue
Wheat	Flour, bran	Wheat cereals, breads, pastas, malt, Postum, breaded products, thickened sauces, gravies, soups, beer, ale
Milk	Fluid milk, cheese, cream	Baked products, scalloped and au gratin, sherberts, ice cream and ice milk, some margarines

ALUMINUM

Traces of aluminum are found in body tissues, although there is no known physiological function for this metal. There has been some concern in recent years that dietary aluminum may lead to Alzheimer's disease or senile dementia in older people. This concern arises from the fact that greater levels of aluminum are found in brain tissue of people dying from Alzheimer's disease than in brain tissue from people dying from other causes. It is now generally agreed that the aluminum deposits in the brain are probably not a cause of the disease, but rather a consequence of it. It is known that cells die in specific regions of the brain in Alzheimer's patients, and the aluminum probably gets deposited on the debris left after a cell dies. Aluminum is relatively abundant in the earth's crust and is widely distributed throughout the world. The levels of aluminum in ground water and drinking water are extremely high in some regions of the world, yet there is no greater incidence of Alzheimer's disease among the residents of those areas.

Aluminum is used topically in several antiperspirant preparations, and is used extensively as an antacid, which accounts for most of the ingested aluminum in the US. Aluminum cookware also contributes substantially to the total amount of aluminum ingested. Very little ingested aluminum gets absorbed through the intestinal tract due to the formation of highly insoluble aluminum salts, especially phosphates. These aluminum phosphates pass through the intestinal tract and are excreted in the feces. For this reason, prolonged use of aluminum-containing antacids can lead to a phosphorus deficiency, or hypophosphatemia, in addition to other digestive complications arising from stomach acid neutralization. Furthermore, the phosphorus deficiency will cause increased urinary calcium excretion, which over time, will result in severe bone loss, or osteoporosis. (See also CALCIUM; OSTEOPOROSIS; PHOSPHORUS.)

AMINO ACIDS

Amino acids are the building blocks of protein. The various proteins in our body and in the food we eat are made up of long chains of amino acids. The amino acids fall into two categories: those which can be manufactured by the body (nonessential) and those which cannot and, hence, must be supplied in the diet (essential). There are eight amino acids which are essential for adults and one more which is essential for the very young infant. The essential amino acids for an adult are: tryptophan, phenylalanine, lysine, threonine, methionine, leucine, isoleucine, and valine. Young, particularly premature, infants, also require cysteine.

Amino acids come from the protein in our foods which is broken down during the digestive process to smaller units of amino acids (peptides) and finally to individual amino acids. These, in turn, are absorbed into the blood stream and carried to the liver. If energy is scarce, the liver can convert some of the amino acids to glucose for use as fuel. Most of the amino acids, however, are used for synthesizing new tissue protein and repairing damaged protein molecules.

Amino acids are also used in the synthesis of substances other than protein. For example, the essential amino acid tryptophan is necessary for the synthesis of an important brain hormone, serotonin.

The quality (biological value) of the proteins that we eat is determined by the number and quantity of the essential amino acids contained within the protein molecule. Egg white is considered the best protein because it contains all of the essential amino acids in abundant quantities. Casein (milk protein) is also of very high quality as is the protein from meat and fish. Plant proteins are usually of lesser biological value because they are lacking in one or more amino acids. The biological value of a plant protein can be enhanced by combining two different types each compensating for the amino acid or acids missing in the other. An example of this is rice and beans. Including a small amount of meat protein can also enhance the biological value of plant protein by supplying the missing amino acid. (See Vegetarian Diets.)

(See also ARGININE; ASPARTIC ACID; CYSTEINE; GLUTAMIC ACID; GLYCINE; HISTIDINE; LEUCINE; LYSINE; METHIONINE; PHENYLALANINE; PROTEIN; TAURINE; TRYPTOPHAN.)

ANEMIAS (NUTRITIONAL)

Any anemia will reduce the oxygen-carrying capacity of the blood. As a consequence, if the anemia is severe enough, the tissues will become relatively oxygen starved. In its severest form, anemia is characterized by pallor, severe lethargy, and a hunger for air. The patient, often a small child, may be breathing rapidly and actually appear to be fighting for air. Fortunately, such severe anemia is quite rare. Far more common is the mild to moderate anemia characterized by tiredness, general feelings of malaise, irritability, and decreased attention span.

New red blood cells are constantly being made in the bone marrow. In order for this to happen smoothly, cell division of immature red cells must occur rapidly and synthesis of new hemoglobin within the maturing red cell must be unencumbered. Both of these processes depend in part on the availability of certain nutrients.

Three nutrients are absolutely essential for cell division to occur—folacin (folic acid), vitamin B_{12}, and zinc. One nutrient is crucial to the synthesis of hemoglobin—iron. A deficiency in folacin, vitamin B_{12}, or zinc will result in a reduced rate of cell division within the bone marrow and, hence, the production of fewer cells. The result is anemia. A deficiency of iron will result in a reduced synthesis of hemoglobin within the maturing red cell and eventually lead to the development of anemia. Thus, the most common forms of nutritional anemia are caused by an inadequate supply of iron, folacin, vitamin B_{12}, or zinc to the bone marrow. The most important factor determining that supply is your diet.

IRON DEFICIENCY

When red blood cells wear out every 120 days, they are broken down and their hemoglobin is picked up by scavenger cells and transported back to the marrow where it is used to form new hemoglobin. Thus, in a healthy adult, very little iron has to be consumed in the diet since reutilization of the iron already in the body is extremely efficient. The adult male who has accumulated adequate iron stores rarely becomes iron deficient. By contrast, the adult female loses blood every month in the menses and so the iron in her blood is similarly lost. This iron must be replaced through the diet, and when dietary sources are inadequate, iron deficiency will result.

During certain stages of life, the need for iron increases markedly. For instance, a growing child of either sex not only increases his or her body mass (bones, muscles, and other organs) but also increases the quantity of circulating blood. To do this, more red blood cells must be manufactured and so more iron must be supplied. Similarly, the pregnant woman has a particularly high need for iron. Her blood volume increases and so she needs more iron to fill her own red blood cells. In addition, the fetus is rapidly growing and requires iron to make hemoglobin. The only source of the additional iron needed to meet these needs is the diet of the woman. During pregnancy, dietary iron may be absorbed up to twice as efficiently as it is in nonpregnant women. However, even with this increased efficiency, iron deficiency will develop if the iron in the diet is too low.

The individual most at risk for iron deficiency is probably the newborn infant. The smaller the infant at birth, the greater the risk. Again, this iron requirement reflects the enormous rate of growth during this period of life and, as a result, the need for dietary iron to keep up with the increasing demand for hemoglobin.

For the reasons outlined above, iron deficiency occurs in our society more often in women and children than in adult men. As you would expect, iron requirements differ according to age, sex, and condition. (See APPENDIX.)

Being careful about our food choices can, in most instances, prevent iron deficiency. For the young infant, breast milk is still the best bet. While the iron content of breast milk is not particularly high, it is present in a readily absorbed form. As a consequence, breast-fed infants rarely, if ever, develop iron deficiency anemia. For those infants who are partly or completely fed on formula, iron has been added to many available products. While infant formulas cannot replace breast milk for overall optimal nutrition for young infants, consumption of iron-fortified products will prevent iron deficiency anemia. Most cereals, particularly those consumed mainly by young children, have additional iron. In the past, this iron has been in a form which was poorly absorbed, but today the situation is improving.

Thus, the staple foods for specific high-risk groups either are naturally rich in available iron or have been fortified with iron. Other groups, if they are to avoid direct supplementation, must consume a diet rich in iron. (See IRON.)

FOLACIN DEFICIENCY

Folacin (folic acid) is a vitamin which is essential for cells to divide normally. The more rapid the rate of cell division, the higher the requirement for folacin. In the adult, the constant replacement of red cells by rapidly dividing marrow cells makes the bone marrow a tissue where cells are dividing more rapidly than anywhere else in the body. Folacin deficiency will therefore manifest itself primarily in the bone marrow by reducing the rate of cell division. When this rate is reduced enough to compromise the marrow's ability to replace lost red cells, the number of red cells in the blood will fall and anemia will occur.

The faster the red cells have to be replaced, the greater the need for folacin. Women are replacing their red cells faster than are men because they must constantly make up for the losses imposed by menstruation. Thus, the folacin requirement is greater in women than in men and anemia due to folacin deficiency is more common in adult women than in adult men. The heavier a woman's menstrual losses, the greater her need for folacin.

Unlike iron, folacin is not stored by the body in any appreciable quantity and so adequate amounts must be consumed on a daily basis. This requirement will increase during periods of great demand for new red cells. Although there is no direct evidence for this it is logical to assume that a woman's requirement for folacin may vary at different times during the menstrual cycle. What is clear, however, is that overall, women must consume more folacin than men do

to keep their bone marrow working at the increased rate necessary to replace their monthly blood loss.

Again unlike iron, almost all of the folacin in a person's diet is absorbed. The excess is simply excreted. Thus, if you are anemic due to folacin deficiency, your body cannot protect itself by absorbing a greater amount of folacin from the food you already eat. Folacin is found in a variety of foods and yet folacin deficiency is still the most common vitamin deficiency in the United States! (See FOLACIN for the Folic Acid Contents of Foods Table.)

In adults, deficiencies are limited almost exclusively to women. This is partly due to their high demand for folacin and to several aspects of their life-styles. As with iron, constant calorie control (dieting) will limit the amount of folacin in the diet. Dieting will also limit the amount of folacin which is available, since your body has no control over the amount absorbed and therefore cannot extract more folacin from the available food if the body's reserves are low.

Even moderate consumption of alcohol will reduce the amount of folacin absorbed and will therefore increase the risk of folacin deficiency. Certain drugs can affect folacin metabolism and result in a deficiency in this vitamin. Perhaps most important in this respect is the contraceptive pill, which may decrease absorption and increase excretion of folacin. The overall result is that many women who use oral contraceptives are at increased risk for folacin deficiency. This is often compounded by the fact that more and more pregnancies are being planned and so women stop taking oral contraceptives immediately before they try to become pregnant. If they succeed quickly, they may enter the early stages of pregnancy relatively deficient in folacin.

Pregnancy, because it is accompanied by rapid cell division in the developing fetus and because both maternal and fetal bone marrow is very active in making new cells, increases a woman's folacin requirement dramatically. Folacin deficiency during early pregnancy may be associated with certain types of congenital malformations of the fetus. Later in the pregnancy, this deficiency may result in anemia in the mother. Therefore, it is currently recommended that all pregnant women take a folacin supplement. This is particularly important if the woman had been taking oral contraceptives for a long time prior to becoming pregnant. In this case she should begin the supplementation as soon as she comes off the pill.

ZINC DEFICIENCY

Zinc is a mineral which, like the vitamin folacin, is necessary for cell division to occur. Thus the demand for zinc will increase when the bone marrow is very active and during pregnancy when cell division is increased in both the woman and the fetus. Zinc is a mineral like iron and is often found in the same foods as iron. Hence, people who are iron deficient are often also zinc deficient. Like iron, zinc is stored in the body and there is some evidence that the state of your zinc reserves will influence the rate at which your body absorbs zinc from your foods. Unlike iron, zinc is not a structural element in hemoglobin or any other major blood protein. Hence, blood loss is not accompanied by the loss of large quantities of zinc. However, the response of the bone marrow to this blood loss increases the zinc requirement. Thus, there is an increased zinc requirement for women of childbearing age, not because the lost zinc has to be replaced but because more red blood cells have to be made.

As with the other nutrients involved in nutritional anemias, zinc deficiency will result from the increased demand not being adequately met by the dietary supply. The amount of zinc supplied in the diet is in turn limited by the quantity and quality of the food consumed and by the life-style of the individual woman. Again, limiting the number of calories means limiting the amount of food and will therefore result in an increased risk of zinc deficiency.

If the diet is low in foods with a high zinc content that risk is compounded. (See ZINC.) Alcohol, by the way, reduces zinc absorption and will therefore increase your risk of deficiency.

Even if your body is deficient in zinc you are not likely to become anemic. There are two reasons for this. First, it takes a greater degree of depletion to result in anemia from zinc deficiency than it does from iron or folacin deficiency. As mentioned, a person with iron-deficiency anemia will often be zinc deficient as well, since the same foods tend to supply both nutrients. The anemia, however, will be caused by the lack of iron and not the lack of zinc (since even moderate iron deficiency will often rapidly result in anemia). This is an important reason why iron-deficiency anemia should not be treated *only* with iron supplements. These do not usually contain zinc, which is undoubtedly also a problem in this case. But, by increasing your consumption of iron-containing foods, you will increase your zinc intake and establish an eating pattern which will prevent subsequent iron or zinc deficiency.

Second, even relatively severe zinc deficiency will often manifest itself by other signs before anemia develops. These signs include skin problems, abnormalities in taste, endocrine problems, and in children, problems with growth and sexual maturation. It is important to remember, therefore, that even if you are not anemic due to a zinc deficiency you may have low enough zinc reserves to be causing other problems. This is particularly important to women of childbearing age because zinc deficiency has been associated with congenital malformations of the fetus. These malformations occur at low serum zinc levels in the mother even in the absence of any other signs of zinc deficiency. Because zinc deficiency is so prevalent in women who are iron deficient, zinc in addition to iron supplementation is strongly recommended in any woman who is pregnant and iron deficient. (See ZINC.)

VITAMIN B_{12} DEFICIENCY

One of the major manifestations of vitamin B_{12} deficiency is anemia. This anemia is identical to anemia which results from folacin deficiency because vitamin B_{12} is necessary for folacin to work properly. In essence, a person who has a deficiency in vitamin B_{12} is deficient in folacin not because folacin is lacking in the diet but because it cannot be properly used by the body. Vitamin B_{12} is found in all foods of animal origin and is required only in small amounts. Hence, with the exception of pure vegetarians *(vegans)*, vitamin B_{12} deficiency as a result of diet almost never occurs. Vitamin B_{12} is also the only water soluble vitamin which is stored in the body. It takes about three years to deplete a person's normal reserves. Hence, the anemia of vitamin B_{12} deficiency takes a long time to develop, and unless there is some abnormality (such as a lack of ability to absorb the vitamin), it should occur only in pure vegetarians. Nutritional anemia due to a vitamin B_{12}–deficient diet is therefore very rare. (See VITAMIN B_{12}.)

OTHER NUTRIENT DEFICIENCIES

Anemia can occur because of a deficiency of other nutrients in the diet but this is extremely rare. Nutrient deficiencies which have been implicated in anemia are *copper* and *vitamin E*. However, the deficiency must be prolonged and severe before anemia results and so only people with extremely unorthodox eating habits are at risk for anemia owing to a lack of these nutrients in the diet.

COMBINED NUTRIENT DEFICIENCIES

Since the conditions which are necessary to develop iron-deficiency anemia and the anemia of folacin deficiency are often similar, some women become anemic because they are deficient in *both* of these nutrients. It is extremely important for such a situation to be identified. Treatment with neither iron nor folacin alone will cure the anemia. Fortunately, the physician will be able to tell if such a combined anemia is present by examining a drop of blood. The treatment of such combined anemias is simple—supplementation with both iron and folacin is given.

Prevention of a recurrence may involve a change in life-style and cer-

---

FACTORS AFFECTING ABSORPTION OF IRON, CALCIUM, FOLIC ACID AND ZINC

Nutrient	Absorption Enhanced by . . . . Found in	Absorption Decreased by . . . . Found in
Iron	Vitamin C . . . . citrus, tomatoes, cantaloupe, strawberries heme iron . . . . meats	Phytate* . . . . bran and germ of cereals (e.g. wheat, rice, corn, oats) tea . . . . commercial black and pekoe tea
Calcium	Vitamin D . . . . fish liver oils, fortified milk, salmon, (exposure to sunlight)	phytate . . . . (see above) oxalates . . . . spinach, cocoa and chocolate, beet greens, tea excess phosphorus . . . . high meat diets
Zinc		phytate . . . . (see above) excess calcium . . . . (see Table 2)
Folic Acid	Glucose . . . . fruits, vegetables, grains	

*Cereals must comprise a high percentage of the diet to cause a significant reduction in available iron.

tainly will involve a change in diet. Making sure one absorbs the key nutrients is obviously just as important as including them in the diet. The table on page 42 describes those factors which enhance or reduce nutrient absorption.

Anemia due to a combination of other nutrient deficiencies is quite rare. Occasionally, a woman who is a pure vegetarian may develop an anemia caused by a deficiency of both iron and vitamin B_{12} in the diet. This is because the best sources of iron are meat and other animal products, and because vitamin B_{12} is found *only* in animal products. However, even small amounts of meat, fish, or dairy products will supply your vitamin B_{12} requirement, and therefore the vegetarian who is anemic is most likely iron deficient and only rarely deficient in vitamin B_{12}.

ANOREXIA NERVOSA

Anorexia nervosa is a disorder with all the symptoms of imposed starvation with one unique difference: starvation is self-imposed. The disorder itself appears to be a paradox, for it is most often seen in young, well-to-do women, starving in the midst of plenty. Its name even appears to be a misnomer, for "anorexia" suggests a loss of appetite, but it appears anorexics don't suffer from a lack of appetite, but rather from a fear of gaining weight. In fact, they are preoccupied with thoughts of food and eating.

Anorexia nervosa most frequently occurs in adolescent girls (85 to 95 percent of the reported cases), with the remainder of cases reported in prepubertal boys. Interestingly, anorexia rarely affects poor people, and it has not been reported in underdeveloped countries. In a study done in England, it was found that one in two hundred young women in private and boarding schools were afflicted with this disorder, while only one in three thousand cases were reported in state run schools.

The weight loss associated with anorexia nervosa is characterized by: (1) age of onset prior to twenty-five years, (2) weight loss of at least 25 percent of original body weight, (3) a distorted attitude toward eating, food, or weight that overrides hunger, admonitions, reassurances, and threats, (4) no known medical illness to account for the anorexia, (5) no other known psychiatric disorders, and (6) at least two of the following manifestations: amenorrhea or irregular menstruation, lanugo hair (a baby-fine hair covering the body), bradycardia or a slow heart rate, periods of overactivity, episodes of bulimia or binge eating often followed by self-induced vomiting.

In an attempt to achieve a better understanding of this disorder, anorexia nervosa has been subdivided into two syndromes—primary and atypical anorexia. While both syndromes are similar in age of onset, duration of the illness, and poor cooperation of patients, there are several differences. In primary anorexia, the overriding characteristic is the "relentless pursuit of thinness." There is a delusional denial of the thinness, preoccupation with food, hyperactivity, and a striving for perfection. Atypical anorexia is best defined by the *lack* of these primary symptoms. In the atypical syndrome, the concern over weight loss appears to be secondary to other problems. Atypical patients claim they don't want to stay thin. They see weight loss as a means of getting what they want by coercing others and also as a way to remain dependent on their parents.

Anorexics appear to manifest many of the same physiological and psychological disturbances that are seen in starvation. Bizarre eating habits, preoccupation with food, irritability, emotional lability, depression, and sexual disinterest appear as common psychological features of both these afflictions. Hilda Bruch, a psychoanalyst who has for many years treated young women with anorexia, defines three areas of psychological dysfunction which make anorexia nervosa unique from starvation. First, there may be a severe disturbance in body image. Anorexics will misperceive their body size, and report themselves to be larger than they actually are. Second, there is a misrepresentation of both internal and external stimuli. For example, there are inaccuracies in the way hunger is perceived. Instead of being a signal to eat, the sensation of hunger becomes positively reinforcing. After just a few bites of food, the anorexic patient will often report feeling full. These individuals are also frequently overactive. Anorexics will often exercise to the point of exhaustion—swimming, running, bicycling—refusing to admit they are tired. Finally, these individuals experience a paralyzing sense of ineffectiveness. They seem to feel helpless and unable to change anything in their lives.

Metabolic changes occurring in this disorder are also similar to those seen in starvation. Most of the physiological functioning altered in this syndrome returns to normal when the patient gains back the lost weight. One interesting difference noted, however, is that 25 percent of the patients destined to become anorexics report amenorrhea prior to the loss of any weight.

Many explanations have been proposed to explain the anorexic's refusal to eat. Hilda Bruch suggests that the rigid behavior associated with eating observed in anorexics is a "struggle for control." Anorexic patients are described as "having been outstandingly good and quiet children, obedient, clean, eager to please, helpful at home, precociously dependable, excelling in schoolwork. They were the pride and joy of their parents and great things were expected of them. When they got to adolescence and were supposed to be self-reliantly independent, they couldn't come to terms with their childhood robot obedience." These children were overcompliant, oversubmissive, and lacked any sense of autonomy. Bruch sees the excessive concern with body size and the rigid control of eating as symptoms of "youngsters' desperate fight against feeling enslaved and exploited and not competent to lead lives of their own." The pubertal growth spurt with the accompanied gain in weight is particularly frightening to these children. It is seen as a time, not only when they become independent, but also a time of having lost complete control over their bodies. Bruch feels the best treatment program consists of normal nutrition and resolution of the disturbed patterns of family interaction and underlying psychological misconceptions.

Psychotherapy alone has not been reported to be very successful in treating this disorder. More success has been achieved when psychotherapy is used in conjunction with other forms of therapy.

Behavior modification therapy has also been employed in treatment of this illness. Patients are deprived of television, visits, books, etc. Positive reinforcement such as attention, conversation, and praise becomes contingent on either eating behavior or weight gain. Feedback is given after each meal as to the number of calories consumed and bites taken. Behavior modification appears to be successful on a short-term basis. Nevertheless, not all professionals would agree that this is the best form of treatment. For example, many psychoanalysts feel behavior therapy can cause problems, as it treats the symptoms without treating the cause. They feel anorexic patients, gaining weight with behavior modification, would then feel that they are losing even more control over their own lives. This could

have devastating psychological effects for these individuals. However, this has not been substantiated, as there have been reports of improved spirits with behavior modification, independent of other therapies employed.

More recently it has been recognized that this illness reflects difficulties in the family relationship. Four characteristic patterns of functioning have been identified in families of anorexic patients. These include enmeshment, overprotectiveness, rigidity, and lack of conflict resolution. The child is viewed as being involved in the parental conflict in such a way as to detour, avoid, or suppress it. In treatment, the family is seen as a unit, and treatment is initially directed at symptom removal (altering eating patterns) using family resources. Later treatment focuses on issues within the family such as marital or parenting problems. A high degree of success has been reported with this therapy, with 88 percent of the patients showing recovery up to four years after treatment.

Optimal treatment for this disorder appears to be a mixed-bag approach. First, an attempt must be made to get the patient to a normal weight. Next, the patient must receive help in resolving those psychological and social issues that have brought on the disorder.

One of the most startling statistics associated with anorexia nervosa is that death rates of up to 20 percent have been reported. Death has been most often attributed to inanition, suicide, infection, and cardiopulmonary disease.

The best outcomes have been observed in patients with high educational achievement, early age of onset and improvement in body image with weight gain. Poor prognosis is associated with late age of onset, continual overestimation of body size after weight gain, premorbid obesity, self-induced vomiting, bulimia, laxative abuse, long duration of illness, males, and marked depression. (See also BULIMIA.)

ANTICARCINOGENS

Anticarcinogens are substances which protect the body from cancer or are effective in treating cancer. Several nutrients have been intensively studied for their ability to act in this capacity, including vitamins C, E, and A, and selenium.

Despite claims to the contrary, megadoses of vitamin C have not been shown to prolong life in terminal cancer patients. However, up to 200 milligrams per day of the vitamin may be protective against the formation of free radicals, which could be one factor causing cancer. More than 2 grams of vitamin C per day reduces the ability of the body to destroy cancer cells.

Vitamin E is a potent antioxidant, which enables it to prevent free radical formation. This may make it protective against certain types of cancer, although there is no proof that this is in fact the case.

Vitamin A has been used therapeutically to treat cancer with some success. As the vitamin itself is toxic in large doses, a number of so-called analogs of the vitamin have been developed which are as effective in treating epithelial cancers but do not have any of the toxic side effects of vitamin A. These analogs can only be obtained by prescription. There is quite a lot of epidemiological evidence to suggest that beta carotene (the nontoxic form of vitamin A found in vegetables) can help prevent cancer. Studies suggest that 30 milligrams a day is sufficient to give a person maximum protection.

Selenium has been shown to help prevent cancer in animals. In addition, epidemiological data shows that people with an adequate intake of this mineral are less likely to develop cancer than those with a low intake. But there is no benefit to taking supplements of the mineral if your diet contains 150 to 200 micrograms of selenium per day, which is characteristic of the average American diet. Supplements can be extremely dangerous and should never be taken in excess of 200 micrograms.

Cruciferous vegetables seem to play a role in protecting you against cancer. These are members of the cabbage family and include cauliflower, brussels sprouts, and broccoli.

To help protect yourself against cancer, be sure to include in your diet, foods rich in beta carotene, such as carrots and green vegetables; vitamin C, such as citrus fruits; and be sure that you get at least ten milligrams per day of vitamin E, found in vegetable oils and nuts. There is no definitive evidence that taking these nutrients as supplements in tablet or capsule form prevents cancer. (See also ANTIOXIDANTS; CANCER.)

ANTIOXIDANTS

Antioxidants are substances which prevent harmful or unfavorable chemical reactions from taking place in the foods that we eat or within our bodies. These adverse chemical reactions usually involve oxygen from the air, and are classified as oxidation reactions, hence the term antioxidant. Antioxidants are added to foods to prevent spoilage during processing, storage, and preparation. Within the body two types of oxidation reactions are constantly occurring: those that burn carbohydrates and fats as fuels, producing energy which is conserved or utilized for work in the body; and those that release oxygen which may damage essential components of the body. Antioxidants prevent the second type of reaction from occurring.

Vitamins C and E and the minerals selenium and zinc are the more common "natural" antioxidants. Many food preservatives, including BHA (butylated hydroxyanisol), BHT (butylated hydroxytoluene), NDGA (nordihydroguaiaretic acid), and EDTA (ethylenediaminetetraacetic acid), act as antioxidants. These substances, when added to the food supply in small quantities, are not harmful, and may in fact be beneficial in prevention of some types of cancer. However, any of these "unnatural" antioxidants may cause harmful side effects if taken in large quantities; amounts far in excess of the allowed levels as food additives.

Even the natural antioxidants should be taken in moderation, because they too can cause harmful side effects when taken in excess. Many people can tolerate large doses of vitamins C and E, with no apparent harmful side effects, but others can develop toxic syndromes from these vitamins. (See VITAMIN C and VITAMIN E for toxicity symptoms and levels.) Selenium can be very toxic at levels that can be easily obtained from commercial supplements, and, indeed, there are regions of the world in which the selenium content of the soil is high enough to cause selenium toxicity from the food consumed by the local residents. Zinc is a relatively nontoxic metal, but excessive amounts of zinc in the diet can lead to complications in absorption and metabolism of other minerals. (See SELENIUM and ZINC for toxicities. See also ADDITIVES; ANTICARCINOGENS.)

APPETITE REGULATION

Throughout history, people have attempted to understand what controls appetite, or the desire to eat. While early research focused on the stomach as the seat of hunger, more recently scientists have centered their attention on a small area of the brain known as the hypothalamus. The hypothalamus appears to be important in a number of regulatory functions aside from hunger, including thirst, body temperature regulation, water balance, and reproductive behavior. The hypothalamus, located at the base of the brain, is ideally situated to act as a way station receiving information from both the environment and the body, ultimately determining when we're hungry.

Over thirty years ago, information obtained from brain-damaged animals, gave scientists their first insights into how this part of the brain controls food intake. Rats with damage in an area of the hypothalamus known as the lateral hypothalamus (LH) ate less food and gained less weight than normal animals. In contrast, rats with damage in a different area, the ventromedial hypothalamus (VMH), ate voraciously and became extremely obese. Animals with LH damage acted as if they didn't know how to initiate a meal, while animals with VMH damage acted as

if they didn't know how to end one. This research led to the Dual Center theory of feeding behavior. Food intake was thought to be controlled by a "feeding" center located in the lateral hypothalamus and a "satiety" center located in the ventromedial hypothalamus. If these areas of the hypothalamus were important to the regulation of food intake, what information did they need to make the decision when to either initiate or end a meal?

ENVIRONMENTAL FACTORS

First, the brain receives information from the environment. The availability of food, its smell, and its taste all appear to be important factors in motivating us to eat. Certain tastes appear to be either inherently pleasing or bad tasting. Almost all animals, including humans, seem to have an innate preference for sweets and an innate aversion to bitter-tasting foods. While some tastes appear to be either universally pleasing or offensive, learning also strongly influences what we eat. Just as individuals may develop a "taste" for certain foods, they may also develop a strong dislike or "aversion" to other foods. Many individuals have had the experience of becoming ill soon after eating. The next time they are offered the same food they were eating when they became sick, they find they have no desire for that food. They may even find the thought of that specific food quite distasteful. This can occur even if the illness was totally independent of the food eaten. This phenomenon is known as a conditioned taste aversion, associating sickness with a specific food. Conditioned taste aversions were first noted when researchers were investigating the effects of radiation on animals during the post-World War II period. They noted that rats made sick by radiation exposure after eating a specific food, would later avoid that food. Two factors appeared important for learning to take place, the food must be novel, one not frequently eaten, and the sickness must be associated fairly close in time with when the food was eaten.

While the availability of food, taste, smell, likes, and dislikes all appear to be important environmental factors that help determine when we are hungry, what information does the brain receive from the body regulating our desire to eat?

METABOLIC FACTORS

One of the classic theories on the regulation of food intake, the glucostatic hypothesis, was proposed by Dr. Jean Mayer. This hypothesis focused on glucose, which is the primary source of energy utilized by the cells of the body, as an important factor in determining when we are hungry. The glucostatic theory proposes that there are receptors in the hypothalamus which are sensitive to the levels of glucose in the blood. When your glucose level falls below some critical value, you become hungry and start to eat, when your level rises above this value, eating stops.

Unfortunately, this theory did not account for the eating behavior of individuals with diabetes. Diabetics have a high level of blood glucose, yet they appear to be in a constant state of hunger. The original theory was soon revised. Glucose was still important in regulating eating, however, it was not the level of glucose in the blood that was the critical factor monitored, but the amount of glucose being utilized by the cells. While diabetics have high levels of glucose in their blood, they have low levels of insulin. Insulin is a hormone released by the pancreas and is necessary for cells to utilize glucose as a source of energy. Therefore, individuals with diabetes have high blood glucose levels but low levels of cellular glucose utilization, resulting in a constant state of hunger.

SATIATION

While both environmental variables and the metabolic factors appear to be important for initiating a meal, what factors are important for ending it? Both humans and animals eat in discrete meals. The end of a meal appears not to depend on the release of energy from the food eaten, for we stop eating long before all the food in a given meal is digested and absorbed. For many years there has been evidence that a blood-borne factor mediates the termination of a meal. For example, it was known that the food intake of a hungry rat could be reduced by up to 50 percent if its blood had been mixed with that of a rat that had just finished a meal. The basic hypothesis was that a blood-borne factor was formed in relation to food intake, and when this factor reached a certain level it would promote satiety. With time the level of this substance would drop, and when it fell below a critical level, the animal would initiate its next meal.

Recently, research has focused on the gastrointestinal hormone, cholecystokinin (CCK), as a possible satiety factor. CCK is released from the upper part of the small intestine. The principal stimuli for its release seem to be the presence of fatty acids and amino acids in the duodenum. CCK has its greatest effects five to fifteen minutes after the onset of a meal. CCK doesn't change the initial reaction to food, but appears to speed up satiation. Studies have found that people infused with CCK stop eating sooner. While they eat less following CCK infusions, they appear as if they

have been normally satisfied.

REGULATION OF BODY WEIGHT

While many of the above factors are important for the short-term regulation of food intake, body weight appears to be regulated over longer periods of time than just a single meal. Individuals maintain stable body weights over days, weeks, and even years. Scientists have proposed the concept of "body weight set point" to help explain how an individual maintains stable body weight over extended periods of time. This theory states that each individual defends a given body weight. The body weight may either be genetically predetermined or a function of early feeding practices. Research on animals has supported this concept. For example, when you give rats palatable foods such as marshmallows, salami, potato chips, and cookies, they overeat and become obese. However, as soon as you put these animals back on a standard laboratory diet, they lose the excess weight they have gained, and weigh no more than animals who never received the good-tasting foods. Similarly, rats who have been reduced by giving them less food than they would normally eat, rapidly "catch-up" in weight when given free access to food again. These animals appear to be defending a preset body weight. This theory does not bode well for dieters, for it suggests that when people lose weight, they are fighting their own set-points.

Our desire to eat appears to be regulated by many factors both in the environment and from within our own bodies. As it is basic to survival, multiple determination of feeding behavior is clearly critical to the organism. (See also DIABETES; DIETARY RECOMMENDATIONS.)

ARGININE

This is a strong, alkaline amino acid (building block of protein). Growing infants and children require good dietary sources of this amino acid because it is not made in the body in sufficient quantity to sustain a normal rate of growth. Foods rich in protein all contain significant amounts of arginine. However, arginine supplements have no value in the human diet. Some bodybuilders take arginine supplements under the mistaken impression that it facilitates muscle growth. However, this is not true. (See also AMINO ACIDS.)

ARTERIOSCLEROSIS

Arteriosclerosis (hardening of the arteries) is a process that develops early in life and progresses as an individual gets older. Fatty materials (lipids) carried in the blood, mainly in the form of a waxy substance known as cholesterol, deposit in the lining of arteries, forming rough plaques that gradually increase in size. This process reduces the opening through which blood can flow. Eventually, the artery may become completely blocked, cutting off the blood flow to those areas of the organ which the artery supplies. If the artery feeds the heart tissue (a coronary artery), the patient suffers what we commonly call a "heart attack." If the clogged artery feeds a portion of the brain, the patient will have a "stroke." Thus, a heart attack or a stroke is not a primary disease of the heart or the brain, but rather a disease of the blood vessels. What do we know about this disease—the most common cause of death in America— and what measures can we take to lower its incidence?

First, and extremely important, is that this disease begins in young adulthood, or perhaps even in childhood, and progresses throughout life. Studies of young American soldiers killed in recent wars have demonstrated that lesions of arteriosclerosis were present in alarmingly large numbers. Moreover, this was a new finding in that during previous wars these lesions were much less frequently seen in our soldiers. These studies, plus other investigations, strongly suggest not only that the disease begins relatively early in life, but also that it is becoming more and more prevalent.

Second, the disease is not "caused" by any one factor; rather it is associated with multiple causes or risk factors. The most important of these are cigarette smoking, hypertension (high blood pressure), high blood levels of certain lipids (primarily cholesterol), and diabetes. Obesity is an indirect risk factor by contributing to hypertension, high cholesterol levels, and diabetes. These major risk factors are additive. Thus, a fifty-year-old man who smokes heavily and has hypertension, high cholesterol levels, and diabetes is at maximum risk of having a heart attack over the next several years. The odds can be progressively decreased by removing each risk factor.

In recent years, a great deal of attention has focused on serum cholesterol levels because these are at least in part under dietary control. Tables have been published giving so-called "normal values," which are dependent on age and sex. For middle-aged men, a value of 250 milligrams per 100 milliliters might be considered the upper limit of normal. This concept is deceiving and may give an unwarranted sense of security. What is really being given are average values for age and sex for Americans. Most Americans, however, consume diets that favor high blood cholesterol levels and hence the average values are too high. This distinction between average and normal is extremely important, since the risk of coronary artery disease increases progressively with the *increase* in blood cholesterol levels regardless of what that blood level is. If the other risk factors are the same, an individual with a level of 300 milligrams per 100 milliliters is more at risk than one whose level is 250 milligrams, who, in turn, is more at risk than an individual whose level is 200 milligrams, and so on. The lower the blood cholesterol levels, the lower the risk.

Cholesterol is manufactured in the body and is also available in the diet. The level in the blood is determined by availability from these two sources. Certain fats in the diet (saturated fats), obtained largely from fatty meats and dairy products, will increase blood cholesterol levels, whereas other types of fats (polyunsaturated fats), obtained largely from vegetable sources, and monounsaturated fats, obtained from fish, peanuts and olive oil, are believed to lower blood cholesterol levels. In general, the "hard" fats are saturated whereas the soft ones are unsaturated.

Cholesterol is carried in the blood attached to protein carriers of different sizes, forming lipoproteins. The low-density lipoproteins (LDL) carry the majority of cholesterol and it is actually high levels of cholesterol in this form that is associated with increased risk of coronary artery disease. Recently, a high-density lipoprotein (HDL) has attracted a great deal of interest. Several studies have suggested that high blood levels of HDL cholesterol (which indicates the amount of cholesterol carried by the high-density lipoprotein) *protect* against coronary artery disease. Thus, while high blood cholesterol in general signals trouble, it is important in such individuals to know the amount of LDL-cholesterol and HDL-cholesterol.

There is very little disagreement among the experts that high levels of LDL-cholesterol, especially when coupled with low levels of HDL-cholesterol, increase the risk of coronary artery disease. There is also general agreement that, since blood cholesterol levels represent a balance between the amount manufactured by the body and the amount consumed in the diet, reducing the dietary intake of cholesterol will only partially lower blood cholesterol. The reason for this is that the body will simply make more and the amount made will vary from individual to individual. What is not agreed upon is how much blood cholesterol can be lowered by consuming a diet low in cholesterol and saturated fat. A good rule of thumb is 15 to 20 percent, but this will vary from person to person and is especially dependent on the initial level. People with very high levels to start with will usually show greater drops with dietary control.

Since arteriosclerosis is a condition that develops over many years, prevention entails a life-style which should begin as early as possible and which must be maintained. As far as the diet is concerned, this means consuming foods lower in saturated fat and cholesterol than what, at present, we generally consume. In addition exercising regularly and not smoking cigarettes will also reduce risk. The earlier these measures are introduced, the better.

Two major risk factors in heart disease—obesity and elevated blood cholesterol—can be avoided by making certain changes in your eating patterns.

One of the earliest projects to identify diet change as a successful means of lowering blood cholesterol was the Anti-Coronary Club in the Bureau of Nutrition, New York City Department of Health. Doctor Norman Jolliffe, the project's director, coined the name "The Prudent Diet." This diet is designed to lower blood cholesterol by limiting the *amount* and the *kinds* of fat that you eat. Fat should contribute no more than one-third of the total dietary calories. The diet should contain at least twice as much polyunsaturated fat as saturated fat. In addition, cholesterol intake should be kept under 300 milligrams per day.

AT THE TABLE

In order to limit the total amount of fat and cholesterol we must limit the main sources of these substances—animal products—in our diet. The maximum amount of meat (*anything* with fins, fur, or feathers) to be eaten per day is 6 ounces if your total intake is 1500 calories, and 8 ounces if your total intake exceeds 1500 calories. This level ensures a cholesterol intake that will be less than 300 milligrams per day. At the same time it limits the amount of fat being contributed by primarily highly saturated fat foods. The red meats (beef, lamb, and pork) should be limited to 16 ounces per week.

To that you must *add* 3 tablespoons (for 6 ounces of meat) or 4 tablespoons (for 8 ounces of meat) of a highly polyunsaturated fat per day. This amount should include what you add as a spread, what is used in cooking (including frying at home), and what is used on salads. These 3 or 4 tablespoons ensure a dietary polyunsaturated to saturated fat ratio of 2 to 1.

Limit egg yolks to two per week whether eaten plain or in prepared foods. Egg whites can be eaten in unlimited quantities. No additional fat-containing foods should be eaten.

All other low-fat foods (such as fruits, vegetables, low-fat dairy products, grains, beans, etc.) can be eaten within limits unless you are watching your weight. In this case, use your discretion on high sugar foods. All together, the amount of fat from the fat in the meat and the added 3 or 4 tablespoons of oil will contribute one-third of your total calories.

Desserts should be low in fat—gelatin, fruit ices, low-fat yogurt, or angel food cake. (See also ALCOHOL; CHOLESTEROL; HYPERTENSION.)

LIPIDS AND POLYUNSATURATES IN SELECTED FOODS, FATS, AND OILS*

100-gm Edible Serving	Total Fat (gm)	SFA† (gm)	MFA† (gm)	PFA† (gm)	Oleic (gm)	Lin-Lin† (gm)	P/S Ratio†	Chol.† (mg)
Beef approx. 6% fat, cooked..	6.10	2.70	2.72	0.48	2.34	0.30	0.2	91.0
Beef approx. 30% fat, cooked	32.00	13.30	15.67	1.33	13.10	1.10	0.1	94.0
Lamb approx. 7% fat, cooked	7.00	2.95	2.69	0.42	2.50	0.33	0.1	100.0
Lamb approx. 30% fat, cooked	29.40	13.70	11.97	1.71	11.25	1.67	0.1	98.0
Veal approx. 6% fat, cooked..	6.70	2.04	1.90	0.67	1.68	0.45	0.3	99.0
Veal approx. 25% fat, cooked	25.20	9.21	8.95	1.26	7.82	1.20	0.1	101.0
Chicken, turkey, Cornish hen, light meat without skin	3.40	0.88	0.76	0.76	0.62	0.56	0.9	78.0
Duck, goose (domestic) without skin	8.20	1.88	3.72	0.74	3.41	0.74	0.4	91.0
Beef, ground, fat unknown	32.00	13.30	15.67	1.33	13.10	1.10	0.1	94.0
Beef bologna	30.00	13.00	15.10	0.90	13.30	0.90	0.1	52.0
Pork, fresh, 30% fat, cooked	30.60	11.68	15.24	3.54	14.02	3.29	0.3	89.0
Frankfurter, all beef, cooked	30.00	12.70	14.80	1.20	13.00	1.20	0.1	51.0
Frankfurter, type unknown	27.20	10.06	13.52	3.17	12.33	3.17	0.3	62.0
Smoked pork, 25% fat, cooked	25.70	8.96	12.17	2.86	11.04	2.60	0.3	89.0
Bologna, salami, cold cuts, 25% fat.	27.50	10.52	13.90	2.13	12.46	2.13	0.2	91.5
Bacon, regular, cooked..	52.00	18.09	22.93	5.47	21.25	5.33	0.3	79.0
Cold cuts, variety unknown	27.50	10.52	13.90	2.13	12.46	2.13	0.2	91.5
Turkey frankfurters	23.76	5.72	9.92	5.78	7.06	5.61	1.0	98.5
Fish, 6% fat	4.00	1.08	1.07	1.55	0.70	0.18	1.4	66.0
Fish, 12% fat	13.40	2.28	3.17	4.56	1.55	0.77	2.0	84.0

Food								
Fish, 20% fat	0.90	0.21	0.17	0.37	0.09	0.02	1.8	66.0
Herring, canned, smoked, pickled	13.60	2.56	8.06	2.16	1.88	0.20	0.8	97.0
Salmon, pink, canned	5.90	0.98	1.75	2.66	1.02	0.30	2.3	35.0
Sardines, canned, drained	11.10	3.00	3.57	3.22	1.66	0.23	1.1	140.0
Tuna, canned, oil packed, drained	8.20	1.63	1.66	4.45	1.66	4.45	2.7	65.0
Tuna, canned, water packed	0.80	0.19	0.13	0.20	0.09	0.02	1.1	63.0
Clams, cooked	2.50	0.48	0.45	0.53	0.14	0.08	1.1	63.0
Crabmeat, cooked, canned	2.50	0.37	0.54	1.02	0.27	0.09	2.8	101.0
Crab, soft shell, steamed	2.50	0.25	0.34	0.55	0.18	0.05	2.2	100.0
Lobster, cooked	1.50	0.14	0.15	0.46	0.11	0.03	3.3	85.0
Oysters, cooked	2.20	0.75	0.42	0.84	0.16	0.09	1.1	45.0
Scallops, cooked	1.40	0.23	0.14	0.53	0.05	0.02	2.3	53.0
Shrimp, cooked	1.10	0.13	0.12	0.44	0.08	0.03	3.4	150.0
Caviar	15.00	3.71	4.65	6.29	3.51	0.03	1.7	300.0
Eggs, whole	11.50	3.40	4.54	1.38	4.16	1.29	0.4	504.0
Egg, yolk	30.60	10.10	13.42	4.11	12.30	3.83	0.4	480.0
Egg, white	0.00	0.00	0.00	0.00	0.00	0.00	0.0	0.0
Egg substitute, brand unknown	9.50	1.21	2.35	5.53	2.34	5.53	4.6	3.4
Creamer, imitation, liquid, frozen, saturated vegetable fat	11.00	8.50	0.10	0.00	0.10	0.00	0.0	0
Creamer—Poly Perx	10.00	1.50	4.60	3.90	3.10	3.30	2.6	0
Cream, light, sweet or sour, 20% fat	20.60	12.80	5.96	0.77	5.18	0.77	0.1	66.0
Buttermilk, 1% fat	0.80	0.50	0.23	0.03	0.20	0.03	0.1	2.3
Milk, 1% fat	1.00	0.60	0.28	0.03	0.25	0.03	0.1	2.9
Milk, 2% fat	2.00	1.20	0.58	0.08	0.50	0.08	0.1	5.8
Milk, whole	3.50	2.20	1.01	0.13	0.88	0.13	0.1	13.5

100-gm Edible Serving	Total Fat (gm)	SFA† (gm)	MFA† (gm)	PFA† (gm)	Oleic (gm)	Lin-Lin† (gm)	P/S Ratio†	Chol.† (mg)
Cheese—grated, dry, creamed	26.50	16.80	7.71	0.58	6.83	0.58	0.0	95.0
cottage, low salt	2.00	1.24	0.58	0.07	0.50	0.07	0.1	8.3
cottage, creamed	4.20	2.60	1.09	0.12	0.91	0.12	0.1	14.7
cream, Neufchâtel, 20% fat	21.18	13.17	6.12	0.78	5.32	0.78	0.1	76.0
cheddar, American, blue, feta, Liederkranz, Camembert	32.20	20.03	9.31	1.19	8.08	1.19	0.1	102.4
Yogurt—part skim, plain	1.70	1.00	0.41	0.04	0.34	0.04	0.0	7.0
part skim, all flavors	0.85	0.53	0.25	0.03	0.21	0.03	0.1	4.6
whole milk, all flavors	3.40	2.20	0.93	0.10	0.78	0.10	0.0	13.2
Ice cream, medium rich, 16% fat	16.10	10.01	4.65	0.60	4.04	0.60	0.1	57.0
Sherbet	1.20	0.75	0.35	0.04	0.30	0.04	0.1	3.5
Ice milk	5.10	3.20	1.42	0.19	1.28	0.19	0.1	14.4
Oil—corn	100.00	12.70	24.74	58.22	24.60	58.22	4.6	0
cottonseed	100.00	26.10	18.88	50.70	18.10	50.70	1.9	0
safflower	100.00	9.40	12.47	73.76	11.90	73.76	7.9	0
sesame	100.00	15.20	39.99	40.46	39.10	40.46	2.7	0
soybean, partially hydrogenated	100.00	13.00	47.00	40.00	31.00	33.00	3.1	0
olive	100.00	14.20	72.47	8.95	71.50	8.95	0.6	0
peanut	100.00	19.10	46.00	30.00	46.00	30.00	1.6	0
coconut	100.00	89.26	6.03	1.83	5.65	1.83	0.02	0
palm	100.00	47.90	38.30	9.30	37.90	9.30	0.2	0
Shortening, household, vegetable	100.00	32.03	42.06	19.60	26.77	16.73	0.6	0

Margarine—% fat unknown—tub	81.00	14.84	29.29	35.88	29.29	35.88	2.4	0
% fat unknown—stick	17.70	35.70	26.00	0.00	0.00	0.00	1.5	0
Mayonnaise, commercial or homemade	79.90	12.00	17.90	46.10	15.90	46.10	3.8	70.0
Peanut butter	50.60	9.66	23.28	15.18	23.28	15.18	1.6	0
Almonds	54.20	4.31	36.84	10.12	36.50	10.12	2.4	0
Cashews	45.70	9.20	26.44	7.42	26.20	7.42	0.8	0
Peanuts	48.70	9.30	22.40	14.61	22.40	14.61	1.6	0
Walnuts	64.00	6.94	9.90	41.81	9.70	41.81	6.0	0
Olives, black	13.80	1.96	10.01	1.24	9.87	1.24	0.6	0
Lard, rendered	100.00	39.60	44.34	11.77	40.90	11.40	0.3	95.0
Butter, sweet or salted	81.00	49.80	23.10	3.00	20.10	3.00	0.1	227.3
MCT oil	100.00	100.00	0.00	0.00	0.00	0.00	0.0	0.0

*Data provided by the Nutrition Coding Center, University of Minnesota. Supported by contract no. 1-HV-6-2941-I of the National Heart, Lung and Blood Institute.

†SFA = Saturated fatty acid. MFA = monounsaturated fatty acid. PFA = polyunsaturated fatty acid. Lin-Lin = linoleic-linolenic. Chol. = cholesterol.
P/S ratio = polyunsaturated/saturated fatty acids.
Reprinted by permission of the Bureau of Nutrition, City of new York.

ASPARTAME

Aspartame is a substance made up of two amino acids, aspartic acid and phenylalanine. Although both of these amino acids are widely found in nature, the chemically combined combination is not. Aspartame is used as an artificial sweetener in many food substances and soft drinks. It is almost devoid of calories because it is many times as sweet as sucrose (table sugar) on a weight basis. Thus very small amounts will give as sweet a taste as much larger amounts of sugar. Most people find aspartame to have much less of an aftertaste than such other artificial sweeteners as saccharin and sucrose. Aspartame has been extensively tested and has been approved by the Food and Drug Administration as a safe food additive. The maximum recommended is 60 packets of Equal or 11 soft drinks sweetened with aspartame. However, the very long-term effects of ingesting large quantities of aspartame are not yet known. Since the body breaks this substance down into its constituent amino acids, aspartic acid and phenylalanine, in any condition where these amino acids are harmful aspartame should be avoided. One such condition is phenylketonuria (PKU), a condition in which the body is unable to metabolize phenylalanine properly. People with PKU must be on a low phenylalanine diet for life, and phenylalanine in aspartame can be very dangerous for them.

At present, for the vast majority of people aspartame seems safe, particularly if consumed in moderate quantities (1.7 grams per day). It may be particularly useful for people suffering from diabetes or obesity, increasing the variety of foods they are allowed to eat. Some people, including certain members of the scientific community have spoken out against the general use of aspartame. A significant number of letters has been received by the FDA describing many and varied side effects of aspartame. Those who believe that they have suffered from the use of this sweetener should refrain from using it. For the vast majority of people it appears to be safe.

ASPARTIC ACID

Aspartic acid is an amino acid which is not essential for humans since it can be manufactured in the body from other compounds. Aspartic acid is one of two amino acids in the compound aspartame, which is currently the most widely used low-calorie sugar sweetener. (See ASPARTAME.)

Aspartic acid by itself or in combination with other amino acids has no known health benefits and therefore should not be taken as a supplement. As with any other single amino acid, large doses of aspartic acid by itself could cause amino acid imbalances. (See also AMINO ACIDS.)

BEE POLLEN

Bee pollen is pollen collected from flowers by honeybees, then mixed with nectar and used as bee food. Before they have a chance to eat it, the pollen can be removed from the bees' legs by special devices placed within the hive. The pollen is then processed and packaged and sold in health-food stores.

Several claims have been made for this pollen. First, it is said that bee pollen is a natural antibiotic; but in fact, it is attacked by bacteria and fungi. Second, it is said to be the richest source of protein when in fact it contains only 5 to 28 percent protein. Compared with soybean curd (tofu), which is 46 percent protein, and brewer's yeast, which is 39 percent protein, bee pollen seems to be far from the richest protein source. Third, it is supposed to have antiaging properties—the centenarians in Russia consume bee pollen, however, the amount they consume is very small. (The more likely reason why these people live so long is that their diet is at least 70 percent complex carbohydrate and very rich in fiber.) Fourth, bee pollen is supposed to fight allergies and asthma. In reality it has been reported to cause serious allergies in susceptible people and not cure them. Finally, there is no truth to the claim that bee pollen improves athletic performance.

There is absolutely no reason to consume bee pollen. Its only claim to fame is that it has a good protein content. But, ounce for ounce bee pollen is much more expensive than the most expensive cuts of fish and meat, which also provide lots of other nutrients and make them of much better nutritional value.

BIOFLAVONOIDS

Self-styled nutritionists claim that bioflavonoids, otherwise referred to by them as vitamin P or hesperidin, are essential for good health and provide resistance to colds and flu. However, bioflavonoids are not essential to humans and cannot be classified as a vitamin. They do not provide protection against colds or flu or against any other disease or condition in humans.

BIOTIN

Except for a few reported cases in people with extremely bizarre eating habits, biotin deficiency does not occur in humans. Yeasts and many bacteria either make or retain biotin. Humans can probably obtain all they need from the numerous microorganisms that are present in foods, or in their own large intestines. In addition, certain foods, for example eggs, liver, kidney, pulses, nuts, chocolate, and some vegetables, are rich in biotin. The human body utilizes a few micrograms of biotin per day. There have been no documented health benefits described from taking large doses of biotin. (See also VITAMINS.)

BREAST-FEEDING

ADVANTAGES FOR THE INFANT

The perfect food for a newborn baby is breast milk. No formula, no matter how "humanized" it has been made, can take the place of human milk. It is designed to support the growth of the infant, to be easily digested and absorbed by the infant's immature gastrointestinal tract, and to supply substances that protect the infant against infection in the period before the child's own immune system develops.

The breasts are fully developed by the time a girl has passed through puberty, but they are only activated into milk production during pregnancy when their size increases. At first they produce only colostrum, which is a yellow fluid high in protein and immune substances. These substances render the infant less susceptible to certain infections, especially ones like gastroenteritis. Colostrum also causes the newborn infant's intestines to grow in size so as to be ready to receive the mother's milk.

The act of suckling stimulates nerve endings around the nipple causing the production of milk by the mother. Milk production reaches a steady state with repeated suckling, and so it is true to say that the longer the time spent in suckling the more milk is produced. Milk production increases when nursings are frequent, and therefore, periods during which full breasts are not emptied should be avoided.

The successful removal of milk from the breast is dependent on the infant's ability to suckle and the mother's "let down reflex." This nerve reflex is responsible for propelling milk from the innermost regions of the breasts to the nipples. After a few minutes of suckling the let down reflex will come into play. However, this reflex may not occur properly if the mother is anxious or distressed, or if the infant sucks poorly because of having recently been quieted down in the nursery with a bottle-feeding.

Beginning the third or fourth day after delivery, a slow transition in the breasts occurs from colostrum to milk production. This means fat and lactose content increases and protein and salt concentrations decrease. Even the best infant formula cannot possibly duplicate this gradual enrichment. By the end of the first month, the amount of milk produced in the mother's breasts is stable—about 600 milliliters each day. This gradually rises to about 800 milliliters by the sixth month. If solid foods are introduced to the infant during this period, then the quantity of milk produced by the mother will decrease, due to the decreased suckling of the infant. However, if suckling continues at the same rate, milk production will continue at this rate, even over a twelve month period.

Human milk is a dilute milk, which means that the body's kidneys can easily handle its waste products. In fact no other fluids need be taken by an infant—not even water. Being a dilute milk with only .9 to 1 percent protein (as opposed to 3 to 4 percent in cow milk) breast milk needs to be fed to the infant frequently. The slower an animal's growth rate, the lower the protein content of its milk. Since it is natural for babies to grow much slower than calves, human milk contains less protein than does cow milk. Similarly, the slower the growth rate, the higher the lactose content, and hence it is not surprising that human milk contains 7 percent lactose while cow milk has only 5 percent.

Fat is the chief form of calories in milk. During the first month of lactation fat amounts to 50 percent of the energy (calorie) requirements. This percentage gradually declines over time. Human milk contains more unsaturated (or vegetable-like) fat than cow milk. Breast milk contains the enzyme lipase, which breaks down fat when activated by bile salts. Therefore, nearly all the fat is absorbed and little is lost in the infant's stool. Both human milk and cow milk are rich in cholesterol. It has been

suggested that the fat content of breast milk actually increases during a feed. Thus "hind" milk would contain more fat than "fore" milk.

The protein found in human milk is also of special composition and so is very difficult to reproduce. When digested, it divides into two fractions, a curd of casein, representing 30 percent, and the remainder as whey, which is in solution. By contrast, cow milk consists of 20 percent whey and the remainder is casein. The actual composition of the casein from cows and humans is also very different—human milk is rich in cysteine and poor in methionine. Studies have shown that certain infants, especially very small ones, may not be able to convert methionine to cysteine and hence require the latter. Finally, the curd from human milk is softer and more easily digested than that from cow milk.

Just as with the major nutrients discussed above, breast milk by itself usually contains adequate amounts of vitamins and minerals to support optimal growth of the infant for the first four to six months of life. However, unlike the protein, fat, and carbohydrate, the quantity of vitamins and minerals in breast milk is affected by the mother's diet. Thus, it is important for the nursing mother to eat a varied diet which will supply adequate amounts of these substances.

Although iron is present in

breast milk in only small quantities it is highly absorbable, hence totally breast-fed infants do not require iron supplementation. Traditionally, breast-fed infants have been supplemented with vitamin D. This is because it was believed that breast milk was very low in this vitamin. Recent studies suggest that vitamin D is present in human milk in a form not previously recognized. However, until more research confirms this, we still recommend a vitamin D supplement (400 international units per day) for breast-fed infants.

Breast milk is not a good source of fluoride. Fluoride decreases the susceptibility to dental caries by as much as 60 percent and so fluoride supplements should be given to all babies living in areas where water is fluoridated less than 60%, whether the babies are breast- or bottle-fed. Teeth begin to develop during early gestation, and by the time of birth calcium is being deposited in both the primary teeth and permanent teeth despite the fact that they are not visible. Fluoride (.25 milligrams) taken daily will strengthen the resistance of teeth to decay.

Breast-feeding imparts benefits to the infant beyond supplying optimal nutrition. Breast-fed infants tend to be less susceptible to disease, especially respiratory diseases and gastrointestinal infections. This is partly because of immune substances in colostrum and breast milk and partly because breast milk contains a substance or substances which discourage the growth of *E. coli,* a bacterium responsible for much of the gastroenteritis found in young infants. Finally, infants rarely become allergic or intolerant to their own mothers' milk, whereas such intolerance may occur to cow milk protein and even to protein derived from soya beans.

Obviously, for any woman who is motivated, breast is best. The longer you can breast-feed the better. However, even if you plan to supplement breast-feeding with an infant formula so as to avoid a major change in life-style (e.g., the working mother who does not wish to pump her breasts), this is far preferable to not breast-feeding at all. Don't be discouraged before you try it. In America today more than half of all women begin by breast-feeding—women from all walks of life with all kinds of life-styles.

ADVANTAGES FOR THE MOTHER

Breast-feeding offers certain advantages to the mother as well as to the infant. These include the initial stimulation of firm contractions of the uterus, which will help minimize postpartum blood loss and restore the uterus to its prepregnancy state more rapidly. Over a longer period, women who breast-feed return to their prepregnancy weight more rapidly. Many women complain that weight problems began after they bore their first child and were aggravated by the birth of successive children. We suspect this may be due in part to the fact that these women did not breast-feed.

Fat is deposited during pregnancy as a reserve for lactation. If the mother nurses for a significant period of time this fat is easily used up. But if she fails to nurse, it is far more difficult to get rid of. Lactation may even be a good time for an overweight woman to lose weight. Energy expended by lactation is like performing vigorous exercise all day long. By moderate dietary restriction and by ensuring the availability of adequate amounts of essential nutrients, a nursing mother may lose significant weight and still provide adequate amounts of high quality milk to her infant. A final advantage of breast-feeding is that it is the cheapest and most energy-efficient way to feed an infant.

There are certain myths which have arisen over the years about breast-feeding that should be dispelled. The serious charge that breast feeding increases a woman's chances of developing cancer of the breast is *absolutely* untrue. Extensive studies have shown that breast-feeding mothers do not get any more cancers of the breast than bottle-feeding mothers. Therefore, fear of contracting cancer is no reason not to breast-feed. A less serious charge is that the aesthetic beauty of the breasts will be compromised—that they may sag later in life. To our knowledge no responsible study has ever shown this. Some people have also said that women with small breasts may not be able to nurse their infant adequately. Ability to nurse does not depend on breast size. With few exceptions, every woman has more than enough active breast tissue to nurse her infant adequately.

MOTHER AND CHILD INTERACTIONS DURING BREAST-FEEDING

There is evidence that a special relationship develops between a breast-feeding mother and her child. There is a constant giving and taking between the nursing pair during the first few months of life such that each receives a great deal of emotional pleasure.

Part of this is psychological and will be shared by both breast-feeding couples and bottle-feeding couples alike. However, breast-feeding mothers may derive extra pleasure due to the release of certain hormones as a result of suckling. Some women have described a feeling of well-being and relaxation, while others describe feelings comparable to sexual orgasm. There are studies which even suggest that the odor from the breasts has a very positive effect on the infant, who shows pleasure in a variety of ways.

Many women who have successfully breast-fed describe nursing as the most pleasurable experience of their lives—an experience that cannot be duplicated and should not be missed.

PRACTICAL TIPS

The earlier you make the decision to breast-feed the better. Discuss the idea with your husband, as it helps to have his support. It makes you feel more confident and less self-conscious when you actually start feeding your baby.

Select an obstetrician and pediatrician who support the practice. The obstetrician will then make sure that you gain sufficient weight to provide for the extra energy you will later need and will also deliver the baby under the minimum amount of sedation and anesthesia. An alert baby will nurse sooner and more vigorously. It is a good idea to start nursing soon after delivery, or even on the delivery table, with no interim bottle-feeding being used at all. The supportive physician will also give you instructions on how to hold the baby and how to breast-feed. If your nipples are retracted it may be necessary to massage them during pregnancy to prepare them for the baby.

Once you start nursing, frequent feeds are good, and you should not try to establish a rigid feeding schedule too soon. Both breasts should be used for feeding. You alternate the starting breast and let the infant suckle ten minutes on one and then five minutes on the other. Later you may extend these periods. Always remember to break the suction with your little finger before taking the baby from your breast to avoid damaging the nipple.

No bottle supplements should be used at the beginning as these reduce appetite and therefore reduce the amount of milk the baby takes from your breast at each feeding. This also leads to a build-up of milk in the breasts, which makes them feel uncomfortable. In addition, different types of suckling confuse the baby. Only after the baby is nursing effectively and your milk production is good should a supplementary bottle be introduced if necessary.

No written account can replace personal experience, but we do hope that these tips will make it a little easier for you by teaching you how to avoid the most common pitfalls women have encountered.

THE MOTHER'S DIET DURING BREAST-FEEDING

If a mother is to be able to produce sufficient milk to satisfy her infant's demands then she must eat a well-balanced diet with special emphasis on critical nutrients, such as calcium, iron, and water-soluble vitamins. This can easily be achieved with very little alteration in the normal diet.

The *composition* of breast milk in regard to most nutrients, namely calories, protein, carbohydrate, and fat, remains relatively constant regardless of the mother's diet. However, if the dietary intake of these nutrients is severely restricted, the *quantity* of milk produced may be reduced. A considerable amount of fat is stored during pregnancy to supply energy to the mother during lactation. After delivery, a woman normally ends up with about nine pounds of extra weight over and above what she weighed before she became pregnant. This, along with an additional 500 calories per day from her diet, should be sufficient to supply all the energy she needs to lactate properly. In order to prevent losing protein from her body, she will also have to eat an extra 20 grams of protein per day, which means that she should be eating about 50 grams per day in all. This is actually very little in American dietary terms.

Breast milk contains a lot of calcium, which is found at a constant level irrespective of how much is found in the mother's diet. If there is too little calcium in the mother's diet it will be removed from her bones. This can weaken her bones and may predispose a woman to osteoporosis (brittle bones) in later life

and so must be avoided. This simply means that a good calcium intake is essential. Milk, cheese, yogurt, and other dairy products are the best sources of calcium.

As the level of phosphorus in the diet rises, the amount of calcium absorbed decreases. Hence, foods like meat and certain carbonated beverages which are rich in phosphorus should be limited. Calcium from vegetable products is difficult to absorb for another reason. It binds to the roughage in the diet called phytate and so is not absorbed very efficiently. Hence, although almonds, collard greens, kale, and tofu are good vegetable sources of calcium, it is still doubtful that a vegetarian excluding dairy products from her diet will get the 1200 milligrams of calcium she needs to produce breast milk at the normal rate without bone losses. If you don't think your diet contains enough calcium, 1000 milligrams of a commercially available calcium supplement should be taken daily. Ask your physician. (See CALCIUM for a list of some good dietary sources of calcium.)

Iron in breast milk is highly absorbable and is the best iron for the infant. As you would expect, iron deficiency is extremely rare in breast-fed infants—but not impossible. If the mother is anemic, this will certainly affect the iron content of the milk. In order to safeguard against such a situation, foods high in iron should be included in the diet in good amounts. (See IRON for a list of foods high in iron.)

The vitamin content of breast milk is extremely sensitive to the maternal vitamin status, especially with regard to the water soluble vitamins. For this reason, plenty of citrus fruits should be eaten for their vitamin C supply and plenty of fortified and whole grains for the B complex vitamins. In addition most physicians recommend the nursing mother continue the prenatal vitamin supplement.

From all this I think you can see that you just have to modify the diet a little to cater to the extra demands of lactation. In fact, if you gain a lot of weight as a result of your pregnancy, you may want to use the nursing period to lose weight. This is perfectly safe as long as you don't try to lose too much too quickly. Check with your physician before you start and if he or she agrees, limit your calorie intake by reducing the starchy foods you eat. Aim to lose no more than a pound a week, and provided that the infant grows normally, you can continue this procedure until you lose those extra pounds. If the infant's growth slows down then you aren't producing enough milk and so you need to eat more. Two groups of mothers who should not diet at this time are teenagers and mothers who were underweight before they became pregnant. (See also CHILDREN; INFANT FEEDING; INFANT FORMULA; PREGNANCY; WOMEN.)

The following menu gives you the kind of diet that a lactating mother should follow.

SAMPLE DIET FOR A BREAST-FEEDING WOMAN

Breakfast
12 oz apple juice
2 slices whole wheat bread
   with 2 oz cheese melted on each slice
2 plums (canned or fresh)

Snack
8 oz flavored yogurt

Lunch
8 oz minestrone soup
8 wheat crackers

3 oz tuna salad on English muffin
1 orange

Snack
8 oz fruit drink*
⅛ cup nuts
⅛ cup raisins

Dinner
¾ cup yellow squash (w/1 tsp margarine)
½ cup string beans (w/1 tsp margarine)
1 small boiled potato (w/1 tsp margarine)
2 chicken cutlets (2 oz each)
12 oz fruit drink*

Snack
10 oz milk (whole or low-fat)
1 cup puffed cereal
1 sliced banana
2 tsp sweetener (optional)
TOTAL: 2650 calories

(Each snack provides approximately 260 calories. Omit any one of them to reduce the total calories.)

**Fruit Drink*
6 oz can apple juice (frozen concentrated)
6 oz can grape juice (frozen concentrated)
4 oz lemon juice
5 cups water
2 tbsp honey (optional)

A nutritious way to increase fluid intake. Combine in a half-gallon container and chill.

BREWER'S YEAST

Brewer's yeast is often used as a nutritional supplement and is especially beneficial to vegetarians. It is a good source of protein and when added to cereals enhances the quality of protein derived from them. This is important for vegetarians who have a fairly low protein intake. It is also a good source of the B vitamins, iron, potassium, and zinc. Brewer's yeast contains the following nutrients (expressed as milligrams per tablespoon): vitamin B_1 (1.25); vitamin B_2 (.35); vitamin B_6 (.2); folacin (.02); iron (1.5); zinc (.5); potassium (152); sodium (10). (See also VEGETARIAN DIETS; specific vitamins and minerals.)

BROMELAIN

Bromelain is a preparation of an enzyme that breaks down protein. It is isolated from the juice of a type of pineapple called *Ananas comosus*. Bromelain is used by physicians to relieve inflammation and swelling and to help wound healing.

BULIMIA

Bulimia is an eating disorder associated with a binge-purge cycle of food intake. Bulimia frequently occurs after an individual has been displaying extreme self-control while dieting. A bulimic episode usually starts with a feeling of increased subjective hunger. This feeling may be accompanied by an inflated metabolism, including breathlessness, sweating, and a racing pulse. At this point, the individual seems to completely lose control, consuming a tremendous amount of food within a fairly short period of time. For example, one young woman reported binging twice a day on a gallon of ice cream mixed with a half gallon of maple syrup, candy, doughnuts, and assorted other sweets. The episode will typically end with self-induced vomiting, which is followed by feelings of depression and guilt and a return to dieting.

Recently the American Psychological Association organized a set of criteria that are now used to diagnose this disorder. These include, (1) recurrent episodes of binge eating, with rapid consumption of a large amount of food in a discrete period of time, usually less than two hours, (2) at least three of the following: consumption of high-caloric, easily ingested food during a binge; inconspicuous eating during a binge; terminations of binge-eating episodes with either abdominal pain, sleep, social interruption, or self-induced vomiting; repeated attempts to lose weight by severely restricted diets, self-induced vomiting or use of cathartics or diuretics; frequent weight fluctuations of greater than ten pounds due to cycles of binging and fasting, (3) awareness that this pattern of eating is abnormal, but fear of not being able to control it voluntarily, (4) depression following the eating binge, and (5) the bulimic episodes are not due to any known physical disorder.

While bulimia is typically seen in normal weight and obese individuals, up to half of all young women with anorexia nervosa are reported to turn to binging and purging as a means of controlling their weight. While bulimics are often compared to individuals with anorexia nervosa, they tend to have a number of differences in mood and personality. Bulimics tend to be more outgoing and more interested in sex than anorexics. Unlike anorexics, bulimic women usually menstruate normally and remain fertile. Bulimics also tend to have increased lability of mood, display more depressive symptoms, and in general are perceived as being at a higher risk for suicide than individuals with anorexia nervosa. Bulimia itself is typically viewed as a more serious condition that is more difficult to treat than anorexia nervosa. The prognosis is also seen as less favorable. In addition to bulimia resulting in social isolation, there are a host of medical complications frequently resulting from this disorder. These range from mild problems such as decay of teeth and gums from the acid brought up when vomiting, to severe electrolytic imbalances which can be associated with seizures and ultimately death.

In general, treatment for bulimia is aimed at interrupting the cycle of overeating and purging, while getting patients to accept a higher weight. (See also ANOREXIA NERVOSA.)

BUTTER

Butter is prepared from cream by allowing it to sour naturally or introducing a bacterial culture (starter) and churning. It contains about 80 percent fat (including 32 milligrams of cholesterol per tablespoon), 2 percent other milk solids, 16 percent water, 1 percent protein, .4 percent lactose, and 1.5 to 4.5 percent salt.

In addition butter contains (per tablespoon) 114 retinol equivalents of vitamin A, a trace of riboflavin, 3 milligrams of potassium, 3 milligrams of calcium, 3 milligrams of phosphorus, .03 milligrams of iron, and 100 calories. (See CHOLESTEROL.)

CAFFEINE

Caffeine is found in the cola nut, coffee bean, certain tea leaves, and in other plants which are not considered food. Caffeine is definitely a drug and is consumed because it produces a stimulating effect; if it did not produce this effect it would not be added to foods and beverages or consumed in its natural form, as tea or coffee. Caffeine is tasteless, odorless, and has no function as a preservative.

The effects of caffeine on the body arise from its stimulating effect on the central nervous system. Positive effects described by people who use caffeine include improved motor performance, decreased fatigue, increased alertness, and enhanced sensory activity. These positive effects go a long way toward explaining why most of us drink coffee as the first drink of the day. However, the same level of intake that produces "positive" effects in many people also induces negative effects in others. These may include irritability, nervousness or anxiety, tremors, restlessness in children, headaches, insomnia, and withdrawal headaches. In adults, these symptoms often appear upon consumption of two or more cups of drip coffee (200 to 300 milligrams of

DIETARY SOURCES OF CAFFEINE

Product	Caffeine (mg)
Coffee	
Drip (5 oz)	146
Percolated (5 oz)	110
Instant, regular (5 oz)	53
Instant, decaffeinated (5 oz)	2
Tea	
One minute brew (5 oz)	9–33
Three minute brew (5 oz)	20–46
Five minute brew (5 oz)	20–50
Canned iced tea (12 oz)	22–36
Cocoa and chocolate	
Cocoa beverage (6 oz)	10
Milk chocolate (1 oz)	6
Baking chocolate (1 oz)	35
Cola drinks (12 oz)	35–45

caffeine) and sometimes after drinking even a single cup of coffee. Children can be even more sensitive. The table above lists some common dietary sources of caffeine.

Soft drinks, which are favorites among children, often have a high caffeine content. Cola drinks made from the cola bean are not the only culprits in this respect. In fact, some noncola soft drinks contain as much as 52 milligrams of caffeine per 12 ounce can, which is even higher than that found in the average cola beverage. Many prescription and over-the-counter drugs, such as cough medicines and cold remedies, contain caffeine—not as their main ingredient, but rather, to give them an extra, stimulating effect.

As you can see, both adults and children are exposed to fairly high levels of caffeine, which has raised some important health questions regarding both short- and long-term use of the substance. Can short-term effects of caffeine result in hyperactivity in children? Does long-term exposure increase the risk of cancer and birth defects? Both questions are currently being investigated in many research centers.

Recent experiments have shown that relatively low doses of caffeine will produce an abnormal behavior pattern in animals which resembles hyperactivity. Such studies have not been repeated in children. However, clinical observations suggest that certain hyperactive children may improve when foods containing caffeine are removed from their diet. It should be emphasized that it is clear from these and other studies that this is not the major cause of this disorder.

The only evidence available which links long-term exposure to high levels of caffeine to cancer is an epidemiologic study relating heavy coffee consumption to cancer of the pancreas. This study, although provocative, is far from conclusive. First of all, pancreatic cancer is fairly uncommon, and so an extremely large population had to be studied to collect a significant number of cases. The larger the overall population, the greater the chance for other variables not considered by the investigators to be important to the effect. For instance, people consuming lots of coffee might have different eating patterns from those who do not. They may smoke or drink more. They may exercise less. Apart from these examples, there is a whole host of other differences which may be present. Only some of these factors were considered in the study.

Second, the increased incidence of cancer was small, which raises the question of the degree of importance of exposure to caffeine (coffee) in the development of the disease. Alcohol is certainly a more important risk factor. Whether coffee and alcohol interact in some way to increase the effect of each other

is a possibility that has not yet been investigated.

Based on this information, caffeine would not seem to be a major health risk. However, the effect of chronic exposure to caffeine (mainly from soft drinks) in children and adolescents has not been studied, particularly with respect to subtle behavioral effects, which may not be obvious but which in aggregate could affect school performance and other important functions.

Another health concern which has recently received a great deal of attention is exposure of pregnant women and their unborn children to large amounts of caffeine. Birth defects can be produced in animals by exposing the mothers to high doses of caffeine early in pregnancy. Even fairly low doses of caffeine later on in pregnancy can retard fetal growth and result in stunted newborn animals. When animals are exposed to caffeine throughout pregnancy both fetal growth retardation and short-term behavioral abnormalities occur. (See page 260, CAFFEINE.)

Few studies have been carried out in human populations. Although the data is inconclusive, there is some evidence to show that the incidence of spontaneous abortions may be higher in women who consume large amounts of coffee and tea. Other studies have indicated a possible fetal growth retardation effect. But there is no evidence of congenital malformations. No one has yet looked at behavioral changes in the offspring of heavy caffeine users.

This evidence would tend to show that caffeine consumed in large amounts, even by heavy users, is not a major cause of birth defects or fetal growth failure. Its contribution to spontaneous abortion also seems to be minimal. So, how then do we translate these findings into realistic recommendations for pregnant women? Moderate coffee or cola drinkers have little to fear. However, anyone consuming more than eight cups of coffee (one or more grams of caffeine) would do well to reduce her intake. This may not only reduce the risk for the complications noted but will also increase a woman's own peace of mind during pregnancy. (See also TEA.)

CALCIUM

Calcium is the most abundant mineral in the body, with 99 percent or more of the total body calcium residing in the skeletal tissues. The average adult body contains 1 to 1.3 kilograms (2.2 to 3 pounds) of calcium. The calcium in bones and teeth forms a crystalline-like matrix known as hydroxyapatite, consisting mostly of calcium and phosphate in a ratio of approximately 3 calcium to 2 phosphorus, with sodium, magnesium, zinc, iodine, fluoride, and other trace elements in small proportions. Although only about 1 percent of the total body calcium is found in the soft tissues and body fluids, it is the third most abundant cation (positively charged particle) in extracellular fluids of the body, following sodium and potassium. Calcium is extremely important for several types of cellular action such as nerve signal transmission, muscle contraction, and hormone secretion. It is imperative to maintain calcium homeostasis in the body fluids in order for these processes to continue. As a result, dietary calcium is inadequate, mechanisms are invoked by the body to utilize the skeletal stores of calcium to maintain serum levels of this mineral. This can lead to excessive bone resorption, especially in the elderly, and to a condition known as osteoporosis.

Calcium levels in the blood are regulated by absorption of dietary calcium from the intestine, resorption and deposition of calcium in bone, and excretion in the urine. Vitamin D and magnesium are important for absorption of calcium and phosphorus from the intestine and for proper bone mineralization. Lactose, a sugar found in milk, improves calcium absorption and further fortification with vitamin D makes milk one of the best sources of calcium. Other milk products, and sardines and other small fish eaten with the bones are rich sources of calcium. Tofu, oysters, and blackstrap molasses are rich in calcium, while other shellfish, beans, and lentils are moderately good sources. Green leafy vegetables are generally considered to have high levels of calcium, however, the presence of oxalates and phytates in some of these vegetables renders the calcium unavailable. Cocoa (and chocolate), soybeans, kale, and spinach are rich in oxalates, while unpolished rice, bran, and wheat meal are high in organic and inorganic phosphates which all decrease the intestinal absorption of calcium. Tetracycline decreases calcium absorption, and conversely, calcium decreases the antibiotic efficacy of tetracycline. Other antibiotics, such as penicillin, neomycin, and chloramphenicol may enhance calcium absorption.

Several factors can cause increased calcium excretion, including high sodium, high carbohydrate and high protein diets, phosphate deprivation, metabolic acidosis, cortisol and synthetic glucocorticoids, thyroid, and growth hormones. Certain bone diseases characterized by rapid bone loss also exhibit excessive calcium excretion. It has recently been suggested that low dietary calcium, rather than high levels of sodium, may account for the high occurrence of hypertension and heart disease in this country. This, however, remains to be confirmed.

The USRDA for calcium is 800 milligrams for adults, although many health professionals recommend a daily calcium intake of 1200 to 1500 milligrams for women and 800 to 1200 milligrams for men. The Food and Agricultural Organization/World Health Organization recommends only 400 to 500 milligrams for adults in underdeveloped countries. The reason for this discrepancy is in the differences in overall diet and physical activity between people of industrialized nations compared to underdeveloped countries. The high sodium, high protein diets of the US cause a more rapid rate of urinary excretion of cal-

cium. The more sedentary life-style in industrialized countries also leads to less bone mineralization and more rapid bone loss, compared to people who must constantly perform more strenuous labor for a livelihood or survival. The greater exposure of people to sunlight in underdeveloped countries leads to more vitamin D formation in the skin, which increases calcium absorption and utilization. We can conclude from these differences, and from other studies, that ample exposure to sunlight, exercise, and moderation of salt and protein in the diet should all contribute to better calcium absorption and bone mineralization for good health in later years.

Calcium supplements are strongly recommended for pregnant and lactating women and for older adults who are not receiving sufficient calcium in the diet, that is, if dairy products are not consumed regularly. Chelated calcium may be absorbed better than nonchelated forms, but the differences are not large and the cost of chelated forms of calcium are generally several times the cost of more readily available forms. Calcium carbonate, obtained from limestone, is the active component of several antacids and a relatively inexpensive source of this mineral. It is generally believed that calcium in this form is absorbed well. Dolomite is a mineral extracted from the earth, consisting of calcium and

CALCIUM SOURCES

(Each portion provides approximately 300 mg calcium)

Food	Weight	Serving
Almonds, chopped	130 gm	1 cup
Buttermilk	245 gm	8 oz
Cheddar cheese	42 gm	1½ oz
Collard greens, chopped and cooked from frozen pkg	170 gm	1 cup
Cottage cheese, creamed or uncreamed	340 gm	12 oz
Evaporated milk, unsweetened	126 gm	4 oz
Fluid milk, whole or skim low-fat milk (with 2% milk solids added)	245 gm	8 oz
Kale, cooked from frozen pkg	260 gm	2 cups
Mackerel, Pacific, canned	100 gm	3½ oz
Tofu (soybean curd)	240 gm	2 pcs
Turnip greens, cooked from frozen pkg	165 gm	1½ cups

magnesium carbonates. Dolomite is often promoted as a good source of calcium because it also provides magnesium, which is essential for calcium absorption and utilization. Some preparations of dolomite have been found to contain heavy metal contaminants, although many scientists question the significance of the trace amounts of these impurities. Bonemeal is prepared by grinding bone, generally obtained from slaughterhouses, into a fine powder. This is often touted as an ideal form of calcium supplement because it provides mineral nutrients in the proper proportions for bone formation. However, the insolubility of the crystalline-like hydroxyapatite results in poor absorption of the calcium in this form. In addition, animals grazing close to highways or other sources of heavy metal contamination, may have lead, cadmium, or mercury in their bones, and this will be passed on to the people eating bonemeal derived from such exposed animals. (See also DENTAL DECAY; OSTEOPOROSIS.)

CANCER

It has been estimated that 50 percent of all types of cancer in women and 30 percent in men are associated with environmental factors. Of those factors, food supply is one of the most important. Recently, concern has been mounting that food additives of various types may be contributing to the rising incidence of certain types of cancer. Such commonly added materials as saccharin, red dye number two, and nitrites have all been implicated. In addition, there is mounting evidence that substances which "contaminate" our food supply, such as pesticide residues or industrial waste products, are also increasing the risk of certain cancers. Even radioactive materials, such as iodine 131 or strontium 90, turn up from time to time in our food supply.

Such data, important as it is, should not be allowed to detract from another aspect of the problem of diet and cancer—that there is a strong association between the kinds of food we eat and the increasing incidence of specific types of cancer. This problem which may be more difficult to deal with since it defies regulation, cannot be laid at the feet of any one product or group of manufacturers. The evidence comes both from studies of large human populations and from experiments on animals. The best data has been collected with two extremely common types of cancer—those of the breast and colon.

BREAST CANCER

Cancer of the breast is the most common cancer striking American women and a leading cause of death in the United States. In other countries, however, the incidence of breast cancer is much lower. If we list countries in the order of their incidence of breast cancer, an important generalization with certain specific exceptions can be made. The more highly developed the country, the higher the incidence of breast cancer. More careful scrutiny of the data gives us certain clues as to what it is about "modern living" which contributes to this problem, as certain westernized countries, for example, Japan, do not show this high incidence of breast cancer.

By contrast, when Japanese people migrate to California, their children have the same incidence of this cancer as other Californians if they adopt a western eating pattern. If, on the other hand, they continue to eat as their parents did in Japan, relatively few have cancer of the breast. Thus, it is something about the food we eat which contributes to the high incidence of the disease. The strongest correlation appears to be with the amount of fat in the diet. The more fat consumed by the population of a particular country, the higher the incidence of breast cancer, regardless of the state of development of the country. The United States, with its high-fat diet, ranks high, but certain countries which consume even more fat, such as Finland, rank even higher.

How does this high consumption of fat contribute to the problem of breast cancer? We know from other studies and from the fact that the disease occurs far more commonly in women than in men that hormones play an important role. Animal studies suggest that a diet high in fat will result in an imbalance of at least two hormones, and it is postulated that this hormone imbalance in some way promotes the occurrence of cancer of the breast.

Women who consume a relatively high-fat diet may alter their hormonal balance and by so doing become more susceptible to developing breast cancer.

COLON CANCER

Colon cancer (cancer of the large intestine) is a very common type of cancer in the United States, and its incidence is increasing. Like cancer of the breast colon cancer occurs more frequently in developed countries and

certain migrating populations demonstrate an incidence of cancer which more closely matches that of their adopted country once they change their eating patterns to resemble those of the native population. Again, the best correlation of cancer of the colon is with dietary fat. The more fat consumed, the higher the incidence of the disease. In the United States particular groups who for one reason or another consume diets relatively low in fat (such as Seventh Day Adventists) show a low incidence of colon cancer.

Unlike breast cancer, colon cancer occurs with equal frequency in men and women. Thus, sex hormones play little or no role in the development of cancer of the colon. How then does this disease occur? While we are not sure yet, animal experiments suggest that a high-fat diet changes the normal bacterial make-up of the large intestine in such a way as to favor the survival of bacteria which can easily transform the fat to other products. One or more of the products of this bacterial transformation may act as a carcinogen (cancer-producing agent) or may promote the activity of carcinogens already present in the large intestine. For example, certain substances normally secreted into the intestine in the bile are known to be carcinogens. It is thought that the high-fat diet may indirectly increase the carcinogenic activity of these substances. In addition, there is data which suggests that the low fiber content in the American diet may further aggravate the problem. (See FIBER).

OTHER CANCERS

While the data is by no means so complete as for cancer of the breast or colon, there is some evidence that cancer of the ovary and of the prostate may also be directly related to dietary fat intake. Other cancers, such as cancer of the stomach, while undoubtedly related to dietary factors, are probably not related to fat. This cancer is much more prevalent in Japan than in the United States, and its incidence *decreases* when Japanese people migrate to California or Hawaii. However, it has been pointed out that the incidence of stomach cancer in Japan is decreasing and that this may be due not to changes in dietary factors per se but to the increased use of refrigeration as opposed to salting for the preservation of food. Thus, the problem of discovering the causes of the various kinds of cancer is a very complicated one and approaching the problem by studying general trends in food intake can sometimes be misleading. (See also ANTICARCINOGENS; ANTIOXIDANTS; CARCINOGENS IN FOOD; CHEMICAL CONTAMINANTS IN FOODS; GLUTATHIONE PEROXIDASE.)

CARBOHYDRATE

About half of the energy in our diet comes from carbohydrate. This dietary carbohydrate can be divided into two groups: the simple carbohydrates such as table sugar or sucrose and complex carbohydrates like starch. All carbohydrates are made up of monosaccharides, or the molecules that go together to make up the various sugars in the diet. These include glucose, a part of table sugar, fructose (the sugar found in fruit) and galactose, which is a part of the sugar known as lactose that is found in milk. The three most common simple dietary sugars are called disaccharides—pairs of monosaccharides joined together. These are sucrose which is found in sugarcane and sugar beets and is composed of glucose and fructose, lactose (milk sugar) which is glucose and galactose combined, and maltose which is formed of pairs of glucose molecules and is formed in plant seeds and grains as they germinate. They are all broken down in the intestine to their monosaccharide units which are absorbed there with the other dietary monosaccharides and used by the body as a source of energy.

The complex carbohydrates in the diet are formed by many dozens of glucose molecules. A single starch molecule may contain hundreds of glucose molecules. A million or more of these molecules are packed together in starchy foods such as grains and potatoes. Beans and peas are another good source of starch. The enzymes in your mouth and intestines break down the starch molecules to single glucose molecules which are absorbed across the wall of the intestines. It takes one to four hours after a meal for all the starch to be digested and passed into the bloodstream as glucose.

Cellulose is another important complex carbohydrate found in the diet. This, like starch, is found in plants and is composed of many glucose units joined together in chains. However, the units are joined together by bonds that the human body cannot break apart. As a result the cellulose passes through the digestive tract largely unchanged and constitutes a major form of fiber in our diet. Pectin and hemicellulose, which are also complex carbohydrates, provide an additional source of fiber in the diet as they, too, are indigestible.

Dietary fiber is very beneficial to health for several reasons. It draws water into the digestive tract and helps to prevent constipation by softening the stool. It exercises the muscles of the digestive tract so that they remain healthy and firm and so do not bulge out into the pouches found in cases of diverticulosis. It speeds up the passage of food through the digestive tract and so reduces the time that cancer-causing substances, both those in the food and those produced in the digestive tract by bacteria, are in contact with the wall of the intestine. It also binds to fats in the diet, such as cholesterol, and carries them out of the body with the feces and so helps to keep blood cholesterol levels low and the risk of heart disease down. (See FIBER.)

You need to take in at least 125 grams of glucose per day from all forms of carbohydrates in your diet. Since every gram of carbohydrate contains 4 calories, at least 500 calories must be in the form of carbohydrate. The ideal diet should contain at least 50 percent of calories in the form of carbohydrates.

Most of these calories should come from complex carbohydrates. For most Americans this means increasing our consumption of complex carbohydrates and reducing our consumption of simple sugars; more whole grains and vegetables and less refined sugar in all forms.

CARCINOGENS IN FOOD

A carcinogen is a substance which is capable of inducing cancer. Certain substances contained in foods may be carcinogens when ingested in large amounts over long periods of time. For example, it is suspected that something in the pickling process in the Japanese diet is responsible for the high incidence of stomach cancer among certain Japanese populations. A specific substance called aflatoxin occurs naturally in a variety of foods and has been shown to have carcinogenic properties when ingested in large amounts. Although foods themselves may contain carcinogens, the greater danger appears to come from food additives and food contaminants. Certain additives have had to be withdrawn from our food supply because they subsequently were shown to be carcinogenic. There is a law, the Delaney Clause, which states that any food additive which in any amount causes cancer in any animal species cannot be used in our food supply. The most recent additive to fall under this law was saccharin.

Food contaminants, such as pesticides, can also be carcinogens. DDT and some other pesticides fall into this category. Unfortunately, banning a pesticide from use once it has been shown to be carcinogenic may be too late for some people. Even certain hormones added to the feed of livestock may increase the risk for various cancers in consumers. Thus, while our food supply is probably the safest in the world we must remain vigilant in protecting it from contaminants. The Food and Drug Administration has the responsibility for protecting our food supply and any reader with specific questions about the safety of a particular food is encouraged to write to them. (See also ADDITIVES; CANCER; CHEMICAL CONTAMINANTS IN FOODS.)

CARNITINE

Carnitine is a substance involved in fat metabolism and is essential for the production of fat in muscle. All muscle in our bodies contains carnitine. It is made from lysine, an amino acid. Carnitine is not a vitamin, although when it was first discovered by G. Fraenkel in 1948 it was called vitamin BT. This was because he found that the mealworm *(Tenesbrio molitar)* could not live without receiving a constant supply in its diet. Its present name comes from the Latin word *carnis* meaning flesh.

Carnitine has absolutely no therapeutic effects and there is no benefit to taking supplements. Even premature babies, who are less able to make carnitine, can obtain sufficient amounts to meet their needs from their normal food.

CELLULASE

Cellulase is an enzyme that breaks down cellulose into glucose and other sugars. It is not present in humans but is present in plants, certain bacteria, single cell animals, and snails. Bacteria with this enzyme enable ruminants like cows and sheep to digest grass, hay, and other vegetation rich in cellulose. The enzyme can be bought in health-food stores and is purported to help people digest vegetables high in cellulose, like cabbage. However, it is readily degraded and inactivated in the stomach and does *not* help in digesting these foods. (See also ENZYMES.)

CHEMICAL CONTAMINANTS IN FOODS

Many environmental pollutants, such as industrial wastes, are absorbed from the soil or atmosphere by living plants and animals. Other chemicals are sprayed onto plants in the form of pesticides. Most of these substances are concentrated by a process known as *biological amplification*. As these substances pass up through the food chain they may be concentrated many times over. One good example is tuna fish, which often contains pollutants at a much higher concentration than they are found in the sea. Another is cow milk, containing much higher concentrations of the contaminants found in animal feeds. This process of biological amplification is particularly efficient if the contaminant is soluble in fat. Here, at the time of ingestion an offending chemical can pass to the fat tissue and remain there for an entire life span. The effect is cumulative, the number and the concentration of these offending substances continue to increase throughout our lives. Most Americans have over ninety different chemical contaminants in their tissues. Most are present in only trace amounts and present no health hazard. Others, however, have already proved to be a significant health hazard.

HEAVY METALS

Some heavy metals, such as lead, mercury, and cadmium, are extremely toxic when ingested in significant quantities. Small amounts of these metals regularly get into our food. For example, lead may enter canned foods from the solder used to seam cans—the highest risk is from acidic foods, which leach out the solder. Such acidic foods would include fruit, fruit juices, tomato products, and any sort of pickled food. The problem is magnified many times over if the food is left in an open can for any period of time. Although the amount of lead consumed in this way at any one meal is very small, over a period of years it could become significant. After a few hours, a can of orange juice in the refrigerator contains about 80 micrograms of lead per ounce and after two weeks about 400 micrograms. This is a great deal when you consider that the FDA recommends that children take in no more than 100 micrograms of lead per day. The problem can be minimized by transferring leftover canned food to glass containers.

PESTICIDES

The United States is the greatest food

producer in the world. This success has been achieved with the aid of the most advanced agricultural techniques, including the use of pesticides and artificial fertilizers (inorganic nitrogen compounds). Fertilizer is added to the soil to increase its nitrogen content, which is essential to maximizing crop yields. Growing plants and soil bacteria extract the nitrogen from the inorganic salts in the fertilizer and incorporate it into their own tissue. These compounds have essentially replaced manure and other fertilizers that have been used for centuries. The use of nitrogen-containing salts has increased the potential for growing foodstuffs in areas of the world where "natural" or organic sources of nitrogen are not readily available. To date, we have no evidence that the use of this type of "artificial" fertilizer has presented any health hazard.

Pesticides do not have such a clean bill of health. They are clearly toxic—at least to the pests that attack our crops—but have significantly increased our ability to raise crops more efficiently. In California recently a type of fruit fly threatened to destroy the food output of our largest agricultural state. The use of pesticides was the only way to avert an inevitable economic disaster. Some might say that the benefits derived from the use of these potentially toxic chemicals outweighed the risks associated with their use. Others would question the validity of this argument.

One of the most effective groups of pesticides, which are also one of the most toxic, are the *chlorinated hydrocarbons,* such as DDT, chlordane, piridine, and dieldrin. These compounds are not easily destroyed by the bacteria in soil and water, and so remain in the environment where they become subject to biological amplification. Approximately 50 percent of the food we eat contains measurable amounts of these substances. What this means in terms of health is not known, although chlorinated hydrocarbons are suspected of being cancer-causing agents. There are alternative pesticides that are less dangerous which could be used without altering crop yields. Their only drawback is that they are a little more expensive—but perhaps a small price to pay for a safer food supply!

Twenty percent of all pesticides used in this country serve merely to improve the looks of the final food product and have no beneficial effects whatsoever in terms of crop yield or nutrient content of the food. When you consider that 1 billion pounds of pesticides are used each year in the United States alone, any reduction in our exposure to pesticides is more than welcome.

ANTIBIOTICS

Antibiotics are legally used in animal

feeds to stimulate growth, and they represent another important food hazard. Fifty million dollars worth of antibiotics are added to animal foodstuffs each year in the US. It has become so cost effective to use antibiotics in the meat industry that in 1980 (the last year for which we have figures) all poultry, 90 percent of all swine, and 70 percent of all beef cattle raised in the United States were being given antibiotics.

This widespread use of antibiotics may be the cause of new types of diseases. The chronic use of small amounts of antibiotics in animal foodstuffs provides the ideal situation for the development of very virulent strains of bacteria. Animals fed such foodstuffs have a constant level of antibiotics in their bloodstreams, which means that those virulent microbes able to survive in a sea of antibiotics develop and multiply, whereas other bacteria, which are unable to grow in the presence of antibiotics, die. Some of the resistant bacteria infect people as well as animals and even those which

do not are able to pass their drug-resistant genes to the types of bacteria that cause human disease. Strains of bacteria that produce pneumonia, gonorrhea, dysentery, and other diseases, which cannot be killed by modern drugs because they have become resistant to such drugs, have developed.

Forty percent of our total antibiotic production today is used in animal husbandry, and problems with drug-resistant bacteria are on the increase. In 1968, 1 percent of salmonella, which causes food poisoning, were resistant to six or more antibiotics. This had risen to 9 percent by 1975 and is now believed to be even higher. Of course, part of this is due to the common use of antibiotics in humans. Nevertheless, it is a major concern, so much so that many international health organizations, including the World Health Organization (WHO), have called for a ban on the use of antibiotics in animal feeds. (See also ADDITIVES; CARCINOGENS IN FOOD; LEAD; MERCURY.)

CHILDREN

FOR THE INFANT: FIVE TO TWELVE MONTHS OF AGE

Complete nutrition can be provided in the first year of life by either human milk or infant formulas, with appropriate vitamin and mineral supplementation. (Most infants will need iron supplements after four months of age.) In the latter part of the first year, some nursing mothers may not produce enough milk, and hence not supply enough energy, protein, and other nutrients to sustain the infant's normal rate of growth. If this should happen, or if the mother decides to wean the child, it is probably best to switch the infant to a formula, instead of introducing solid food as the mainstay of the diet. New solids are introduced one at a time in small amounts, so that each can be evaluated for any allergies or adverse reactions. The mother must not overfeed the child at this time, however, as large amounts of solid foods introduced in rapid succession may cause an imbalance of nutrients, and a dangerous overload on the kidneys and other immature organs throughout the body.

When solids are introduced, the recommended sequence is:

1. Iron-fortified cereals (between four and six months of age)
2. Baby (pureed) foods
3. Junior (ground) foods (by approximately eight months of age)

Ground meat or other soft table foods may be included when the child is between nine and twelve months, as long as they meet the infant's nutritional needs. Egg whites and whole milk should be avoided until after the first year, since they may cause allergic reactions. Low-fat milks are not suitable for infants until two to three years of age, since the infant needs a high fat intake to provide the fat needed for the growth of all cells and the child's kidneys cannot yet handle the waste products yielded from metabolizing such a concentrated form of protein.

FOR CHILDREN OVER TWELVE MONTHS OF AGE

After twelve months of age, the nutrient demands of a growing child are somewhat reduced. Parents should make sure the infant is continuing to grow at a normal rate by consulting growth charts. These charts show how big a child should grow based on birth weight. If the child was born on the fiftieth percentile, she or he was right in the middle of the range of all babies born in America at that time. If the child was born on the ninetieth percentile, then only ten percent of all babies were born bigger. Now, if a baby was born on time and was not immature at birth because of some complication during pregnancy, it should stay more or less on its percentile line. It may go up a few percentiles or down a few, which is perfectly normal, but it should not consistently go up or down. If weight does go down this means either the child is not eating enough of the right foods or not absorbing the food for some reason. If the weight goes up on the percentiles, then the child is getting too much to eat and a lifelong obesity problem could be developing.

Several things are very important to remember about this period of growth. The child must eat good quality protein, which generally means animal protein. Meals should not be missed as this is detrimental to a child's performance in school. There is no question about the fact that children who go to school without eating a good breakfast perform significantly poorer than children who eat a good breakfast, one which contains both carbohydrate and protein. A morning meal of cereal and milk is just right. Iron-rich foods are also essential, in order to prevent anemia. (See also ADDITIVES; ADOLESCENT; ALLERGY; ANEMIAS; BREAST-FEEDING; DENTAL DECAY; INFANT FEEDING; INFANT FORMULA; JUNK FOOD; PROTEIN-CALORIE MALNUTRITION; VEGETARIAN DIETS.)

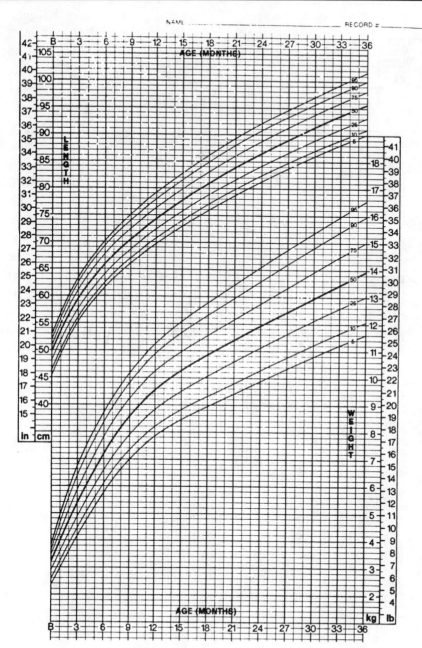

Figure A-4. Physical growth NCHS percentiles for girls aged 0 to 36 months. (Adapted from National Center for Health Statistics: NCHS growth charts, 1976. Monthly Vital Statistics Report. Vol. 25, No. 3, Suppl. (HRA)76-1120. Rockville, Md.: Health Resources Administration, 1976. Data from the Fels Research Institute, Yellow Springs, Ohio.)

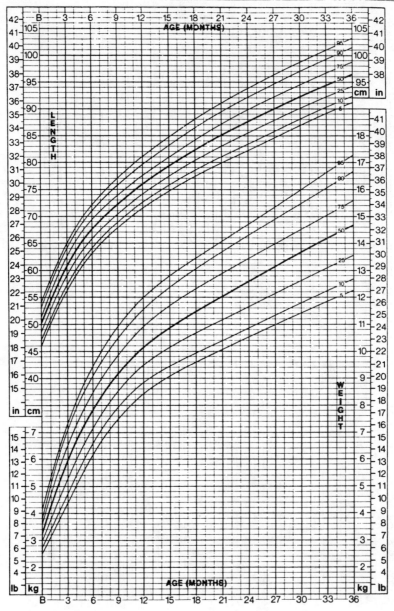

Figure A-2. Physical growth NCHS percentiles for boys aged 0 to 36 months. (Adapted from P.V.V. Hamill et al., Physical growth: National Center for Health Statistics percentiles. Am. J. Clin. Nutr. 32:607, 1979. Data from the Fels Research Institute, Yellow Springs. Ohio.)

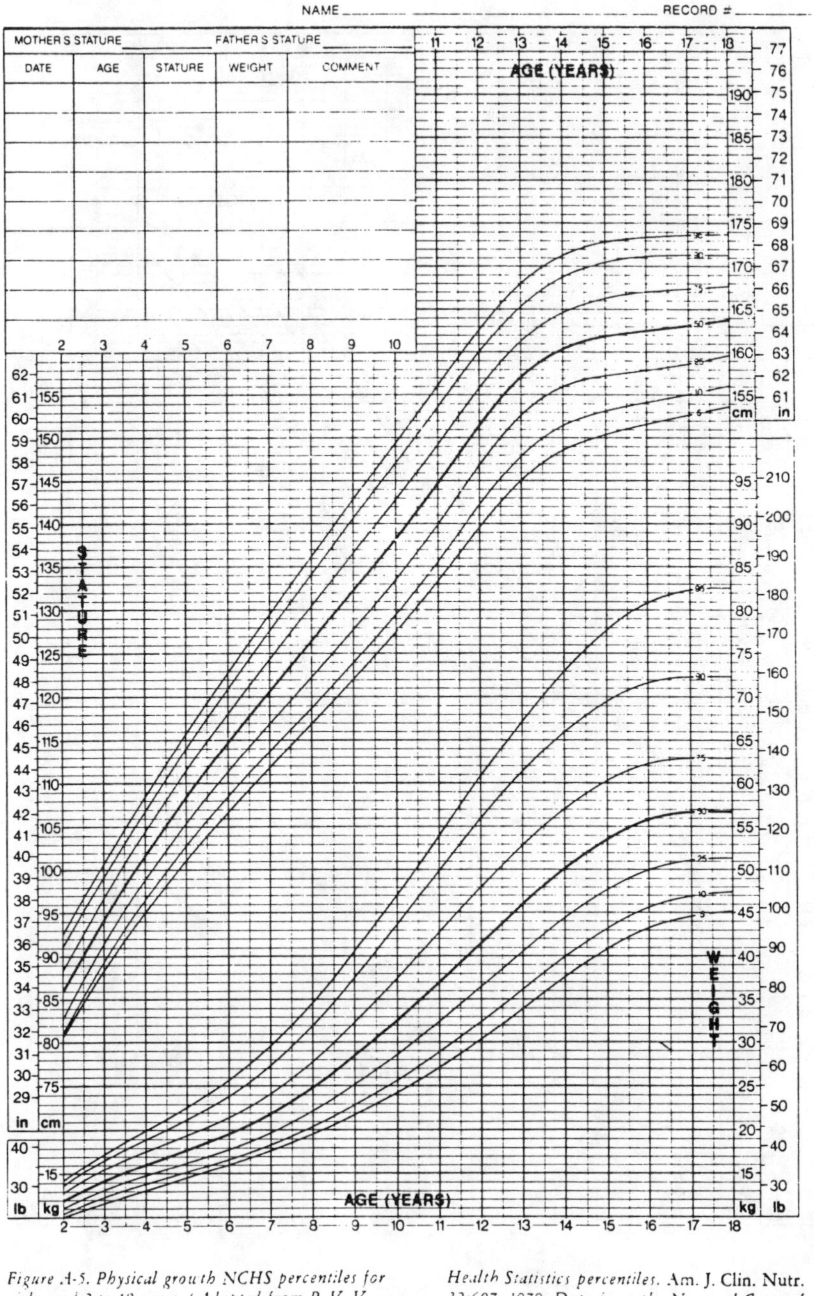

Figure A-5. Physical growth NCHS percentiles for girls aged 2 to 18 years. (Adapted from P. V. V. Hamill et al., Physical growth: National Center for Health Statistics percentiles. Am. J. Clin. Nutr. 32:607, 1979. Data from the National Center for Health Statistics, Hyattsville, Md.)

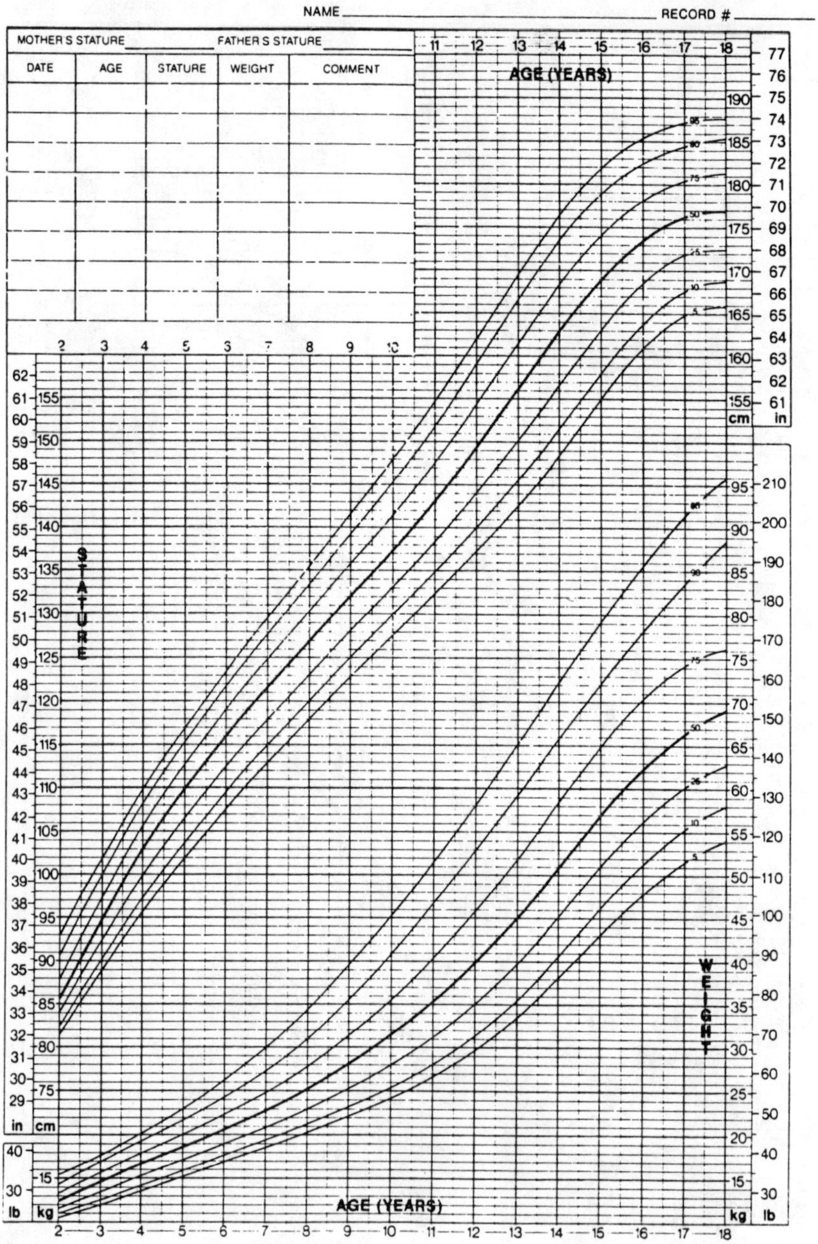

Figure A-3. *Physical growth NCHS percentiles for boys aged 2 to 18 years. (Adapted from P. V. V. Hamill et al., Physical growth: National Center for Health Statistics percentiles, Am. J. Clin. Nutr. 32:607, 1979. Data from the National Center for Health Statistics. Hyattsville, Md.)*

CHLORIDE

Chloride ions are an important constituent of all body cells and also play a big part in maintaining the acid-base balance of the body. In the stomach they are an integral part of the hydrochloric acid molecules that are a key factor in digestion. There is no recommended dietary allowance (RDA) for chloride but the safe dietary range is from 70 to 5100 milligrams. Excesses or deficiencies of this nutrient are extremely rare, but when they occur they upset the acid-base balance of the body. If the body fluids become too alkaline or acidic metabolism is impaired. All foods containing salt (sodium chloride) have a significant chloride content. (See also SODIUM.)

CHOLESTEROL

Cholesterol is a soapy-looking yellowish substance. It is essential for life, being a building block of all cell membranes. Each day 1000 milligrams are needed for this purpose and for the manufacture of bile (which helps you absorb fat), sex hormones (estrogen, progesterone, and androgen), vitamin D, and myelin (the fatty sheath that insulates the nerves). Despite its importance, cholesterol is not a dietary essential for adults, as it is made in the liver and the intestines at a rate sufficient to meet the body's needs. We make from .5 to 1 gram per day depending on the body's needs and the amount consumed in the diet. Men consume about 450 milligrams per day and women, 266 milligrams per day. In most people, the more cholesterol consumed, the less the body makes. This system seems to work well up to a dietary intake of 150 to 300 milligrams of cholesterol. More than this leads to an increase in body, and hence blood, cholesterol levels and increases the risk of atherosclerosis.

ATHEROSCLEROSIS— CHOLESTEROL, HEART ATTACK, AND STROKE

Cholesterol was first implicated as a causal factor in atherosclerosis— hardening of the arteries—when doctors performed autopsies on heart attack victims and found that their arteries were clogged and hardened by deposits of cholesterol. This was later found to be true of stroke victims as well. When you run upstairs or are harassed by your boss, the coronary arteries supplying the heart are forced to supply the heart muscle with larger volumes of blood than at rest. This causes angina, or heart pain, if the arteries are clogged. The narrowed artery also facilitates the formation of blood clots which can suddenly cut off the blood supply to a part of the heart muscle, causing a heart attack. Similarly, an occluded artery in the brain leads to a sudden loss of blood supply to a part of the brain and results in a stroke.

Since these original studies, comparisons between countries have also suggested a link between dietary cholesterol and heart disease. In countries like Greece, Yugoslavia, and Japan, where both the intake and blood levels of cholesterol are lower than in the US, the incidence of heart disease is also lower. However, the final proof that cholesterol was linked to heart disease did not come until 1984, when the results of a ten-year study (costing $150 million) were published. This study showed that by reducing blood cholesterol levels the incidence of fatal heart attacks could be reduced.

Fifty percent of all people who suffer from a heart attack have had no prior symptoms. The other 50 percent may suffer from chest pain, shortness of breath, swelling in the ankles, and irregular heart beats. This disease, which is the most common cause of death in the US, accounts for 50 percent of all fatalities, or some one million people. Of those deaths two-thirds are due to coronary artery disease and one-third are due to stroke. Deaths from cardiovascular disease are about two-and-a-half times as prevalent as those from the second leading cause of death, which is cancer. All this costs the nation over $50 billion a year in terms of lost productivity, expenses for medical care, disability, and death. The relative importance of cardiovascular disease, in terms of percent of all deaths for a given age group, rises steadily with age (26 percent of all deaths at thirty-five to forty-four years as opposed to 68 percent in the over seventy-fives). This reflects, in part, the progression of the disease with age.

Cardiovascular disease is caused by several factors, including high blood pressure, high blood levels of fats (notably cholesterol), diabetes, obesity, cigarette smoking, a "type

A" personality, physical inactivity, and a family history of atherosclerosis. These factors are additive, so a person who is overweight and smokes is more at risk than an obese nonsmoker.

BLOOD CHOLESTEROL LEVELS AND YOUR DIET

Blood cholesterol levels are very much related to the diet. The following table gives a list of the average serum cholesterol values for white males and females in this country.

The lower the blood cholesterol level, the lower the risk for heart attack, so it would be desirable to have even lower values than those expressed in the table and some suggest that we should all reduce our cholesterol levels to below 180 milligrams per 100 millimeters of blood serum.

In the diet, cholesterol is provided by eggs (42 percent); meat, poultry, and fish (38 percent); dairy foods (15 percent); and fats and oils (5 percent). As cholesterol is found in all animal cell membranes, it is

HOW MUCH CHOLESTEROL IS IN YOUR BLOOD?
(SERUM CHOLESTEROL: MG PER 100 ML)
AVERAGE VALUES BY AGE GROUP

Age (yrs)	White Males	White Females*
0–4	155	156
5–9	160	164
10–14	158	160
15–19	150	157
20–24	167	164
25–29	182	171
30–34	192	175
35–39	201	184
40–44	207	193
45–49	212	203
50–54	213	218
55–59	214	231
60–64	213	231
65–69	213	233
70–74	208	229
75–79	205	231
80+	206	221

*Values are for white women who do not use oral contraceptives.

distributed throughout the meat, lean as well as fat, and cannot be trimmed off like visible fat. In milk, much of the cholesterol is dissolved in the fat, so low-fat products contain less cholesterol than whole milk and cream. The cholesterol content of some common high-cholesterol foods is given in the following table.

SATURATED AND UNSATURATED FATS AND THE CHOLESTEROL LEVEL

It has been discovered that the levels of both cholesterol and fat in the blood seem to be altered by changing the composition of fat in the diet. In general, saturated fats increase the

CHOLESTEROL CONTENT OF SOME COMMON HIGH-CHOLESTEROL FOODS

Food	Serving	Cholesterol (mg)
Beef, lean, trimmed of fat (cooked)	3 oz	77
Kidney	3 oz	690
Lamb, lean, cooked	3 oz	83
Liver (beef, calf, lamb), cooked	3 oz	372
Pork, lean, trimmed of fat (cooked)	3 oz	77
Veal, lean, cooked	3 oz	86
Chicken, breast and skin	3 oz	74
Chicken, breast (skinless)	3 oz	53
Chicken, drumstick and skin	3 oz	80
Chicken liver	3 oz	480
Turkey, light meat (skinless)	3 oz	51
Turkey, dark meat (skinless)	3 oz	64
Brie	1 oz	28
Butter	1 tsp	12
Cheddar cheese	1 oz	28
Cottage cheese (low-fat)	1 oz	13
Cream cheese	1 tbsp	16
Egg, yolk	1 med	240
Egg, white	1 med	0
Ice cream	1 cup	56
Margarine, all vegetable fat	1 tsp	0
Milk, whole	1 cup	34
Milk, 2% fat	1 cup	22
Milk, skim	1 cup	5
Sour cream	1 tbsp	8
Whipped cream	1 tbsp	20
Yogurt, low-fat	1 cup	17

level in the blood while polyunsaturated fats decrease the cholesterol level, as do monounsaturated fats, but to a very minor extent. But what do these terms, saturated and unsaturated, mean? Basically, if you eat soft margarine rather than butter, then you are choosing unsaturated fat in preference to saturated fat. But what is the exact difference between these two types of fat?

Almost all of the fat in our diet is in the form of chemical compounds containing specific fatty acids. Fatty acids are a simple group of chemicals that may be saturated, monounsaturated, or polyunsaturated. The term "saturated" refers to the number of hydrogen atoms in the fat. If the fatty acid has enough hydrogen atoms, it is saturated; if there is room for two more hydrogen atoms, it is monounsaturated; and if it can accept four or more hydrogen atoms, it is polyunsaturated. This differing ability to deal with hydrogen atoms accounts for the very different properties of saturated and unsaturated fats in the body.

All natural fats contain mixtures of saturated, monounsaturated, and polyunsaturated fats, but these mixtures vary widely in composition. For example, butter contains an average of about 66 percent saturated fat. In contrast, soybean oil contains about 15 percent saturated fat and 66 percent unsaturated fat. Similarly, safflower oil contains

about 75 percent polyunsaturated fat.

Generally speaking, polyunsaturated fats are derived from liquid vegetable oils—corn, cottonseed, safflower, and soybean oils are good examples. Walnuts, almonds, filberts, fish, and margarine are other good sources. Margarine is made by bubbling hydrogen through vegetable oil. The more hydrogen the oil absorbs, the firmer it becomes. Consequently, soft margarines contain less hydrogen and more polyunsaturated fats than do hard margarines. Saturated fats, on the other hand, tend to be naturally solid and of animal origin. This is frequently the visible type of fat that we eat everyday— lard, butter and other dairy products, meat fats, chicken, coconut, egg yolk, and vegetable shortening fall into this category. Monounsaturated fats fall somewhere in between and include avocados, cashews, olives, and peanuts.

A diet containing equal quantities of the three different kinds of fat is ideal. An excess of polyunsaturated fat may be as bad as an excess of saturated fat. Studies have linked such an excess to an increased incidence of various forms of cancer and to the formation of gallstones. So you see, you really can have too much of a good thing. The golden rule of nutrition is moderation in all things.

The vegetable oils contain large amounts—as much as 50 percent—

of linoleic acid, a polyunsaturated fat that is essential to the body for healthy skin and proper growth. About 60 percent of the human brain is composed of fat, of which a considerable portion is made from substances derived from linoleic acid. It is particularly important in terms of heart disease, as it seems to reduce the tendency of the blood to clot in the final stages of the obstruction of blood vessels. Apparently it does this by preventing the tiny disc-shaped blood cells called platelets from sticking together and causing a blood clot. It is absolutely vital that the diet supplies sufficient linoleic acid, because our bodies cannot manufacture it themselves.

CHOLESTEROL AND PROTEIN: HDL VS LDL

Cholesterol circulates in the blood attached to specific blood proteins, the two main ones being low-density lipoprotein (LDL) and high-density lipoprotein (HDL). LDL carries cholesterol from the liver to the tissues. The higher the level of LDL, the greater the risk of atherosclerosis. HDL carries cholesterol from the tissues, including the lining of the arteries, back to the liver and reduces the risk of heart disease.

The ratio of total cholesterol to HDL cholesterol in a person's blood seems to be the best predictor of a future heart attack. This ratio explains why so many people who remain free of heart disease have a level of total cholesterol that in others results in a heart attack. Even if your cholesterol level is relatively low, you could still have a bad ratio and suffer a heart attack. Three-quarters of the heart attacks in this country occur among people with blood cholesterol levels between 150 and 300 and half occur in men with levels below 250.

Based on recent studies, anyone whose ratio of total cholesterol to HDL cholesterol is higher than 4.5 to 1 should be treated to lower the ratio. This means that if a person has a total cholesterol level of 250 and an HDL level of 75 the ratio will be 3.3 to 1, which is associated with only half the usual rate of heart disease in this country. But a person with a total cholesterol level of 200 and an HDL level of 35 would have a ratio of 5.7 to 1, the ratio typically found in Americans who develop heart disease.

This ratio seems to go a long way toward explaining why men have so many more heart attacks than women do. Males and females start out with the same cholesterol levels, but at about the time of puberty boys experience a 20 percent to 25 percent drop in protective HDL, leaving men with an average HDL level of 45 milligrams per 100 milliliters of blood serum as opposed to the average 55 milligrams per 100 milliliters of blood serum for women. This difference is believed to be the reason there are 60 percent fewer deaths from heart attacks in women than men in the US.

After menopause, women lose this advantage when their HDL levels fall and their total cholesterol levels go up. By looking at the table on page 101 you might even think that women after menopause are at higher risk than men, as their total cholesterol levels are higher. (Indeed, 30 percent of women in this country and only 25 percent of men have levels above 240.) However, this is not the case. It merely means that there are more older women living than older men. As their blood cholesterol levels do not go up until after menopause it takes some time before the elevated levels cause sufficient atherosclerosis to cause death due to heart attack or stroke.

Although estrogen seems to maintain HDL at a high level in premenopausal women, too much estrogen seems to be very harmful, as women taking oral contraceptives are at greater risk for suffering a heart attack than women who do not. This is because oral contraceptives tend to cause blood clots in the blood vessels, leading to heart attacks and strokes. There is evidence to show that the risk of clotting increases with higher estrogen doses. It is therefore important to keep the dose of estrogen as low as possible, provided a sufficient amount is given to prevent pregnancy and any menstrual irregularities. Too little estrogen is also

harmful. When women go into menopause, estrogen levels drop and blood cholesterol levels increase significantly. The risk of heart attack becomes similar to that of men of the same age. Cigarette smoking on the part of oral contraceptive users increases the risk of serious adverse effect on the heart and blood vessels. The risk increases with age and with the degree of smoking. Fifteen cigarettes or more a day has a serious effect, especially in women over the age of thirty-five.

Runners, skiers, and other individuals who are very active have been found to have very high HDL levels. Thus, one of the benefits of exercise seems to be an increase in the levels of this protective substance. But it needs to be strenuous exercise—at least 20 minutes of vigorous aerobic exercise taken four times a week.

Overweight people tend to have low levels of HDL and weight loss in their cases raises their HDL levels.

Several types of fiber seem to lower LDL levels and raise HDL levels. Pectin, which forms the pith of oranges and the major portion of the flesh of apples and root vegetables, is one such fiber. One to two ounces of pectin can reduce some people's cholesterol by up to 10 percent. To get this amount of pectin you would have to eat five good-sized apples each day. Hence, it is easier to buy the pure compound in the pharmacy and add it to desserts.

REDUCING YOUR CHOLESTEROL LEVEL

Regular use of oatmeal, oat bran, and beans can also help reduce blood cholesterol levels by up to 10 to 20 percent, especially in people with high cholesterol levels. (The following table shows the high risk groups for each age range. A 1 percent drop in serum cholesterol reduces the risk for coronary heart disease by 2 percent; fiber-rich diets reduce the risk by 20 to 40 percent!)

To prevent atherosclerosis, the best plan for the general population is to follow the dietary guidelines of the American Heart Association, American Medical Association, and the Food and Nutrition Board, which will often reduce cholesterol levels by up to 20 percent. These guidelines are outlined below. It takes three to six weeks before any significant change occurs. If this diet doesn't work and your cholesterol level is still above 265 you might want to dis-

cuss the possibility of drug therapy with your physician.

CHOLESTEROL LOWERING DIET

1. Eat *lean* meat (no more than two or three times a week), fish, poultry without the skin, dry beans and peas (lentils, kidney beans, chick peas, and tofu), and shellfish.
2. Trim excess fat off meats.
3. Restrict your intake of eggs (no more than three yolks per week), organ meats (liver and kidneys), cold cuts, sausage, hot dogs, bacon, spare ribs, canned meats, duck, fatty cuts of beef, lamb, pork, and nuts.
4. Limit your intake of butter, cream, hydrogenated margarine, vegetable shortenings, coconut and palm oils (and nondairy creamers containing them), Half & Half, and sour cream.

RISK RATINGS FOR HEART DISEASE BY AGE GROUP

Age	Moderate Risk*	High Risk*
2–19	greater than 170	greater than 185
20–29	greater than 200	greater than 220
30–39	greater than 220	greater than 240
40+	greater than 240	greater than 260

*Milligrams of cholesterol per 100 milliliters of serum.

5. Use polyunsaturated vegetable oils such as corn, safflower, soybean, and sunflower oils and soft margarine containing these oils, diet margarine, imitation mayonnaise, and salad dressings containing the polyunsaturated oils or diet dressings.

6. Use low-fat dairy products. Eat fewer hard cheeses and semisoft cheeses such as brie and cream cheese. Concentrate on lower fat cheeses such as low-fat cottage cheese, part-skim ricotta, part-skim mozzarella, farmer cheese, and those labeled low fat. Cut down on whole milk, ice cream, and whole milk yogurt. Use instead skim milk and 1 percent fat milk, low-fat yogurt, ice milk, and buttermilk made from skim milk.

7. Accent whole grain breads and cereals, rice, pasta, and noodles.

8. Decrease your intake of pies, cakes, cookies, and doughnuts.

9. Broil, bake, or boil rather than fry.

10. Eat more fruit, fresh, frozen, canned (in their own juice rather than in syrup), and dried fruits, and fresh and frozen vegetables.

11. Read manufacturers' labels to determine both the amounts and types of fat contained in foods.

12. Reduce your intake of salt, especially if you tend to retain water or have a history of high blood pressure in your family.

13. Exercise regularly. Vigorous exercise at least two times a week seems to diminish the risk of suffering a heart attack. But because sudden heavy exercise is dangerous, you must begin your exercise program gradually, and might want to discuss the type of program which is right for you with your physician.

Perhaps the crucial question is "If I follow these suggestions can I reverse the process of atherosclerosis?" The verdict is not in on this yet but all evidence collected to date, both in animals and humans, would tend to show that following these suggestions will not only help prevent the condition from getting any worse but may begin to clear the arteries. (See also ARTERIOSCLEROSIS; EICOSAPENTAENOIC ACID; EXERICISE; NUTRITION AND EXERICISE.)

CHROMIUM

Chromium is required for normal glucose absorption. It makes it possible for the hormone insulin to do its work in helping the cells in the body to absorb glucose from the blood. When chromium is lacking in the diet of animals insulin works inefficiently and a diabeteslike condition develops. The ability to absorb glucose has been improved by chromium supplements in some people with adult onset diabetes. Some elderly people who have difficulty in absorbing glucose have also shown improvement when given chromium supplements. Chromium is best absorbed from foods where it's found as glucose tolerance factor (GTF), a compound containing niacin, glycine, glutamic acid, and cysteine in addition to chromium. The richest source is brewer's yeast but it is found in meats, cheeses, and whole grains in the form of GTF. Adults require 50 to 200 micrograms per day. (See also DIABETES.)

COPPER

The average adult has a total body store of copper in the range of 100 to 150 milligrams. Most of this mineral is distributed in vital organs such as the heart, liver, kidney, and brain. Hair also contains significant levels of copper, as well as zinc. It should be pointed out that hair analyses are sometimes used to measure the body's status of these metals, but such analyses are very unreliable because the hair is exposed to harsh treatments and environmental factors which will alter its mineral content considerably.

Copper is transported in the blood by a protein called ceruloplasmin. This copper protein appears to be involved in iron absorption and metabolism, and a copper deficiency can lead to iron deficiency and resultant anemia. Copper is also a component of numerous enzymes in the body, most of which are involved in oxygen utilization in metabolism. Milk is a poor source of copper (as well as iron) and anemias responding to copper administration have been reported in premature infants and infants fed a milk diet without additional nutrients.

Hypocupremia, or low blood copper, has been associated with some human diseases, such as sprue, but apparently these diseases are not due to a copper deficiency. Elevated blood copper levels are often seen in viral infections, rheumatoid arthritis, myocardial infarction, leukemia, and in certain other cancers, although the causes for the increased levels of copper are unexplained.

An acute excessive dose of copper produces nausea, vomiting, abdominal pains, diarrhea, headache, dizziness, and a metallic taste in the mouth. Severe toxicity can cause death. Chronic copper intoxication is not well documented in humans, although cases of toxicity in livestock may be instructive. Animals exhibit no apparent ill effects from excessive copper consumption until a threshold is exceeded, at which time severe liver damage, red blood cell destruction (hemolytic anemia), and kidney damage ensue. A copper intake in excess of 20 milligrams per day could therefore be dangerous.

There is no recommended dietary allowance (RDA) for copper, although the Food and Nutrition Board has established a provisional recommended dietary range of 2 to 3 milligrams per day for adults. Several nutrients interact with copper, affecting its absorption and making it difficult to set a reliable RDA. The average American diet contains 2 milligrams of copper or more per day and copper deficiency is rare in this country. Rich sources of the mineral include shellfish, liver, kidney, legumes, nuts, and raisins. The copper content of soils will affect the levels of copper in crops grown in those soils. Copper deficiencies may occur from eating only foods, including meat, grown in a copper-deficient region.

Animal studies have revealed that excessive intake of zinc, cadmium, or molybdenum can result in a copper deficiency. Likewise, excessive copper intake can lead to zinc or molybdenum deficiency. (See also ANEMIAS; HAIR ANALYSIS; IRON; MOLYBDENUM.)

CYSTEINE

Cysteine is an amino acid which belongs to a class of amino acids containing sulphur atoms. Cysteine is not essential for adults since it can be made from another amino acid which is essential, methionine. Cysteine may be essential, however, for premature infants who are unable to manufacture it from methionine. A wide variety of both animal and plant proteins contain cysteine and therefore there is no reason to take supplements. Supplementation with large amounts is potentially dangerous since it could produce an amino acid imbalance. (See AMINO ACIDS.)

CYTOTOXIC TESTING

The cytotoxic test is used by some health professionals to test for allergic reactions to certain foods. A sample of blood is taken from a patient and the white blood cells are isolated from the sample. Extracts from foods are added to aliquots of the white cells. If the cells change in shape then the person is said to be allergic to the particular food extract added. This test is totally invalid as there is absolutely no correlation between having a positive result in the test to a given food and being allergic to that food. (See ALLERGY.)

DENTAL DECAY

Cavity, one of the most common afflictions of modern times, is a relatively late stage in the progressively destructive bacterial disease process known as *dental caries.* The bacteria involved are concentrated in the form of a gelatinlike mat that adheres to specific sites on the teeth. This mat is referred to by dentists as bacterial plaque. The plaque may contain hundreds of millions of bacteria on a single tooth surface and produces dental decay.

This teeming community of germs uses sugar as its main source of energy. In the course of making this vital energy by a process of fermentation, bacteria liberate a variety of acids, some of them strong enough to dissolve the very substance of the tooth. In a sense teeth become victims of our own environmental pollution. Repeated cycles of acid formation can in time cause decay of the tooth, which shows as a white or brown spot beneath the plaque layer; with continued dissolution of the tooth mineral, a clinical cavity develops.

In the United States today, each person consumes approximately 58 kilograms (128 pounds) of sugar per year; 43 kilograms (95 pounds) in the form of sucrose and the remainder as corn syrup and minor caloric sweeteners. The trend in the twentieth century has been toward a modest but steady increase in the total consumption of carbohydrates; even more important is a change in form and frequency of consumption—less starch and complex carbohydrates and much more sugar. Most of this sugar is already added by food and beverage processors, while less is added to foods at home; less of the sweet foods are eaten at meals, and more as snacks between meals.

A large body of animal experimental data, human clinical studies, and observations of eating patterns and the development of dental caries strongly support the idea that the form and frequency of sugar ingestion is even more important than the amount of sugar consumed. When sucrose is markedly restricted, few cavities develop. This has been observed in patients with hereditary diseases that require the avoidance of sugar—in clinical experiments in which sucrose products were replaced by approximately one hundred specially prepared materials with *xylitol,* a nonfermentable sugar alcohol which has a sweet taste, and in special institutionalized populations.

A number of different kinds of sugar (sucrose, glucose, fructose, maltose, lactose) can promote the energy needs of plaque bacteria and lead to the formation of plaque acids. Studies in experimental animals show that they all produce some dental decay. In addition, starch, because it is converted to the sugars maltose and glucose by enzymes in the mouth, can also cause decay. But there are clear-cut differences in the *amount* of decay the various sugars and starch can produce. Sucrose is undoubtedly the most conducive to dental decay. Recent studies on the types of bacteria in plaque and on the mechanism by which plaque forms on teeth suggest some of the reasons for the special role of sucrose.

One particular bacterium, *Streptococcus mutans* seems especially adapted to stick to the teeth and begin the process of plaque formation. The current view is that this bacterium comes close to being the "specific" germ associated with decay on the smooth surfaces of the teeth. Other kinds of bacteria *(Lactobacillus, Actinomyces)* appear to share with *mutans* the responsibility for decay on the biting surfaces of back teeth and along the gum line. Sucrose, and not the other sugars or starch, can actually be used by *Streptococcus mutans* to manufacture a sticky substance (glucan) which adheres itself to the tooth surface. Sucrose, therefore, is more than just a source of energy and acid; it enables specific decay-producing bacteria to build up on tooth surfaces.

It makes good sense to regulate your sugar intake in general, especially that of sucrose, to reduce the risk of dental decay. Sweet, gooey foods are especially dangerous as they stick to the teeth and maintain a high concentration of sucrose close to the tooth surface, thereby providing a long lasting supply of sucrose for the bacteria. The process by which starch is converted to sugar is usually slow enough so it doesn't constitute a major threat, but here too some moderation is advisable. It is therefore obvious to us all that dietary control is one of our major weapons against tooth decay.

EARLY NUTRITIONAL INFLUENCES

It is clear that diet has a profound effect on the bacteria that stick to the teeth. What about the teeth themselves—how can they be influenced and protected?

The major impact of food and water intake on teeth occurs during their development, well before they emerge through the gums into the oral cavity. For the primary (baby) teeth this occurs largely before birth. The jaw bones of the fetus begin to calcify by the fourth month of pregnancy and the primary teeth show evidence of calcification (deposition of calcium in the teeth) soon thereafter. At birth, calcification of the primary teeth is well advanced and the first permanent molar has begun to calcify. An adequate intake of calcium, phosphorus, and vitamin D is necessary for the pregnant woman to ensure adequate calcification of the total fetal skeleton, including the jaw bones and teeth. The recommended dietary allowance for calcium during pregnancy is 1200 milligrams per day. Good sources of this nutrient are milk, yogurt, cheese, and green leafy vegetables. The average diet is usually adequate for phosphorus (1 gram per day) and vitamin D (400 IUs per day).

Proper diet during infancy and early childhood is important to ensure the normal development of the portion of the primary teeth formed after birth and of the permanent teeth which develop throughout this period.

Defects in tooth structure *(enamel hypoplasia)* can be caused by deficiencies of vitamins A, C, or D, or by severe protein deficiency during pregnancy or early childhood. These nutritional defects are rare in countries like the US, but are quite common in the less-developed countries like Nigeria or Guatemala. *Enamel hypoplasia* in the US is usually the result of diseases resulting in high fevers or from the use of tetracyclines, a commonly prescribed antibiotic. Pediatricians are now fully aware of the effect of tetracyclines on teeth and do prescribe alternate medications. Hypoplastic teeth are probably no more susceptible to the start of tooth decay than normal teeth, but once decay begins it progresses more rapidly through the defective areas.

FLUORIDES AND TOOTH RESISTANCE

It is generally agreed that the most important factor in determining the resistance of a tooth to subsequent attack by the acids generated by bacterial plaque is a proper level of fluoride during tooth formation. Ideally this is achieved by the normal use of drinking water, which contains one part per million of fluoride. Approximately half of the population of the US enjoys this benefit. In the rest of the country fluoride can be prescribed as a dietary supplement and produce a level of protection similar to that afforded by fluoridated water. The burden, however, is on the parent, to make sure that the supplements are taken regularly until all the teeth (except for the wisdom teeth) have emerged into the oral cavity.

The Council on Dental Therapeutics of the American Dental Association recommends that no supplementation be given if the water contains more than 60 percent of the recommended level. In other words, if your water supply contains .6 or more parts per million of fluoride you don't need a supplement. This information is available from your local board of health. If the level is less ask your dentist or pediatrician to prescribe fluoride drops or tablets, or a vitamin-fluoride combination. The doctor can recommend a supplement that will provide a level similar to the amount ingested from fluoridated water (.25 milligrams of fluoride per day for children older than three). The proper dosage is important. With too high a dose the teeth will develop white spots or discolorations called *fluorosis*. There need be no concern when these simple instructions are followed. There are no side effects to the proper use of fluorides, and no effects other than fluorosis with elevated levels of fluoride. More than thirty-five years of research in many countries of the world attest to the safety and value of fluoridated water and fluoride supplements. The cancer scare, recently introduced by organized antifluoridationists, has been found to be groundless by the National Cancer Institute in the US and by the Royal College of Physicians in England.

Once the teeth have emerged through the gums, dietary fluorides still have an effect for a few years on a "topical" basis. There is a benefit to be gained from direct contact between the tooth surface and fluorides in water or dietary supplements in juice or other liquids (preferably not milk, since its high calcium level reduces the fluoride effect). The fluoride secreted in saliva is also helpful. This surface benefit wanes within a few years after the teeth are in the mouth because of the low concentration of fluoride, a concentration designed primarily for incorporation into the teeth during formation.

Further reduction in decay can be anticipated, however, from the use of fluoride toothpaste, fluoride mouth rinses, or topical application by a dentist or hygienist. Remember that these types of fluorides are in much higher concentration than in water or dietary supplements and are not meant for swallowing on a regular basis. With a combination of dietary and topical fluorides, decay can be reduced 60 to 80 percent. For virtually a 100 percent reduction in decay use a combination of fluorides and dietary control. Increase your tooth resistance in this way and decrease attacks by bacterial acids. Good oral hygiene will add an additional margin of safety. (See also CALCIUM; FLUORIDE.)

DIABETES

Six million Americans suffer from diabetes, a disease in which there are insufficient amounts of the hormone insulin made in the body to meet its needs. Since this hormone, which is produced in the pancreas, is needed for the tissues to take up glucose from the blood for use as fuel, a deficiency will result in high blood levels and low tissue levels of glucose. Theoretically, a person may be diabetic because the pancreas is unable to make insulin or because the tissues are not able to respond properly even though insulin is present. Both of these types of diabetes do occur.

The first type, which appears early in life and which is therefore referred to as juvenile diabetes, is an *absolute* deficiency of insulin. The beta cells of the pancreas, which are the cells that produce insulin, are destroyed. As a result, little or no insulin is made, blood sugar rises, and the tissues are starved for fuel. This type of diabetes occurs almost exclusively in certain people who are genetically disposed to it and may be due to a virus that invades the pancreas. There is no nutritional pattern which increases a youngster's chances of developing juvenile diabetes.

By contrast, the type of diabetes which occurs in later life (usually in the fifties or sixties) is not asso-ciated with any abnormality in pancreatic beta cells. Insulin is produced in normal amounts (sometimes even in increased amounts) but the tissues of the body have somehow become resistant to the action of insulin. Again, the blood sugar will rise and the tissues will be starved for fuel. This type of diabetes also has a genetic basis. It is more common in certain families than in others. However, unlike the juvenile form, there is a nutritional component in the cause of maturity onset diabetes. It is much more common in obese people than in lean people. Thus, to the extent that diet is involved in obesity, consumption of too many calories is a contributing cause of diabetes. While the increased consumption of calories regardless of the source will increase a person's risk of contracting diabetes, ingestion of sugar, per se, will not. The increased amount of fat tissue increases the body's resistance to the action of insulin. For this reason, weight reduction alone may control this kind of diabetes. (See OBESITY.)

Although nutrition plays only a limited role when it comes to the causes of diabetes, it plays a major role in the management of diabetes. Treatment of any patient with diabetes, regardless of the type, will have

---

COMPLICATIONS OF DIABETES

Macrovascular	**Microvascular**
Atherosclerosis	Kidney disease
Heart attack	Blindness
Stroke	
Gangrene of the extremities	

---

two major aims—to control the level of blood glucose and to prevent the serious complications of the disease. While insulin therapy may be of primary importance in treating people with diabetes, proper nutrition will make it easier to achieve these aims. The main complications of diabetes are listed in the table above.

Diabetes is often associated with high levels of lipids (fats) in the blood, which increase the risk of atherosclerosis. These high serum lipid levels can often be brought down by reducing the amount of total fat, saturated fat, and cholesterol in the diet. Thus the person suffering from either form of diabetes should be on a prudent diet which is lower in total fat, saturated fat, and cholesterol and higher in polyunsaturated fat than the usual American diet. Lowering the percentage of total calories derived from fat will, of necessity, increase the percentage of calories derived from carbohydrates. Therefore, the best diet for an individual suffering from diabetes will be one that is relatively high in carbohydrates.

At the same time, we wish to limit the amount of carbohydrates in the form of simple sugars since these are absorbed very rapidly and will therefore raise blood sugar to very high levels before the insulin which has been administered can bring the levels back into the normal range. As a consequence, the preferred diet for a person with diabetes is a low-fat diet which has a normal protein content, a reduced content of simple sugars, and a very high content of complex carbohydrates (starches). In addition, there may be a benefit derived from consuming relatively large amounts of fiber (nondigestible carbohydrate). The following table compares the composition of the typical American diet to that of a diet recommended for a person with diabetes.

In addition to the composition of the diet, the frequency of meals is extremely important, particularly for the juvenile diabetic. The pancreas is unable to respond properly to the glucose derived from a meal by secreting more insulin. Therefore, insulin must be given by injection. Even though the modern insulin

COMPOSITION OF THE TYPICAL AMERICAN DIET VERSUS A DIABETIC DIET

	Typical American Diet	Recommended Diabetic diet
Carbohydrate	40% (high in simple sugars)	50–60% (high in complex carbohydrates, e.g., starches and vegetables)
Fat	40% (high in saturated fat)	20–30% (1:1:1 ratio of polyunsaturated to mono-unsaturated to saturated fat)
Protein	20%	20%
Fiber	low	high

preparations can release insulin slowly from the injection site, it is important to avoid periods of feast (when blood sugar may rise too high) or famine (when blood sugar may fall too low). There is some evidence to show that by avoiding these wide swings in blood glucose levels the microvascular complications of diabetes can be reduced. Thus, the juvenile onset diabetic or the maturity onset diabetic requiring relatively large quantities of insulin for control should consume five or even six meals during the day.

In summary, a person suffering from diabetes should follow certain simple but extremely important nutritional guidelines:

• Calories should be aimed at achieving an ideal weight (in the juvenile diabetic, this often means gaining weight; in the maturity onset diabetic, this usually means losing weight).

• Fat should be limited to 25 to 30 percent of the total calories consumed.

• Saturated fat should supply 10 to 15 percent of the total calories, and vegetable fat (polyunsaturated and monounsaturated), the other 15 percent.

• Protein can range from 12 to 24 percent of all calories (not critical).

• Simple sugars should be kept to 10 to 15 percent of all calories consumed and only a small amount of this should come from refined sugars.

• The remainder of the calories (around 40 percent) should come from complex carbohydrates (usually starch).

Although diabetes is a very serious illness, with proper insulin replacement and careful attention to the diet, any person who suffers from this disease can expect to lead a useful and productive life.

DIETARY FIBER

While the evidence that the low-fiber diets consumed by western societies contribute to the high incidence of diabetes in those populations is still indirect and circumstantial, recent evidence does suggest that an increased intake of dietary fiber may have a role in the management of diabetes.

Several recent studies have demonstrated that adding fiber (20 grams of crude fiber) to the diets of diabetic patients, reduced blood sugar and reduced the amount of insulin that was necessary to maintain good control. There are several possible explanations for the results which were observed. The one which seems to have the most support currently is that fiber delays the absorption of simple sugars from the gastrointestinal tract. This may be due to an actual binding of the sugar molecules by the fiber or to a direct effect of fiber on the gastrointestinal tract. For example, dietary fiber might delay emptying of the stomach, thereby slowing the entrance of the meal into the small intestine where absorption must take place. Alternatively, dietary fiber might in some way affect the cells which are responsible for breaking down and absorbing simple sugars, and therefore, glucose absorption might be slower.

Whatever the exact mechanism, the result is a slower and more sustained release of glucose from the gastrointestinal tract into the blood stream. This is a very desirable consequence, since it will prevent the wide swings in blood sugar which may occur when simple sugars are ingested in the absence of fiber. In addition, the amount of insulin necessary to control blood sugar is often reduced.

From a practical standpoint, this means that, for the diabetic person, consumption of natural sugars should be in a form as close to the natural state as possible. An apple is better than apple sauce or apple juice. In addition, there is no reason why a person with diabetes should not increase the fiber content of her or his regular diet and even add fiber to the diet in the form of bran or raw vegetables. (See FIBER.)

DIETARY GUIDELINES

There is good evidence to show that a high-starch, low-fat, controlled energy diet can be used with success in the treatment of diabetes. Such a diet results in decreases in blood cholesterol levels and reduces the incidence of atherosclerosis. Although rigid carbohydrate restriction no longer appears advisable for the diabetic, simple sugars should be avoided. Individualized dietary therapy is essential with regard to weight control, meal spacing, and intake of cholesterol and saturated fat, and the following guidelines should give you some idea of how to go about it.

Calculating Your Diabetic Diet. Estimate your ideal body weight in pounds by allowing 105 pounds for the first 5 feet of height and five pounds for each additional inch over 5 feet. If you have a medium or heavy frame, add 5 to 10 pounds. Hence, a person with a medium frame, who is 6 feet tall, should have an ideal weight of approximately 171 pounds. Convert this weight to kilograms by dividing the pounds by 2.2.

Now, calculate the amount of energy you need per day for each kilogram of ideal body weight on the basis of body weight and activity.

You now need to figure out the composition of the diet.

Protein: You need 1.5 grams per kilogram of ideal body weight.

Carbohydrate: This amount should be 50 to 60 percent of the calories.

Fat: The remaining calories should be in the form of fat, with saturated fat making up about 10 percent of the total calories and polyunsaturated fats about 10 percent of the calories.

Translating the Diet as Food Servings. Now using the exchange lists which follow, translate the diet into food servings and distribute them among three meals plus any extra snacks. Anybody getting insulin must have a bedtime feeding. Children need midmorning and midafternoon snacks, too.

The foods in the exchange lists are grouped according to their nutrient similarities: vegetables, fruits and juices, and starchy foods (breads,

WEIGHT AND ACTIVITY LEVEL*

	Sedentary (kcal)	Moderate (kcal)	Marked (kcal)
Overweight	20–25	30	35
Normal	30	35	40
Underweight	35	40	45–50

*From Goodhart and Shils, *Modern Nutrition in Health and Disease*, 6th Edition, p. 992.

EXCHANGE LISTS

List 1. Free Foods

Bouillon	Gelatin, unsweetened	Mustard	Chicory	Lettuce (all kinds)
Clear Broth	Lemon, Lime	Pickle, sour	Chinese Cabbage	Parsley
Coffee		Pickle, dill-	Endive	Radishes
Tea		unsweetened	Escarole	Watercress
		Vinegar		

List 2. Vegetable Exchanges = ½ cup cooked or 1 cup raw
One exchange of vegetables contains about five grams of carbohydrate, two grams of protein and 25 kcal.

Asparagus	Carrots	Mushrooms	Tomatoes – 1 cup raw
Bean Sprouts	Catsup (2 tbsp.)	Okra	½ cup cooked
Beans (green or wax)	Cauliflower	Onions	Tomato or Vegetable juice-6 oz.
Broccoli	Celery	Peppers (red or green)	All leafy greens
Beets	Cucumbers	Rutabaga	
Brussels Sprouts	Eggplant	Sauerkraut	
Cabbage (all kinds)		Summer Squash	

List 3. Fruit Exchanges
One exchange of fruit contains 10 grams of carbohydrate and 40 kcal.

FRUITS:

			JUICES:
Apple – ½ med.	Cantaloupe – ¼ med.	Peach – 1 med.	Apple, Pineapple – ⅓ cup
Applesauce – ½ cup	(6" dia.)	Pear – 1 small	Grapefruit, Orange – ½ cup
Apricots, fresh – 2 med.	Cherries – 10 large	Pineapple – ½ cup	Grape, Prune – ¼ cup
Apricots, dried – 4 halves	Dates – 2	Prunes, dried – 2	
Bananas – ½ small	Figs, dried – 1 small	Raisins, 2 tbsp.	
Blueberries – ½ cup	Fruit cocktail, canned –	Strawberries – ¾ cup	
	½ cup	Tangerine – 1 large	
	Grapefruit – ½ small	Watermelon – 1 cup cubed	
	Grapes – 12		
	Honeydew Melon – ⅓		
	(7" dia.)		
	Mango – ½ small		
	Nectarine – 1 small		
	Orange – 1 small		
	Papaya – ⅓ med.		

List 4. Starch Exchanges (cooked servings)
One exchange of starch contains 15 grams of carbohydrate, two grams of protein and 70 kcal.

BREADS:	CRACKERS:	CEREALS:
Any loaf – 1 slice	Graham (2½" sq.) – 2	Hot Cereal – ½ cup
Bagel – ½	Matzoh (4" x 6") – ½	Dry flakes – ⅔ cup
Dinner roll – 1 (2" dia.)	Melba Toast – 4	Dry puffed – 1½ cups
English Muffin – ½	Oysters (½ cup) – 20	Bran – 5 tbsp.
Bun, Hamburger or Hot dog – ½	Pretzels – 8 rings	Wheatgerm – 2 tbsp.
Cornbread (1½") – 1 cube	Rye Krisps – 3	Pastas – ½ cup
Tortilla (6" dia.) – 1	Saltines – 5	Rice – ½ cup
VEGETABLES:		DESSERTS:
Beans or Peas (plain) cooked – ½ cup		Fat-free sherbet – 4 oz.
Corn – ⅓ cup or ½ med. ear		Angel Cake – 1½" square
Parsnips – ⅔ cup		
Potatoes, white – 1 small or ½ cup		
Potatoes, sweet or yams – ¼ cup		
Pumpkin – ¾ cup		
Winter Squash – ½ cup		

List 5. Meat Exchanges (cooked weight)
One exchange of lean meat contains seven grams of protein, three grams of fat and 55 kcal.

Beef, dried, chipped – 1 oz.	Poultry without skin – 1 oz.	Lobster – 1 small tail	Egg – 1 med.
Beef, lamb, pork, veal	Fish – 1 oz.	Oysters, Clams, Shrimp –	Hard Cheese – ½ oz.
lean only – 1 oz.		5 med.	Peanut Butter – 2 tsp.
Cottage Cheese, uncreamed –		Tuna, packed in water – ¼ cup	
¼ cup		Salmon, pink, canned – ¼ cup	

List 6. Milk Exchanges
One exchange of milk contains 12 grams of carbohydrate, eight grams of protein, and 80 kcal.

Buttermilk, fat free – 1 cup	Skim milk – 1 cup
Yogurt, plain, made with nonfat milk – ¾ cup	1% Fat Milk – 7 oz.

List 7. Fat Exchanges
One exchange of fat contains five grams of fat and 45 kcal.

Avocado (4" dia.) – ⅛	French dressing – 1 tbsp.	Peanuts – 10
Bacon, crisp – 1 slice	Mayonnaise – 1 tsp.	Walnuts – 6 small
Butter, Margarine – 1 tsp.	Roquefort dressing – 2 tsp.	
	Thousand Island dressing – 2 tsp.	
	Oil – 1 tsp.	
	Olives – 5 small	

LIST	Number of Portions Allowed for Various Calorie Levels			
	1000 Calories	**1200 Calories**	**1500 Calories**	**1800 Calories**
List 1 – Free Foods	. . . . Unlimited			
List 2 – Vegetable Exchanges	2	2	2	2
List 3 – Fruit Exchanges	3	3	3	3
List 4 – Starch Exchanges	3	5	7	9
List 5 – Protein Exchanges	6	6	7	7
List 6 – Milk Exchanges	2	2	2	3
List 7 – Fat Exchanges	2	2	6	7

For a person following a 1500 calorie plan, the exchanges can be allotted in this way:

BASIC PLAN	SAMPLE MENU	FREE FOODS
Morning		
List 3 = 1	½ small grapefruit	coffee, artificial
List 5 = 1	1 medium egg	sweetener
List 4 = 2	1 slice whole wheat bread & 1½ cup puffed cereal	
List 7 = 1	1 tsp. margarine	
List 6 = 1	1 cup (8 oz.) skim milk	
Noon		
List 5 = 2	½ cup tuna (in water)	lettuce, pickles,
List 4 = 2	2 slices bread	lemon juice,
List 7 = 3	2 tsp. mayonnaise & 1 tsp. oil	vinegar
List 2 = 1	3 slices tomato	
List 3 = 1	½ cup diced pineapple	
Evening		
List 2 = 1	½ cup string beans	lettuce, radishes,
List 5 = 4	4 oz. chicken (no skin)	soy sauce, parsley
List 4 = 2	½ cup mashed potato & 4 oz. fat-free sherbet	
List 7 = 2	2 tsp. margarine	
List 3 = 1	2 dates	
Snack		
List 6 = 1	8 oz. skim milk	coffee
List 4 = 1	1½ in. square sponge cake	

cereals, beans) are each grouped together. Within each list, foods are described in specific quantities or units. The term "exchange" is used because a serving of a food within a list can be exchanged for another food within the *same* list. For example, on the fruit list, you can exchange ten cherries for half a cup of orange juice, should you prefer the orange juice. Or you can make two exchanges, in a case where ten cherries and half a cup of orange juice would equal a whole medium apple (since half an apple equals ten cherries and half an apple also equals half a cup of orange juice).

The total number of servings allowed for each calorie level is given below. At all levels, the protein intake will be adequate and vitamin and mineral supplements should not be necessary if selections are made from a variety of foods.

The use of these exchange systems are designed to permit you to put together a diet that takes into account your individual food preferences. If you take insulin, obviously you must adjust your eating habits as well as your calorie intake. Your meals should be spaced in such a way as to take into account the insulin you have given yourself and your level of physical activity. Otherwise, you will suffer from periods of low blood glucose. If you fall into this category, check with your physician.

Since diabetes is often accompanied by other medical problems which require special diets, the basic diet may have to be further modified. Salt restriction may be a necessity for a person with heart or kidney disease. For those people with gastrointestinal problems, such as gall bladder disease, colitis, or peptic ulcers, the consistency or composition of the diet may have to be changed. Those with gall bladder problems may have to reduce their fat intake even further than advised here, and people with kidney or liver problems may need to reduce the recommended protein level. It is very difficult to sort these problems out on your own, and so you should seek the advice of your physician under these circumstances. (See also HYPOGLYCEMIA.)

DIETARY RECOMMENDATIONS

The last decade has witnessed an increasing interest in the way we look at the food we eat. We have become more and more aware of the importance of our eating habits to our health. Scientific evidence has also shown that certain components of our diets may be directly implicated in diseases like coronary artery disease and cancer. The public interest in nutrition has prompted several institutions to publish and advertise a whole range of "dietary recommendations." These recommendations are aimed at educating the public to making the proper food choices in order to prevent several diseases which have been shown to be directly or indirectly caused or aggravated by the kinds of food we eat.

The best known of these dietary recommendations (and the ones that have been most widely advertised) are:

    a. *The Prudent Diet,* published by the American Heart Association,
    b. *The Dietary Goals for the United States,* prepared by the Senate Select Committee on Nutrition and Human Needs,
    c. *Toward Healthful Diets,* published by the Food and Nutrition Board of the National Academy of Sciences.

In reality, all these recommendations are very similar. Although there are a few points of discrepancy, which we will describe below, they all point out a "sensible" way to eat based on what we have learned from a multitude of studies. We will summarize the most important recommendations and what they mean.

EAT A VARIETY OF FOODS

Although this may sound obvious to everyone, it is amazing how we tend to restrict the foods we eat to the ones we like best. There are about forty different nutrients that have to be supplied continually by the diet, and it is impossible to get them unless the diet is composed of a large variety of items.

REDUCE THE CONSUMPTION OF ANIMAL FAT AND CHOLESTEROL

A high consumption of animal fats (which are mostly saturated) and of cholesterol has been associated with high blood cholesterol levels, which in turn is associated with a high incidence of heart disease. Fats coming from vegetable sources, or poly-unsaturated fats, tend to lower blood cholesterol. It is recommended that we lower the total intake of fat (from our current intake of 40 percent of our caloric intake down to 30 percent), and that we increase the proportion of polyunsaturated fat to about 30 to 35 percent of our total fat consumption. Although some institutions (like the Food and Nutrition Board) do not find it necessary to lower cholesterol intake, we (and the other two institutions mentioned previously) feel that the scientific evidence is such that we should indeed lower our intake of cholesterol to about 300 milligrams per day, from our average intake of 600 milligrams per day. In practical terms, these recommendations mean that we have to reduce the intake of food of animal origin—whole milk, butter, meat (liver, for instance), and eggs. Very simple alterations in our diet can achieve the desired purpose. (See CHOLESTEROL.)

REDUCE THE INTAKE OF SODIUM

High sodium intake has been associated with the development of hypertension. The average sodium intake in our country (which comes mainly from salt) is 6 to 18 grams per day. Unfortunately, much of this sodium is either "hidden" in processed foods (canned food, cakes, etc.) or

inherent to certain natural foods, so it is difficult to reduce the intake unless we go through a considerable amount of food preparation. We do recommend, however, stopping the excessive salting of foods when cooking or right before eating. Your palate can be trained to require less salt and this practice will effectively diminish your total intake of sodium. (See SALT; SODIUM.)

INCREASE YOUR CONSUMPTION OF COMPLEX CARBOHYDRATES AND FIBER

The consumption of carbohydrates in our diet has steadily decreased since the turn of the century. Conversely, our fat consumption has increased. Also, simple carbohydrates (like sugar) have gradually replaced more complex carbohydrates (like starch). The recommendation here is to increase the intake of complex carbohydrates. There is evidence that a diet high in these nutrients may reduce the risk of heart disease and diabetes. In addition, fruits that contain complex carbohydrates usually also contain a high amount of fiber, which may reduce the incidence of diverticulosis and colon cancer. Lastly, increasing the intake of these carbohydrates may reduce fat intake and hence total caloric intake. This may help to maintain body weight. (See CARBOHYDRATE; FIBER.)

MAINTAIN AN "IDEAL" BODY WEIGHT

Excessive body weight has been shown to increase the risk of several chronic disorders, including high blood pressure, diabetes, and increased blood cholesterol. Although the concept of ideal body weight is rather undefined, some approximations can be made. The table Suggested Body Weights indicates the range of acceptable weights according to your height. Do take into consideration that if you have a heavy frame, your ideal body weight will be higher, but if your weight is much higher than the ideal you should reduce it. The only way to achieve this goal is to reduce the amount of calories you eat. If at the same time you increase your energy use, that will surely help. (See NUTRITION AND EXERCISE.)

SUGGESTED BODY WEIGHTS
(range of acceptable weights*)

Height* (feet-inches)	Men (pounds)	Women (pounds)
4'10"		92–119
4'11"		94–122
5'0"		96–125
5'1"		99–128
5'2"	112–141	102–131
5'3"	115–144	105–134
5'4"	118–148	108–138
5'5"	121–152	111–142
5'6"	124–156	114–146
5'7"	128–161	118–150
5'8"	132–166	122–154
5'9"	136–170	126–158
5'10"	140–174	130–163
5'11"	144–179	134–168
6'0"	148–184	138–173
6'1"	152–189	
6'2"	156–194	
6'3"	160–199	
6'4"	164–204	

*Height without shoes; weight without clothes.
Source: HEW Conference on Obesity, 1973.

ALCOHOL

Most recommendations agree on the fact that if you do drink alcohol you should do it in moderation. Alcoholic beverages are quite high in calories. Excessive drinking will curtail your appetite for foods which contain nutrients that you need and increase the incidence of some serious conditions such as cirrhosis of the liver. We recommend that if you drink alcohol, do not exceed 10 grams of alcohol per day (the equivalent of approximately one highball or one light beer per day). (See ALCOHOL.)

The recommendations outlined above are not intended to suggest that you drastically change your eating habits. Rather, they are aimed at pointing out to you which eating customs should be changed gradually in order to improve your diet and overall health. (See also FOOD BALANCING.)

DRUG-NUTRIENT INTERACTION

The use of drugs in our society for the treatment of specific diseases and for the relief of perceived ailments has reached unprecedented levels. Drugs are used without prescriptions to relieve pain, calm one down, perk one up, dry sinuses, induce sleep, relieve constipation, soothe an upset stomach, neutralize excess acid, and for many other purposes. Billions of capsules and tablets are consumed each year by the American public. Certainly, drugs can cure certain diseases, reduce the symptoms of many others and promote better health, and to these ends they must be used. However, their excess use has created many problems. One such problem, only recently recognized, is that many drugs can alter the manner in which the body handles essential nutrients.

Certain segments of our society, because of their high consumption of medications and because of their own special nutritional requirements, are particularly at risk for drug-induced nutrient deficiencies. At the top of the list are the elderly. The table on page 128 is a list of drugs, commonly taken by older people, which can cause alterations in nutrient metabolism.

ASPIRIN

Aspirin (acetylsalicylic acid) in one form or another is perhaps the most common self-prescribed medicine in America today. It is used as an analgesic for almost all types of pain. Aspirin also has a specific anti-inflammatory effect, which makes it the drug of choice in treating certain kinds of arthritis, a common affliction in older people. Thus many older people are chronic users of aspirin in high doses (1 to 3 grams a day). Such use can cause microscopic bleeding of the gastrointestinal tract with concomitant loss of iron. Since iron needs may be increased, the older person who is a regular aspirin user is in double jeopardy and must consume a diet high in iron.

There is also evidence that aspirin may compete with folacin (folic acid) for a place on the protein molecule in blood which transports this vitamin to the tissues. Thus, less folacin is able to reach the sites where it is active. In addition, some data suggests that aspirin may increase the rate of folacin loss in the urine. For these reasons, a person who is consuming large doses of aspirin over a long period of time should pay par-

DRUG-NUTRIENT INTERACTION

COMMONLY USED DRUGS THAT AFFECT NUTRIENTS

Drug	Nutrient	Mechanism
Alcohol	folacin	decreases absorption
	thiamine	increases requirement & decreases absorption
	vitamin B$_6$	impairs conversion to active form
	zinc & magnesium	increases excretion
Antacids	phosphorus	inhibits absorption
Anticoagulants	vitamin K	inhibits utilization
Anticonvulsants	vitamin D & folacin	inhibits utilization
Aspirin	iron	increases bleeding
	folacin	competes for transport
Cholestyramine (cholesterol-lowering agent)	fats and fat-soluble vitamins (A, D, E, K)	inhibits absorption
Corticosteroids	vitamin D	increases utilization
	vitamin B$_6$	increases requirements
	zinc	increases excretion
Diuretics	potassium	increases excretion
	calcium	increases excretion
Laxatives	fat-soluble vitamins (A, D, K)	inhibits absorption
	phosphorus	depletion from bones
Nicotine (cigarettes)	vitamin C	uncertain
	vitamin B$_6$	uncertain
	vitamin B$_{12}$	uncertain

ticular attention to consuming foods rich in folacin. Finally, although the data is not conclusive, several studies suggest that chronic use of aspirin increases the need for vitamin C.

LAXATIVES

Constipation is a very common problem in certain groups, especially the elderly. Although probably the best treatment is increased dietary fiber, many older people are, instead, chronic laxative users. Some laxatives may decrease vitamin D absorption and, if they contain mercury, may deplete phosphorus from the bones. Both of these actions can aggravate the tendency toward osteoporosis. Mineral oil, a widely used remedy for constipation, interferes with the absorption of fat-soluble vitamins, particularly vitamins A, D, and K. Again, the ensuing vitamin D deficiency may adversely influence an already precarious calcium balance.

ANTACIDS

While there is rarely a need for antacids, particularly in older people who generally have decreased stomach acidity, many elderly adults regularly use these preparations. If large amounts are used for long periods of time, and if aluminum hydroxide is one of the ingredients, phosphate deficiency can result. Dietary phosphate reacts with the aluminum and forms aluminum phosphate, which is passed in the stool. As a result, blood phosphate is kept at a normal level only by phosphorus released from bone. Again, the older individual already suffering from bone demineralization is at particular risk.

DIURETICS

In our society, where relatively much salt is consumed, the incidence of high blood pressure increases with age. Therefore, many older people suffer from this ailment. One of the most common treatments for high blood pressure is the administration of diuretics. These drugs induce sodium and water loss through the kidney. Diuretics are also used to treat people with chronic heart disease who may tend to accumulate water in their tissues (edema). Along with the sodium loss, a desirable effect, many diuretics also promote potassium loss, an undesirable effect. The potassium, an essential mineral, must be replaced. Foods rich in potassium should be consumed daily, or else a potassium supplement should be taken.

Some diuretics may also increase calcium excretion, a particularly unwanted side effect, and a few can cause the depletion of other minerals. Any person regularly consuming diuretics should be under the care of a physican who will recommend appropriate mineral supplementation when indicated.

ORAL CONTRACEPTIVES

Oral contraceptive drugs, which usually are a mixture of synthetic estrogen and progesterone, are estimated to be used by about fifty million women all over the world. Oral contraceptives have been shown by some studies to decrease the levels of folacin in the blood. Furthermore, some women appear to be particulary susceptible to oral contraceptive agents and can develop a type of anemia due to a deficiency of folacin. (See ANEMIAS.) It appears that in these women the absorption of certain forms of the vitamin present in the diet is impaired. Although the proportion of "highly susceptible" women seems to be rather small, it is advisable to keep in mind that prolonged use of oral contraceptives may cause a slight folacin deficiency. Since the screening of blood levels of folacin is difficult and there are few laboratories that carry out the procedure, we recommend an increase in the intake of dietary folacin.

Some studies have also suggested that oral contraceptives may produce a mild deficiency of vitamin B_6, characterized by a general malaise. Although the data is not conclusive, it would be advisable to increase the intake of vitamin B_6 during oral contraceptive use to prevent the occurrence of borderline deficiency. Vitamin C levels in plasma and white blood cells (a commonly used measurement to assess vitamin C status) have also been shown to be decreased in women taking oral contraceptives. This appears to be due to an increased breakdown of vitamin C. Therefore, a diet rich in vitamin C is advisable. Although the requirement for riboflavin also seems to be increased by the use of oral contraceptives, this vitamin is so prevalent in our food supply that supplementation is unnecessary.

FOODS THAT INTERFERE WITH DRUG METABOLISM

Some foods (or compounds in them) interfere with how effectively a drug functions in the body. For example, calcium and iron interfere with te-tracycline and vitamin K interferes with the action of anticoagulants. Try to limit foods containing those nutrients until two to three hours before or after taking those medications.

Another important factor involved in ensuring a totally nourishing diet is appetite. Many illnesses and chronic conditions—particularly those associated with constant pain—produce a loss of appetite, called anorexia. In some instances, the drugs alone will suppress appetite or compound the anorexia caused by the condition. Those drugs that are known to suppress appetite in some people are

cough medicine	amphetamines
antihistamines	alcohol
caffeine	antacids
narcotics	cancer chemotherapy
digitalis	

If you must take a drug which will suppress your appetite, here are some tips to keep your food intake up.

• Consume smaller, more frequent meals.
• If milk is tolerated, use it (in fluid or powdered form) to boost the nutrient content of a meal by adding it to soups and beverages. Powdered milk blended with peanut butter until the mixture is stiff makes a tasty nibble.
• If sweets are preferred, consume milk-rich puddings, flavored yogurt, shakes (without egg), and dried fruit.

EICOSAPENTAENOIC ACID (EPA)

Japanese fishermen and Eskimos who eat a great deal of fish rarely die of coronary artery disease. These groups seem to be protected by the high amount of fish oil in their diets, or rather the eicosapentaenoic acid (EPA) that it contains. Nobody knows how EPA protects against heart disease. It appears to reduce the amount of low-density lipoprotein (LDL) in the blood and raise the level of high-density lipoprotein (HDL) at the same time. It may also prevent the disk-shaped cells (platelets) from sticking to the walls of the blood vessels at the sites of cholesterol deposition, which makes atherosclerosis worse. The moral here is that it might be very healthful to devlop a taste for fish—the fattier the fish the better. Mackerel is especially rich in EPA. The much-maligned shellfish have also come out on top. Original analysis showed them to be rich in cholesterol and hence off limits for heart patients. Newer analytical methods have shown that what was once thought to be cholesterol may in fact be EPA.

ENTERAL NUTRITION

Enteral nutrition is a very special form of nutrition used when a person is unconscious or unable to swallow because of some serious disease. It is always prescribed by a physician and usually administered through a tube passed into the patient's stomach through the nose and esophagus. The food is usually a liquid containing protein, fat, carbohydrate, and all of the essential vitamins and minerals. Patients can be fed and maintained in good nutritional status in this manner for indefinite periods of time. (Also see PARENTERAL NUTRITION.)

ENZYMES

Enzymes are substances which promote a chemical reaction within the body without themselves being acted upon. Every cell in the body contains thousands of enzymes necessary for promoting the numerous chemical reactions needed for essential life processes. Enzymes are proteins and are manufactured by cells in a manner similar to the synthesis of other proteins. One of the many functions that enzymes have is to help in the chemical breakdown of foods; the process known as digestion. For this reason some people have advocated taking enzymes with their foods to aid digestion. Unfortunately, for the most part this does not work. The enzyme itself will usually be destroyed by the acid in the stomach and will be useless thereafter. Enzymes can be useful in food processing and may convert some foods to a more digestible form *before* they are ingested. An example of this is yogurt which may contain enzymes produced by naturally occurring bacteria which break down the lactose. However, this occurs before you eat the yogurt. While the bacteria may survive the passage through the stomach and continue to produce the enzyme in the lower gastrointestinal tract the enzymes themselves will be destroyed.

There is no reason for a healthy individual to take enzymes to help digestion. It is expensive and will not accomplish the purpose. (See also CELLULASE; MOLYBDENUM; PAPAIN; PROTEIN; TRYPSIN.)

EXERCISE

Along with the increasing interest in distance running has come an equal fascination with the diet necessary for optimum athletic performance. Nutrition and exercise have become inseparable topics. In fact, it might even be said that the current interest in exercise has increased the average person's awareness of the importance of good nutrition. Until five years ago, few people were aware of the phenomenon of carbohydrate loading. Now, every keen jogger is well aware of the pros and cons of such practices. The foods, or more specifically the nutrients within those foods that we consume, represent the fuel necessary to generate and sustain any exercise which is being undertaken.

FUELS UTILIZED DURING EXERCISE

Athletes have to adjust their energy intake according to their physical activity. Usually this occurs automatically: As physical activity increases, food intake will also increase. During training and competition, the energy requirements can increase all the way up to a level of 6000 calories a day depending on the type of exercise. When training stops, food intake must be decreased to avoid gaining weight. Incidentally, when exercise is used as a means of reducing weight, energy (food) intake should be less than the energy spent on exercising.

The fuels used will vary depending on the intensity and duration of exercise. During moderate exercise (like walking at a relatively fast pace for short periods of time), fat provides most of the energy. As the intensity and the duration of the exercise increases, carbohydrates become the major fuel. At maximum capacity, carbohydrates become the exclusive source of energy.

Carbohydrates are stored in the liver and muscles in a large molecule called glycogen. When circulating in the blood, carbohydrate is in the form of the simple sugar glucose. The amount of glycogen stored in the muscle becomes a critical factor during extended performance.

During prolonged exercise muscle glycogen is depleted. This glycogen is converted to glucose, which circulates in the blood and is extracted by the tissues as a major fuel. As the exercise proceeds, tissues, primarily muscle tissues, increase their use of circulating glucose, and blood sugar values fall, eventually causing a condition known as hypoglycemia (low blood glucose) when the available liver and muscle glycogen stores become depleted. To avoid depletion of the carbohydrate stores in the body during intense exercise, many athletes will use a carbohydrate-loading diet (also called glycogen-loading). This technique is discussed below. (See CARBOHYDRATE.)

Proteins are not an important source of energy during exercise. However, during prolonged training, athletes will increase their muscle mass and this will require synthesis of new proteins. Athletes may require four times as much protein as nonathletes. This increased need is usually met by the increase in food intake due to the increased energy demands.

DIET DURING TRAINING

The dietary requirements of ongoing training are different from those during the actual competition. The bulk of an athlete's diet should be made up of complex starches and other carbohydrates. A person in training will generally consume 3000 to 5000 calories per day. Unlike sedentary people, training athletes use the excess carbohydrates to cater to their high daily energy output. These calories do not become a source of stored energy in the form of fat because they are quickly used up.

Special mention should be made of the athlete who trains in hot cli-

mates. In addition to salt (sodium) depletion, which results from excessive sweating, the body may become deficient in potassium through losses in saliva and sweat. Symptoms of low blood potassium may develop if the person fails to replenish the total body potassium stores. Foods like oranges, tomatoes, and bananas are good sources of potassium. Supplementation with potassium chloride pills is not necessary and may be dangerous.

THE CARBOHYDRATE-LOADING DIET

Since, as we have seen, reserve energy is stored in the muscle in the form of the complex carbohydrate, glycogen, and there is a limit to how much glycogen can be stored in the muscle, a theory has developed which says that by enlarging the stores of glycogen, performance can be improved. Studies show that glycogen stores can be raised, particularly in muscle, by a diet that removes carbohydrate completely from the diet for a period and then replaces it at a high level. This is the so-called carbohydrate-loading diet that is the prime topic of distance runners' conversations before a marathon. It is also the cause of domestic strife and job dysfunction, as runners subjecting themselves to the diet undergo personality changes compounded by fatigue and an inability to concentrate on anything but food.

The diet is usually preceded by an initial emptying of muscle and liver glycogen stores, accomplished by a 10 to 15 mile run at a near maximal effort, six days before a marathon. Following the depletion run, the individual lives on a carbohydrate-free, high-protein, and high-fat diet for the next three days while continuing to train. This will further deplete muscle glycogen stores. If successfully accomplished, this leads to fatigue, short temper, and light headedness—all signs of hypoglycemia.

During the remaining three days before the race, the individual eats a high-carbohydrate diet. The traditional prerace steak and potato dinner has been replaced by pasta and beer. This system of depletion, followed by loading, leads to a build up of glycogen in the muscle beyond the normal level. It has been shown both in Sweden and in the US that there is a very good correlation between the increased muscle glycogen stores achieved in this way and the length of time an athlete can sustain maximal exercise performance. Glycogen tends to cause water retention and critics of the technique point out that increased muscle glycogen stores may impair performance by increasing the water stored in, and hence the weight of, muscle. This can produce some stiffness. We do not recommend carbohydrate-loading to the "weekend athlete." For the trained athlete it may provide a useful means of maintaining endurance.

STARTING AN EXERCISE PROGRAM

There is currently very little doubt about the benefits of a well-designed exercise program. Besides improving physical fitness in general, it will diminish the risk of obesity, coronary artery disease, and hypertension.

We will show you here how to design an exercise program that will assist you in achieving and maintaining your optimum weight for good health. Bear in mind that to be effective an exercise program has to become so thoroughly ingrained in your life-style that you feel a little uncomfortable without it. It cannot be viewed as a temporary procedure.

An appropriate exercise program must take into account your age, sex, weight, health, and objectives. If you have some physical disability you must be careful to discuss your objectives with your physician in order to proceed prudently and attain the maximum benefits from your program. Even if you have no known disability you must remember that shifting your life-style from mainly sedentary to even moderately active puts a strain on the body, especially the heart and lungs—not to mention the muscles! For this reason it is simply not a good idea to launch into an exercise program without consulting your physician, no matter how healthy you think you are.

An exercise program consisting of a trip to the gym where you hook yourself up to a fancy machine that shakes you up is not going to be effective. Surprisingly, even stationary exercise involving strenuously working small groups of muscles (such as lifting weights, shoveling snow, or digging) is not very helpful and can even be dangerous, for it places a greater strain on the heart than dynamic exercise does. Dynamic exercise includes such activities as running, swimming, and bicycling, which involve the entire body, especially the large muscles of the legs. The following table gives you some idea of how much energy you use during various physical activities.

The type of exercise you choose should be one that you enjoy and can maintain for 20 to 30 minutes. To achieve fitness you may want to exercise from four to six days a week; to maintain fitness it is usually necessary to exercise only on alternate days. Remember, too much too fast is the quickest way to get discouraged.

You don't have to work at your maximum to get a training effect. Your physician will administer an exercise stress test to establish the max-

---

CALORIE EXPENDITURES PER HOUR FOR DIFFERENT ACTIVITIES*

Activity	Calories Expended per Hour of Continuous Exercise
Bicycle riding	200–600
Walking moderately fast	200–300
Football	560
Soccer	560
Frisbee	200
Basketball	500
Tennis	500–700
Volleyball	300
Swimming	300–600
Dancing	200–400
Jogging	400–500
Skiing, cross country	650–1000
downhill	350–500

*Based on an individual weighing approximately 130 to 150 pounds. Add on more calories if the person is heavier.

imum heart rate (number of beats per minute) for a person of your age, sex, and physical condition. Never push your heart rate beyond 85 percent of your maximum. On the other hand, it should not drop below 70 percent of your maximum during exercise. As you begin to get into condition you will notice it takes a little more effort on your part to push yourself to that 70 to 85 percent range, so you should be prepared to check your heart rate periodically to monitor your progress. Your program should be structured as follows:

1. Warm-up period—five to ten minutes. Count your pulse for 10 seconds and multiply by six to find out your heart rate. Heart rate during warm-up should not exceed 50 percent of the maximum established by your physician.
2. Exercising period—start exercising slowly for 3 minutes. Count your pulse: If heart rate is still below 70 percent, increase the exercise for another 3 minutes and again count your pulse. Continue until it is up to 75 percent of your maximum. Continue for another 3 to 5 minutes. If your heart rate exceeds the 85 percent maximum, slow down. You may not be able to keep the rate in the 75 to 85 percent range for a full 20 minutes when you first start your program, but within a few days you'll be able to do so with no difficulty.
3. Cool-down period—continue exercise very slowly for at least 5 minutes. This helps the blood return to your heart while your heart rate is slowing down. If your pulse is not fewer than 100 beats per minute 10 minutes after you stop, the exercise was too strenuous. Keep a record. Conditioning takes from 6 to 10 weeks.

All people should be careful not to push themselves in hot weather. However, if *any* of the following characteristics apply to you, be sure to consult your physician before embarking on any exercise program.

High blood pressure
Smoking
High cholesterol count
Family history of heart disease
Overweight
Over forty years old

To maintain the health benefits of an exercise program you must make a lifetime commitment to a regular physical conditioning program; to eating a well-balanced, nutritious diet; to moderation in smoking and drinking; and to avoiding undue stress and emotional strain. Remember—physical fitness rapidly deteriorates with the resumption of sedentary habits.

NUTRITION AND EXERCISE

Nutrition training is as fundamental to athletic performance as physical training. The amount and kind of food most suitable to the athlete varies with the demand of the task. Both the serious athlete and the dedicated exerciser can benefit from nutritional awareness. With an appropriately balanced diet some of the difficulties of physical activity may be eliminated. (See NUTRITION AND EXERCISE.)

In the exercising arena carbohydrates shed their stigma of being fattening and become the principal source of fuel (energy) during train-ing and performance. Chemically, this category of nutrients consists of sugars in either a simple or complex form. Protein, although available for fuel, is used for building and replacing body tissue. Fats, too, are useful sources of fuel and help transport fat soluble nutrients. The following table is a summary of the nutrients and their sources.

Ideally, the total calories in the diet should be distributed as follows:

- 50 to 60 percent from carbohydrates
- 15 percent from protein
- 25 to 30 percent from fats

NUTRIENTS AND SOURCES

Nutrient	Composed of	Calories per gm	Sources
Carbohydrates	simple sugars	4	Fruits, honey, cane sugar, syrups, milk. Varying amounts in vegetables, grains, nuts, and legumes.
	complex sugars (starch)	4	Grains, legumes, vegetables, tubers, nuts.
Protein	amino acids	4	Meats, fish, poultry, milk and milk products. Combinations of grains and legumes or nuts.
Fat	fatty acids	9	Meats, fish, poultry,* whole milk and whole milk products (e.g. cheese), nuts, spreads, seeds, and cooking fats.

*Poultry has about half as much fat as lean red meat in a serving of equal weight.

The other three categories of nutrients of concern to the athlete are water, vitamins, and minerals. Water is particularly important during extended periods of rigorous exercise. Among other functions, water is responsible for the regulation of body temperature. Excessive losses of body fluid may result in decreased muscle strength and reduced cardiac efficiency. As odd as it seems, drinking to satisfy thirst will, in many cases, not be sufficient to replace fluid losses. Therefore, be sure to take in abundant water before, during, and after exercise.

Supplemental vitamins have not been proven to enhance either training efforts or performance. Replacement of the minerals sodium and potassium has been discussed. With the exception of iron, any additional need for vitamins and minerals will be met by the increase in food intake required to supply the necessary increase in calorie consumption. Women may need a low dose (18 milligrams) of iron supplementation during intensive training and performing.

The current approach to diet in exercise is a major departure from the traditional training meal of steak and buttered potatoes. The main criticisms of that regimen are that it is too high in fat and needlessly high in protein. A good diet for an individual who engages in regular, moderate exercise (under 5 miles of jogging per day) should emphasize abundant complex sugars, at least 1 quart of fluid per day, and an amount of food which matches the appetite while maintaining the weight (if the body weight is already at a desirable level). Meals should be spaced so that exercising is never performed sooner than 2 hours following the meal. The four sample meals that follow illustrate the amount and kind of food needed at various stages of training and competition.

We have tried to emphasize foods with a greater nutrient density. The nutrient density is loosely defined as the amount of necessary nutrients present in a food compared to the number of calories. Examples of high nutrient dense foods compared to their less dense counterparts are: fruit juices rather than fruit drinks or soft drinks; whole wheat bread rather than white bread; low-fat milk rather than whole milk; and dried fruit rather than candy. Try to use salt only in cooking. Use herbs and spices as desired.

Menu 1 is designed for an average adult taking regular exercise. The amount of food will vary with the size and sex of the individual but the basic composition is the same. It contains 2400 calories and 97 grams of protein.

Menu 1

Breakfast *(520 calories)*
1 cup puffed wheat
1 cup low-fat (1%) milk
2 slices whole wheat toast
2 tsp margarine or butter
1 fresh pear
6 oz orange juice

Lunch *(570 calories)*
Turkey sandwich
2 slices bread
2 oz turkey
1 tbsp mayonnaise
lettuce
2 pineapple slices
1 cup vegetable soup
8 oz fruit punch

Midmorning or Midafternoon *(330 calories)*
1 oz peanuts
1 tbsp raisins
8 oz apple juice

Dinner *(750 calories)*
1 baked potato
2 tsp magarine
2/3 cup carrot-raisin salad on lettuce
4 oz boiled chicken
1 cup fruit-flavored yogurt

Snack *(230 calories)*
2 cups popcorn
1 tsp margarine or butter
12 oz unsweetened lemonade

For the person undergoing rigorous training, the diet must have a significant increase in the quantity of nutrients over Menu 1. The amount of protein in this diet should be enough to meet the needs of growing muscle (lean body mass). Menu 2 provides 3000 calories and 125 grams of protein.

Menu 2

Breakfast *(600 calories)*
¼ cup low-fat milk
¾ cup oatmeal
2 slices whole wheat bread
2 tsp margarine or butter
1 cup citrus sections
1 poached egg
8 oz apple juice

Lunch *(870 calories)*
1 hamburger roll
4 oz lean beef patty
12 oz orange-apricot juice
½ canteloupe melon
1 cup cream of tomato soup
8 crackers

Midmorning or Midafternoon *(260 calories)*
6 dried apricot halves
6 cashews
8 oz orange juice

Dinner *(930 calories)*
1 cup rice with herbs & mushrooms
1 tbsp butter or margarine
1 small tomato (sliced)
1 tbsp french dressing
3 oz roast turkey with green pepper
1 cup spinach
1 cup ice cream

Snack *(340 calories)*
2 Dutch twisted pretzels
12 oz tangerine juice

The preevent schedule for many athletes may include the start of a glycogen-depleting diet. If the event is on a Saturday, for instance, begin the preceding Sunday, continuing through Tuesday, following the low-carbohydrate diet given in Menu 3. This menu provides 2200 calories, only 15 percent of which are from carbohydrates.

Menu 3

Breakfast *(500 calories)*
coffee or tea (black or with cream)
2 eggs scrambled with ½ oz Swiss cheese
3 oz ham (lean)
½ grapefruit

Midmorning *(430 calories)*
2 oz American cheese
¼ cup peanuts

Lunch *(340 calories)*
clear consomme
1 cup tuna fish salad on lettuce
cucumber sticks
coffee or tea

Midafternoon *(120 calories)*
4 oz cottage cheese*
coffee or tea

Dinner *(700 calories)*
7 oz fried chicken (include skin)
mushrooms
1 green pepper ring
2 oz sweet chocolate

Snack *(110 calories)*
cream cheese* stuffed in celery sticks
tea or coffee

*Dairy products such as these can be made more appealing with the addition of a light sprinkle of chili powder, cinnamon, seasoning salts, sesame seeds, or dill.

On Wednesday, when your energy and glycogen levels should be pretty low, start eating a high carbohydrate diet such as that given in Menu 4. This plan provides a maximum 1900 calories of which 75 percent is carbohydrate.

Menu 4

Breakfast *(400–500 calories)*
12 oz pineapple juice
1 cup cornflakes
8 oz low-fat milk
1 cup grapes
2 slices whole wheat bread
2 tsp margarine or butter

Lunch *(400–500 calories)*
1½ cups spaghetti
1 cup tomato sauce
1 cup gelatin dessert

Midmorning or Midafternoon *(250–300 calories)*
½ cup sherbet
5 wafers

Dinner *(500–600 calories)*
1 cup green peas
3 oz veal cutlet
angel food cake
8 oz grape juice

However, some athletes may wish to increase the percentage of carbohydrate with the addition of low-milk sugars such as jelly beans or soft drinks. A half cup of jelly beans (approximately 38 small candies) will provide an additional 400 calories and an additional 100 grams of carbohydrate. Twelve ounces of a flavored soft drink will provide 150 calories and 39 grams of carbohydrate.

On the day of the event, the athlete should have a light meal at least two hours prior to the start of the physical exertion. The meal should consist mostly of carbohydrate foods and should be low in protein and fat. Protein and fat will not enhance the upcoming performance. In addition, fat will delay the emptying of the stomach and could result in a sluggish feeling at the starting line. The following meal is an example of a preevent breakfast.

---

8 oz. pineapple juice
1 slice whole wheat bread with 1 tsp jelly
½ cup cornflakes
4 oz low-fat (1%) milk

FASTING

Fasting is the process of abstaining from eating any food for a given period. During times of fasting the body must draw on energy reserves to maintain essential functions. At the initial stages of a fast (for instance, in the first few hours) glycogen and fat stores are used to supply glucose and energy, respectively. Although most cells in the body can use fat as a source of energy, brain cells depend on glucose as a source of energy. As fasting goes on for longer periods of time (1 to 2 days), glycogen stores are exhausted and amino acids from protein are transformed into glucose. The result is loss of body protein tissues, an unwanted effect. When the fast is prolonged even longer (1 to 2 weeks), the fat in the body reserves is transformed to ketones, which can also serve as fuel for some brain cells. However, many areas of the brain rely exclusively on glucose, so proteins in the body are always utilized. The body adapts to long-term fasting through a series of processes that are intended to reduce energy consumption. This adaptation allows us to maintain life for prolonged periods. Nevertheless, a series of changes take place during fasting that are potentially dangerous, including sodium and potassium depletion, cardiac problems, and high uric acid levels.

Some people have advocated prolonged fasting as a way to reduce weight. This practice is very dangerous since the effect that prolonged fasting will have cannot be predicted. Therefore, a fast that is not supervised by a physician should not be undertaken. (See also REDUCING DIETS.)

FAT

Fat is a general name for a class of organic compounds which are insoluble in water. A mixture of these compounds is present in the adipose (fat) tissue. (See OBESITY.)

In the body, fat serves several different functions: an insulator (subcutaneous fat), a reserve of energy in periods of low caloric intake, a support for some organs, a vehicle for fat-soluble vitamins, and a structural component of cell membranes. In food, fat provides more energy than both carbohydrate and protein (one gram of fat provides 9 calories while a gram of protein or carbohydrate provides 4 calories). Fat also provides taste and odor to foods.

FIBER

Dietary fiber itself has no nutrient value and is not even absorbed into the body and yet it has been assuming more and more importance in the past few years as a crucial component of our diet. Is this new importance justified and if it is, why is fiber so important? Fiber is important for three basic reasons: it provides bulk without calories, it is a constituent of foods which have a high nutrient density, and it has certain beneficial actions while it is passing through the gastrointestinal tract. Before discussing the importance of each of these characteristics of dietary fiber, let us define what we mean by this component of our diet. Fiber is a complex carbohydrate similar in its molecular make-up to starch but differing radically from starch in the way in which these molecules are held together. The human intestine contains enzymes which can cleave the starch molecule into its component sugars. Hence this complex structure remains intact as it passes through the gastrointestinal tract. It is not absorbed and hence has no inherent nutritional value. By contrast, the gastrointestinal tract of other mammals does contain enzymes capable of splitting certain types of fiber and so animals such as cows or sheep or goats can digest this material and ab-

sorb the released sugar. Thus what is nondigestible fiber to one animal is a source of usable carbohydrate to another.

Nondigestible fiber in the human diet comes from two main sources: fruits and vegetables in the form of cellulose, and hemicellulose and grains in the form of bran. Thus a high-fiber diet is one rich in raw fruits and vegetables and in whole grain cereals. What are the advantages of such a diet?

HIGH BULK—LOW CARBOHYDRATE

A diet which is high in fiber will provide enough bulk to keep your appetite under control while at the same time keeping your caloric intake relatively low. The use of high-fiber foods to replace the traditional much higher calorie snacks is a good example of this principle at work. At many cocktail parties today raw vegetables are served as an alternative to cold cuts, fried foods, cheese, and other high calorie foods. (The average person will take in several hundred fewer calories in the course of an evening.) Much more important than the use of these foods at specific occasions is their incorporation into the regular diet. If this can be done, the amount of food consumed can remain the same, or even be increased somewhat, and the number of calories can be cut significantly. Many of the most successful weight reduction programs employ this principle by allowing unlimited amounts of high-fiber foods, particularly raw vegetables.

HIGH NUTRIENT DENSITY

While fiber alone supplies no nutrients, the company it keeps in most high-fiber foods will result in a rich supply of vitamins and minerals being available on a high-fiber diet. Thus fruits may be a good source of vitamin C and certain minerals. Vegetables may be rich in some of the B vitamins such as folacin, and in some cases, in minerals like iron. Whole grains are our richest source of many of the B vitamins such as thiamine, niacin, riboflavin, and pyrodoxine. These foods, then, are supplying generous quantities of vitamins and minerals and at the same time providing relatively few calories. This is what we mean by foods of high nutrient density—a food providing the maximum amount of nutrients at the minimum amount of calories. Since fat is the most concentrated source of calories, foods of high nutrient density are usually low in fat. This is particularly true of high-fiber foods. Therefore a diet high in fiber will generally be low in fat. Since most Americans eat too much fat, increasing the fiber content of the diet can be beneficial.

SPECIFIC BENEFITS OF A HIGH-FIBER DIET

The gastrointestinal tract is not simply a conduit through which food passes and is digested and absorbed. It is a highly efficient pump that continuously forces the food in one direction at a rate which will allow for maximum digestion and absorption and at the same time will efficiently move the waste products out of the body. The longer it takes to move the contents of the intestines, the firmer the stools which are eliminated; the firmer the stool, the harder the muscles of the gastrointestinal tract must work and the greater the pressure which must be generated. One of the properties of fiber is that it traps water inside the gastrointestinal tract thereby softening its contents. The result is that the muscular wall of the intestine can work less hard and move the intestinal contents more rapidly and at a lower pressure. In the short term then, a high-fiber diet will result in a softening of the stool, which is very important particularly among older people where constipation is very common. In the long term, however, a high-fiber diet will result in a reduction of the amount of pressure generated within the intestines. There is a condition, again more prevalent in older people, called diverticulosis in which small outpouches of the intestine appear. It is caused by constant high pressure within the intestines which results in a ballooning out of areas where the intestinal wall may be weak. A diverticulum is an outpouching of the intestinal wall and diverticulosis results when many of these have occurred. Food and bacteria can stagnate in these diverticula and cause infection, which is called diverticulitis. There is strong evidence that by consuming a high-fiber diet over a long period of time (for most of one's lifespan) diverticulosis and diverticulitis can be avoided. The preventive properties of the high-fiber diet are due to the fact that such a diet will keep the pressure inside the gastrointestinal tract at low levels. However, in order to achieve this benefit the diet must be consumed regularly as part of your normal eating pattern. The earlier you begin, the better.

✓ Fiber not only traps water, but it also can trap other intestinal contents. There is some evidence which suggests that some of the constituents of bile, which normally is secreted into the intestine, are trapped by fiber and are thereby prevented from being reabsorbed into the body. One such constituent is cholesterol. In certain individuals, a high-fiber diet has been shown to lower serum cholesterol levels. It has been suggested that this cholesterol binding mechanism in the small intestine is the explanation for this effect.

Finally, fiber may also bind other constituents of the diet releasing them more slowly for digestion and absorption. One such substance may be simple sugars. Such a slow release of simple sugars may have important implications in the dietary management of diabetes.

Perhaps the most important role played by fiber in the diet from a health standpoint is an indirect one. Evidence has been accumulated over the past few years which indicates that by increasing the rate at which food moves through the gastrointestinal tract, fiber may reduce the risk for cancer of the colon (large intestine). The theory is as follows. Cancer of the colon is caused by the presence of some substance or substances made within the colon which, after prolonged contact with the wall of the colon, *induces* cancer. Fiber has no effect on the production of these cancer producing substances. However, it will reduce the time the intestinal contents, and hence these substances, can be in contact with the wall of the colon. A high-fat diet seems to be involved in the actual production of these cancer inducing substances. Reducing your fat intake will also lower your risk for colon cancer. A high-fiber diet is usually lower in fat. Thus increasing dietary fiber offers a double benefit.

WHO WILL BENEFIT?

Some benefits of a high-fiber diet occur over a short period of time and others require long-term compliance. For an older person who has consumed very little fiber during his or her lifetime, a gradual change to a high-fiber diet will offer certain benefits. The stools will become softer and constipation with all its accompanying discomforts will often be relieved. While this may have no effect on prolonging life or avoiding major illnesses, it can materially improve the quality of life. A person of middle age will not only derive this benefit, but if a high-fiber diet is maintained, may derive certain long-term benefits. Weight control, often a problem in middle-aged people of both sexes, will be easier to accomplish. At the same time, the lower fat content inherent in such a diet will decrease the risk of coronary artery disease and certain cancers. Finally, the risk of certain problems in the gastrointestinal tract, such as diverticulosis, will also be reduced. For young adults, particularly young women, a high-fiber diet with its high nutrient density, offers a way to control appetite, consume fewer calories, and at the same time take in adequate amounts of needed vitamins and minerals. During the growing years, instituting a high-fiber diet will have all of the benefits mentioned above, and in addition, will help establish certain eating patterns at a time when they may be most useful. There are many studies which suggest that the way we eat in later life is influenced to a great extent by our eating patterns in adolescence and even before. Since the maximum benefits to be derived from a high-fiber diet will only be derived if such a diet is consumed for a very long time, the earlier it can be instituted and the longer it is adhered to, the better. Who will benefit from a higher fiber diet? Most of us. When should we begin? Now.

HOW TO INCREASE THE FIBER CONTENT OF YOUR DIET

For anyone who wishes to increase the fiber content of their diet, the first rule is to do it gradually. A person who is accustomed to consuming a diet in which there is very little fiber (the average American diet) will often feel bloated and may sometimes experience considerable gastrointestinal discomfort if large amounts of fiber are suddenly introduced. Therefore, institute the necessary changes slowly; over a period of weeks or months. The second rule is to incorporate the necessary changes into your existing diet. This will allow you to consume more fiber without radically changing the way you currently eat. For example, if your usual breakfast is juice, cereal,

FIBER CONTENT OF SOME COMMON FOODS

Food	Amount (measure)	Fiber (gm)
Almonds	½ cup	1.8
Apple, unpeeled	1 medium	1.5
Asparagus pieces, cooked	½ cup	0.3
Bananas	1 med	0.9
Beans, green, cooked	½ cup	0.6
Bran, wheat	2 tsp	1.0–2.0
Bread, white or French	2 slices	0.1
Bread, whole wheat	2 slices	0.9
Broccoli, chopped, cooked	½ cup	1.2
Bulgar wheat, cooked	½ cup	0.5
Cabbage, cooked	½ cup	0.6
Cabbage, raw, shredded	½ cup	0.3
Carrots, cooked	½ cup	0.7
Carrots, raw	1 med	0.5
Celery	1 stalk	0.3
Corn, on cob, cooked	1 ear	1.0
Cornflakes	1 cup	0.2
Cucumber	½ med	0.8
Lettuce, iceberg	⅛ head	0.3
Lettuce, romaine	2 leaves	0.4
Macaroni, cooked	½ cup	0.1
Mushrooms	10 small	0.8
Noodles, cooked	½ cup	0.1
Oatmeal, cooked	½ cup	0.1
Orange	1 med	0.9
Orange juice	½ cup	0.1
Peanuts, roasted	½ cup	1.7
Peas, cooked	½ cup	0.5
Popcorn	3 oz	2.0
Potatoes, baked in skin	1 med	0.6
Potatoes, mashed	½ cup	0.4
Rice, brown, cooked	½ cup	0.3
Rice, white, cooked	½ cup	0.1
Soybeans, cooked	½ cup	1.0
Spinach, cooked	½ cup	0.5
Squash, summer, cooked	½ cup	0.6
Squash, winter, cooked	½ cup	1.4
Strawberries, raw	½ cup	1.0
Tomato	1 med	0.8
Walnuts	½ cup	1.1

toast, and coffee, try a half grape-fruit, bran cereal, and whole wheat toast. For lunch if you eat a sand-wich, use whole wheat bread and have perhaps a small salad of raw vege-tables. For dinner: salad with raw vegetables, baked potato including skin, fruit, cheese, and whole wheat crackers. As the amount of high-fiber containing food increases, the quan-tity of other foods will gradually come down by itself. You will soon find yourself filling up with smaller por-tions of meat, fish, dairy products, and their many combinations. You can still enjoy all your gourmet de-lights; the only change will be that the size of your portions will go down and the fiber will allow you to ac-complish this without feeling hun-gry.

The third rule is to provide your increased fiber from as large a vari-ety of foods as possible. This will not only ensure that you get the maxi-mum amount of all the necessary vi-tamins and minerals, but it will also ensure that your meals do not be-come monotonous and it will allow you to experiment with many differ-ent recipes. The table on page 151 is only a partial list of foods which are rich in fiber.

For those of you who have de-cided to try a diet higher in fiber, let us assure you that not only can add-ing fiber to your diet be healthful but it can also be fun. After all, most of the world's population has been eat-ing this kind of a diet for centuries. (See also Gastrointestinal Dis-ease.)

FLUORIDE

The human body contains a very small amount of fluoride. However, it has been shown that where the diet is high in fluoride the crystalline deposits in the teeth and bones are larger and more perfectly formed. When teeth and bones are first calcified, calcium and phosphorus are laid down as hydroxyapatite. As development continues, fluoride replaces the hydroxy parts of the crystal, which makes it harder and the teeth more resistant to decay.

Most Americans get the major portion of their fluoride from drinking water, although fish and tea contain quite a lot. When fluoride is present in the drinking water at a level of one part per million, the incidence of dental caries is significantly reduced. (See also DENTAL DECAY.)

FOLACIN (FOLIC ACID)

Folacin is one of the B-complex vitamins. The recommended dietary allowance (RDA) for adults is 400 micrograms per day. The RDA during pregnancy is 800 micrograms a day, which reflects the role of the vitamin in cell multiplication. Good sources of folacin include liver; green, leafy vegetables; beets; cabbage; oranges; canteloupe; corn; green peas; pumpkin; sweet potato; whole wheat bread; wheat germ; and milk. However, folacin is readily destroyed in cooking.

A deficiency of folacin will affect all cells that are rapidly dividing as folacin is required to make new DNA. The more rapidly dividing the cells, the greater will be the effect. The cells lining the gastrointestinal tract are replaced every three days and in times of folacin deficiency the surface of the tongue becomes sore and cracked and the wall of the intestine becomes thinner than normal and less able to digest and absorb food, leading to diarrhea. Millions of new blood cells are made every minute and if there is folacin deficiency both red and white cells fail to form normally. The reduction in numbers of red cells leads to anemia. This is known as megaloblastic anemia (See ANEMIAS.) In addition, as white blood cells are principally responsible for the body's defense against disease a reduction in their numbers makes the body more susceptible to disease. Folacin deficiency also affects the brain causing fatigue, depression, abnormal reflexes, disorientation, confusion, and a reduced ability to carry out mental tasks. Folacin deficiency is probably the most widespread vitamin deficiency in the world. Many Americans get less than the RDA for folacin in their diet but do not show any signs of folacin deficiency. It has been estimated that as many as 30 percent of all premenopausal women fall short of the 400 microgram daily requirement. Oral contraceptives impair folate absorption and may be partly responsible for this. Alcohol also increases a person's need for the vitamin as do a number of other drugs. Anything that requires cell multiplication, such as pregnancy, cancer, skin destruction as occurs in burns and measles, and blood loss, raises folacin needs. (See also ANEMIAS; PREGNANCY.)

FOLIC ACID CONTENT OF FOODS
IN MICROGRAMS (mcg) PER SERVING

5–20 mcg/serving

carrot	1 med.
ear of corn	1 med.
mushrooms	3 large
potato	1 med.
apple	1 med.
hard cheese	1 oz
grapefruit	½ med.
milk	8 oz
bread	1 slice
sesame seeds	1 tbsp
lean beef, veal or pork	6 oz

20–50 mcg/serving

green beans	1 cup
cucumber	1 small
squash	⅔ cup
strawberries	1 cup
egg	1 large
kidney	3 oz
shellfish	6 oz
yogurt	8 oz

100–150 mcg/serving

liver (all)	3 oz
broccoli	2 stalks
orange juice	6 oz

200–300 mcg/serving

brewer's yeast	1 tbsp
spinach	4 oz

FOOD BALANCING

The concept of a balanced diet is one of the pillars of good nutrition. No food is perfect. However, by combining foods of different varieties all of the required nutrients can be consumed without taking in too much of those nutrients whose excess is undesirable. Thus a balanced diet is a pattern of food choices which will promote good health. In the past we grouped foods based on their nutrient content and then constructed a diet composed of a certain number of foods from each category. Perhaps one food from the meat, two from the cereal, one from the milk, and three from the vegetable groups. Most nutritionists have given up the use of the four or seven food groups because people usually do not eat that way and because very good diets (e.g., vegetarian diets) may exclude one or more of these food groups completely. (See VEGETARIAN DIETS.) Instead nutritionists encourage variety and high nutrient density.

Variety, of course, means trying lots of different types and classes of food. High nutrient density means choosing foods which are rich in nutrients but low in calories. Thus, very high calorie foods (particularly those high in fat, which is the most concentrated form of calories) are used only occasionally especially if they are low in other nutrients. A good example would be the use of whole milk or low-fat milk. A glass of each has the same amount of calcium and vitamin B_2 but the low-fat milk has many fewer calories allowing you to consume other nutritious foods without overloading your system with calories. For most of us then who want to eat a balanced diet eating a variety of foods and concentrating on those of high nutrient density will accomplish our goal. (See also DIETARY RECOMMENDATIONS.)

FOOD PROCESSING

In the past sixty years the kinds of foods we eat have changed dramatically. In 1900, 60 percent of the US population was involved in food production, whereas today only 5 percent of our population has direct participation in the growing and production of the foods consumed. Food is now grown and processed in just a few places and then transported to the rest of the country. The time involved in transporting these food items makes it necessary to preserve them. Preservation of foods also has allowed us to be more independent of geographical or climatic changes, making available all year fresh fruits and vegetables that would otherwise be difficult to obtain.

Unfortunately, the major trade-off in the processing and preservation of foods is the loss of some specific nutrients. It is important to know which nutrients are most affected by processing, in both the foods we buy and the ones we prepare at home. The major preservation methods currently employed in the food industry can be divided into five major groups.

I. Heat Processing is done for the purpose of increasing storage life (by destroying microorganisms or inactivating enzymes) or to increase palatability (for example, baking or broiling).

Blanching is one type of heat processing that is commonly used prior to the canning and freezing of fruits and vegetables. This procedure inactivates enzymes that may destroy nutrients or produce changes in color or taste, and also softens the food to facilitate canning. The process is usually performed by heating water to temperatures close to boiling or steaming. Losses of nutrients like minerals, vitamins, and proteins may occur in blanching. These losses vary with the conditions used in the process. As much as 50 percent of the vitamin C content can be lost, mainly in the blanching water. But this figure varies a great deal according to the kind of food; for example, vegetables with a large surface area to volume ratio (such as peas and sliced carrots) tend to lose more vitamin C than those with a small surface area to volume ratio (such as potatoes and sprouts).

Loss of folacin during this process of blanching is also considerable and can reach up to 45 percent depending on the method used (usually with steam-blanching the loss is half of that with water at 212 degrees Fahrenheit). Other vitamins can also be affected by blanching (and by any process involving heating) since, except for vitamin B_{12} and niacin, all vitamins are unstable when exposed to high heat. However, the percent of loss can vary a great deal depending on the vitamin content and temperature.

Pasteurization of milk or other foods involves mild heat treatment. This will kill all disease-causing organisms but will not destroy all bacteria and spores. Sterilization is required to kill all of the living organisms but requires higher temperatures for longer periods of time and often ruins the food product in the process. Pasteurization will extend the storage life of foods but usually for only a short period. Hence, although pasteurization protects us from disease-causing organisms, the remaining bacteria can cause the milk to sour within a day or two at room temperature.

II. Refrigeration and Freezing The cooling-down of foods in the main chamber of the refrigerator is used to either delay ripening or to store foods for relatively short periods of time in their raw state. At these low temperatures microorganisms grow much slower than normal and spoilage is inhibited. This effect is accentuated during freezing.

From the nutritional point of view, freezing is probably the best method to preserve foods. The major loss of nutrients in frozen foods does not occur during freezing but during the blanching prior to freezing. The loss during freezing itself is minimal. Furthermore, when foods are frozen immediately after harvesting the nutritive value may be higher than when bought at the market (where they may have been for several days). Prolonged storage in the freezer and thawing before use can also produce vitamin losses in both vegetable and animal products.

III. Drying Removal of water markedly inhibits the deterioration of foods as bacteria cannot grow in the absence of water. Drying can be done in several ways, using moderate temperatures. This results in some minor loss of proteins by heat destruction. As in other methods involving heat, vitamin C is destroyed in substantial amounts (up to 30 percent), depending on the moisture content. Vitamin A is partially lost during this process. Another consideration in drying is the interaction between nutrients, like the Maillard Reaction, which causes the combination of sugar with protein in such a way as to make these nutrients indigestible.

IV. Fermentation is a process by which many foods can be preserved without significant nutrient losses. It creates conditions in the food that are not compatible with the growth of microorganisms. Fermentation is widely used in the production of alcoholic beverages and dairy products.

V. Chemical Preservation The addition of chemicals to foods in order to preserve them is a subject discussed under food additives. (See ADDITIVES.) More than being concerned with the losses of nutrients caused by these chemicals, we have to focus our attention instead on their relative degree of safety.

Processed foods have long been labeled as being of inferior nutritive quality. While in some instances this is true, in other cases the nutrient losses are the same or even less than the ones in home-processed foods. From a realistic point of view, food processing is a necessity in a society where the majority of the population resides in an urban environment to which it would be extremely difficult, if not impossible, to make available all completely fresh produce and animal products.

Recently, the baby food industry has taken a step which was designed to protect our infant population from the possible long-term effects of early exposure to sugar and salt. They have removed the added sugar and salt from all of their products. This decision was reached partly because of mounting scientific evidence that early long-term exposure to either of these substances may contribute to the problems of obesity and hypertension, respectively, and partly because of consumer demand for products with no added salt or sugar.

Many of our processed foods today contain added sugar. This is particularly true of desserts, but it can occur in a variety of different products and thereby increase the caloric content of many of the foods we eat. While no doubt the flavor of the food is enhanced, the public must be aware that this enhancement is at the risk of higher calories. Adults can make a choice—if they are calorie-conscious they can compare brands—infants cannot. Since 80 percent of infants consume commercial baby foods, the decision to add no sugar has resulted in fewer calories for the majority of young infants. While we have no assurance that this will result in a reduction in the incidence of childhood obesity, it is a step in the right direction.

The decision not to add salt may be even more important than not adding sugar. Infants show no preference for salty foods. The salt that was previously added was for the benefit of the mother. Baby foods were catering to maternal taste, and infants were exposed to high concentrations of salt in early life. While there is no direct evidence linking early exposure to sodium with subsequent hypertension (high blood pressure), animal experiments suggest that such a link is possible, especially in genetically susceptible populations. Thus there was no reason to add salt and a potentially good reason not to. The baby food industry responded properly.

As a result of this action baby food manufacturers have demonstrated how the food industry can respond positively to issues concerning nutrition and health. We hope that as further issues relating elements in our food supply to long-term health problems become clarified, infant food manufacturers as well as other food companies will continue to respond as well.

PROCESSING METHODS, NUTRIENTS AFFECTED,* AND SHELF LIFE

Method	Nutrients Reduced	Nutrients Unaffected	Typical Foods	Shelf Life†
Canning	vitamin C; thiamine	vitamins A, D; minerals	fruits, vegetables, milk, meats, beverages	2–5 yrs
Freezing	vitamin E, proteins (from denaturation)		vegetables, meat, fruits	6–12 mos
Dehydrating	vitamins A, C, E, protein, fiber‡	iron	milk, vegetables, fruits, grains & cereals, meats	
Milling	thiamine, riboflavin, niacin, choline, iron, fiber	carbohydrates, protein	wheat (similar processes for corn and rice)	6–12 mos
Baking	thiamine, proteins	fat, minerals	grains & cereals, meats, snack foods	2–12 wks
Fermenting		all	vegetable products, milk products	6 wks–6 mos

*Trace minerals such as zinc, magnesium, and copper are reduced with most methods of food processing.
†Nutritional quality decreases with time. Based on ideal home-type storage.
‡Fiber is not a nutrient but has been found to be important for health maintenance.

SOURCES OF NATURALLY OCCURRING NUTRIENTS

Nutrient	Sources	Availability	Best Form
Vitamin A	carrots	fresh: all year	
	leafy greens	fresh: summer & fall	cooked in small amounts of water
		frozen: all year	
B vitamins thiamine, riboflavin, niacin, biotin, folacin, pantothenic acid, B_{12}	grain products	all forms: all year	whole grain (e.g. brown rice, whole wheat bread, stone ground cornmeal products)
	yeast	dried: all year	brewer's yeast
	legumes	all forms: all year	cooked (any method) or sprouted (mung and soybeans)
	nuts	unshelled: winter & all year	unsalted, raw (most varieties) or dry roasted
		shelled (packaged): all year	
	leafy greens	fresh: summer & fall	cooked in small amounts of water
		frozen: all year	
B_{12} only	milk products, meat, eggs	all forms: all year	all forms
Vitamin C	citrus fruit & juices	all forms & varieties: all year	fresh
	potatoes	all forms: all year	baked or boiled in the skin*
	green peppers, broccoli, leafy greens, cabbage	fresh: all year	steamed* or fresh
	tomatoes†	fresh: all year	fresh
	melons, strawberries†,	fresh: summer	fresh
	sprouts	fresh and canned: all year	fresh

Nutrient	Sources	Availability	Best Form
Vitamin D	fortified milk, egg yolks, salmon, tuna	all forms: all year	any form
Vitamin E	germ of grains	whole grain products: all year	untoasted wheat germ
	leafy greens	fresh: summer & fall frozen: all year	cooked in small amounts of water
	legumes	all forms: all year	cooked (any method) or sprouted (mung and soybeans)
	nuts	unshelled: all year	unsalted, raw (most varieties) or dry roasted
		shelled (packaged): all year	
Vitamin K	leafy greens	fresh: summer & fall frozen: all year	cooked in small amounts of water
	liver	all forms: all year	any form
Calcium	leafy greens	all forms: all year	any form
	legumes	all forms: all year	cooked (any method) or sprouted (mung and soybeans)
	nuts	unshelled: all year	unsalted, raw (most varieties) or dry roasted
		shelled (packaged): all year	
	milk products	all forms: all year	all forms
	clams, oysters	frozen or canned: all year	any form
		fresh: proximity to coast	any form

Nutrient	Sources	Availability	Best Form
Iron (Best absorbed when taken with a food high in vitamin C)	leafy greens	fresh: summer & fall frozen: all year	cooked in small amounts of water
	liver	all forms: all year	any form
	legumes	all forms: all year	cooked (any method) or sprouted (mung and soybeans)
	meat	all forms: all year	all forms
	grain products	all forms: all year	whole grain (e.g., brown rice, whole wheat bread, stone ground cornmeal products)
	oysters	frozen or canned: all year	any form
		fresh: proximity to coast	any form
	dried fruit	all year	any form
Magnesium	leafy greens	all forms: all year	any form
	legumes	all forms: all year	cooked (any method) or sprouted (mung and soybeans)
	nuts	unshelled; all year shelled (packaged): all year	unsalted, raw (most varieties) or dry roasted
	grain products	all forms: all year	whole grain, (e.g., brown rice, whole wheat bread, stone ground cornmeal products)
	water	all year	all sources

Nutrient	Sources	Availability	Best Form
Potassium	leafy greens	all forms: all year	any form
	citrus fruit	all forms & varieties: all year	fresh or frozen (not canned)
	bananas	all year	any variety
	milk, meat	all forms: all year	all forms
Zinc	seafood, oysters	frozen or canned: all year	any form
		fresh: proximity to coast	any form
	liver	all forms: all year	any form
	wheat germ yeast	fresh or dried: all year	any form

*These foods should be placed directly into the hot cooking environment.
†These foods are more costly when out of season.

GASTROINTESTINAL DISEASE

Most people will suffer from some sort of gastrointestinal upset during their lifetimes. The most common complaints are minor—indigestion, nausea, or an occasional bout of diarrhea. Other problems are more serious, such as peptic ulcers and diverticulosis. A great deal of research has gone into how the diet can prevent or reduce the symptoms of gastrointestinal disorders. Obviously, anything that alters gastrointestinal function alters the intake, digestion, and absorption of foods and the nutrients they contain.

Digestive disturbances very often result from emotional upsets. We often attribute indigestion or diarrhea to anger or anxiety. In children, excitement (even over receiving a treasured gift) can cause vomiting. In the same way, neuroses and psychoses can give rise to gastrointestinal symptoms in both children and adults.

Symptoms exhibited in the gastrointestinal tract may be due to problems in other parts of the body. Many diseases are accompanied by symptoms of digestive disorders. Some good examples of this are severe congestive heart failure, renal disease, brain tumors, pneumonia, and tuberculosis.

The following sections review the current dietary therapy advised for the most common disorders of the gastrointestinal tract.

PROBLEMS OF THE UPPER GASTROINTESTINAL TRACT

Heartburn. This is a burning pain which occurs when the contents of the stomach are pushed up into the esophagus (the tube leading from the mouth to the stomach). The pain usually occurs behind the sternum and often spreads to the neck and back of the throat in waves. The pain may be so intense that it can awaken a sleeping person. Heartburn is most likely to happen when the pressure in the stomach exceeds that in the esophagus, which occurs for the most part when a person lies down or bends over. If this happens frequently, the acid in the gastric contents will irritate and inflame the lining of the esophagus.

The treatment of heartburn involves avoiding foods that weaken the tension in the band of muscle around the base of the esophagus (called the cardiac sphincter), which prevents the movement of foods upward. This means limiting fat in the diet, which decreases the tension in the cardiac sphincter, and concentrating on foods rich in protein which tends to increase sphincter pressure. Caffeine-containing beverages and foods (see CAFFEINE), alcohol, peppermint and spearmint, and cigarette smoking also decrease cardiac sphincter pressure. These also tend to increase the secretion of gastric acid which will increase the irritation of the esophagus, as will decaffeinated coffee and red peppers.

Foods which are likely to irritate an already inflamed esophagus are also best avoided. These include acidic fruit juices such as orange, grapefruit, and tomato. It is advisable to eat smaller, more frequent meals, as this reduces the degree of distention of the stomach. Whenever the stomach becomes overdistended, the pressure in the stomach exceeds the pressure in the esophagus and increases the chance of reflux. Drinking liquids during the hour before and/or after meals will have the same distending effect.

People with heartburn should also avoid lying down or bending over for three hours after eating, as these actions can increase the pressure in the stomach. Tight-fitting clothing can also have the same effect. It is best to elevate the head of a person's bed so that the chest is higher than the stomach to prevent reflux during sleep. Although the mechanism is not well understood, heartburn occurs quite frequently in obese people and improves when they lose weight.

As well as changes in diet, heartburn sufferers are advised to use antacids frequently to neutralize the acidity of their gastric juices. Drugs which reduce acid secretion may also be prescribed by a physician.

Indigestion. In common usage, indigestion means any discomfort in the gastrointestinal tract. It may be a symptom of a whole host of disorders, either in the digestive tract or in other parts of the body. As well as being caused by various medical conditions, indigestion can be triggered by emotional tension, by eating too much or too rapidly, or by chewing poorly.

When indigestion occurs occasionally, it is not necessary to modify the diet. However, when it happens frequently, due to emotional factors or poor eating habits, simple changes in the dietary routine can be extremely helpful. Eating slowly, at regular times, in a relaxed atmosphere is a good idea. Avoiding fatty, highly spiced and seasoned foods, alcohol, and caffeine-containing foods and beverages can also be helpful.

However, when indigestion is persistent, it may be an indication of more serious problems—such as gastritis or peptic ulcers.

Gastritis. This is an inflammation of the lining of the stomach. The complaint of indigestion from a person suffering fom gastritis may take the form of a lack of appetite, nausea, vomiting, belching, a feeling of fullness, or stomach ache.

When gastritis appears suddenly (acute gastritis) it is often caused by taking aspirin or other drugs which irritate the stomach wall. Overindulgence in alcohol, a food allergy, food poisoning, stress, or infections can also cause gastritis. In these cases, the solution is simply to eliminate the offending substance from the diet, or to find tension-relieving activities, as well as avoiding the foods and beverages previously mentioned which can cause excess acid secretion. If the person cannot eat due to nausea or vomiting, food can be withheld for a day or two, after which time the diet is built up from liquids to a bland diet (see the table below). A bland diet eliminates all foods which could conceivably irritate the lining of the stomach, stimulate the secretion of gastric acid (coffee, tea, alcohol), or distend the stomach (carbonated beverages). It is low in fiber, contains little or no salt, pepper, or spices, and no highly acidic foods.

The symptoms associated with acute gastritis may persist for long periods of time. This condition is called chronic gastritis and can lead to a loss of the cells lining the stomach with a consequent reduction in the secretion of gastric digestive juices. No one is sure of the cause of chronic gastritis, although several things have been suggested—overeating, eating too quickly, eating when emotionally upset, eating certain foods, drinking alcohol or coffee, smoking, infections, and nutrient deficiencies. As the cause of the disorder is unclear, so is any treatment except for a bland diet, which seems

---

Foods to be Avoided on a Bland Diet

Fried or fatty foods.

Smoked and preserved meats and fish, or pork.

All raw vegetables and all cooked vegetables, *except for* potatoes, peas, squash, asparagus tips, carrots, tender string beans, beets, and spinach.

All fruits and juices, *except for* orange juice, ripe bananas, avocados, baked apples (without skin), applesauce, canned peaches, pears, apricots, white cherries, and stewed prunes.

All pastries, preserves, and candies.

All alcoholic beverages and carbonated drinks.

Pepper, spices, vinegar, ketchup, horseradish, relishes, gravies, mustard, and pickles.

to help many people. In some patients with chronic gastritis, there develops a vitamin B_{12} deficiency, as the loss of cells lining the stomach and the intrinsic factor they produce impair B_{12} absorption. (Intrinsic factor is a carbohydrate required for normal absorption of this vitamin.) Hence, people with chronic gastritis should be sure to include foods rich in vitamin B_{12}—such as seafood, meat, eggs, dairy products, and enriched vegetable products—in their diets.

Peptic Ulcers. The term peptic ulcer includes ulcers found in the stomach (gastric ulcer) or the duodenum (duodenal ulcer). An ulcer itself is the wearing away of the lining of the stomach or duodenum. Eventually, it proceeds through the small blood vessels within the walls of the gastrointestinal tract causing bleeding, which can be fatal. If a hole is made in the wall, a major infection known as peritonitis quickly develops, which can also be fatal.

Under normal circumstances, the inside wall of the gastrointestinal tract is protected by a covering of mucous. If this covering becomes thin, or is destroyed, an ulcer develops, causing a burning pain. Stress, which causes excess acid secretion, along with cigarette smoking, poor nutrition, insufficient sleep, excess caffeine, and the use of drugs (like aspirin) that irritate the stomach wall all can exacerbate or cause ulcers.

All of these things should be avoided by the patient with ulcers in an attempt to limit gastric acid secretion and give the ulcer a chance to heal. Antacids can be very beneficial by neutralizing gastric acid and should be taken one hour after meals. However, drug therapy is the main effector in the current treatment of ulcers. Drugs like cimetidine (Tagamet) and ranitidine hydrochloride (Zantac) are taken, which inhibit acid secretion. Bland diets are unnecessary when a person is symptom-free but may be beneficial during a flare-up. Peptic ulcer can be an indication of the presence of a serious disorder, and so anyone with this ailment should consult their physician.

COMMON DISORDERS OF THE DIGESTIVE TRACT

There are several other gastrointestinal problems which affect the digestive tract that we all can suffer from once in a while—including gas, diarrhea, and constipation.

Gas. Many people complain of belching, others of abdominal distension and cramping after they eat certain foods. Although the public commonly believes that belching is caused by gas formed from foods in the stomach, it is really the result of expelling air that has been swallowed or sucked in, often unconsciously as a result of tension. Rarely, it is a symptom of a more serious disorder. People with gallbladder pain, colonic distress, or an impending obstruction of a coronary artery often belch frequently.

Intestinal gas has a number of causes. Some gas is derived from swallowed air and other gases are produced by bacteria in the gut. We may lack the necessary enzymes to digest specific forms of carbohydrate found in certain foods, such as lactose in milk, which are broken down by bacteria in the intestine producing gas. Foods suspected of causing gas can be omitted one at a time for a trial period until the offending substance is identified. The following table lists the possible causes of gas problems and the way they can be treated.

Diarrhea. When the intestinal contents move too quickly through the intestines for fluid to be absorbed from the stool or excess water is added to the stool from the cells lining the intestinal tract, diarrhea results and bowel movements are more liquid and frequent than normal.

A number of factors can cause diarrhea, including stress, nervous

POSSIBLE CAUSES AND SOLUTIONS TO MILD GAS PROBLEMS

Possible Cause	Solution
carbonated beverages	herb teas, fruit juices, water
chewing gum	omit on a trial basis
gulping or swallowing air	relax, take small sips and bites
beans and peas	smaller portions; try different variety
cabbage family (sulfur-containing vegetables)	cabbage, broccoli, brussels sprouts, cauliflower. Cook *without* placing a lid on the pot
excess bulk	reduce added bran (if used) or amounts of salad-type vegetables and/or fruits
intolerance to milk sugar	smaller portions of milk, yogurt, and cheese; omit when discomfort is persistent
specific sensitivity	omit *on a trial basis* any one (at a time) of the following: carrots, raisins, bananas, apricots, prune juice, pretzels, bagels, wheat germ, pastries, potatoes, eggplant, apples, citrus fruits and bread.

tension, overeating, and certain drugs, foods, and spices that irritate the gastrointestinal tract. Spoiled food and bacterial infections in the gastrointestinal tract can also be the cause of diarrhea. Usually, an acute bout of diarrhea lasts less than twenty-four hours. If this is the case, eliminating the irritant food or other cause and drinking clear liquids is all that is necessary or beneficial.

Chronic diarrhea for periods lasting longer than forty-eight hours is much more serious and may result from some serious medical condition. Under such circumstances, help from a physician should be sought.

Constipation. Everybody has different toilet habits. Some people have a bowel movement twice a day and others only once every two or three days. Provided that when you do have a bowel movement there is no pain or discomfort then you are not constipated and there is absolutely no need to take laxatives or any other measures to give yourself more frequent bowel movements. However, if a bowel movement is hard and is passed with difficulty, discomfort, or pain, then you are constipated.

An increase in the bulk in the diet is usually the safest remedy for constipation. This means increasing the servings of foods rich in fiber. (See Fiber.) Fiber absorbs a lot of water and softens the stool. It also adds a lot of bulk to the stool as it

is not digested, which increases the speed at which it passes through the gastrointestinal tract. The average American takes only 4 to 5 grams of fiber per day, instead of the ideal level of 12 to 15 grams. Cereal fiber is the most effective form for increasing stool bulk. Bran contains 2 to 4 grams of fiber per rounded teaspoon and is an effective way of increasing dietary bulk. But, to be effective it should be taken with at least 6 ounces of fluid per teaspoon of bran.

Prunes contain a natural laxative. Prunes or prune juice taken at night will ensure defecation in the morning for most people. Constipation may also sometimes be relieved by adding fat to the diet.

Another cause of constipation is the lack of physical activity. The muscles that are responsible for propelling food down the gastrointestinal tract are improved by any activity that increases the muscle tone of the entire body. You don't have to embark on an extensive exercise program to improve the condition, as even making a habit of walking up stairs instead of always taking the elevator can be of help in this respect.

Diverticulosis. People who follow a low-fiber diet for many years can develop diverticulosis. This is a condition in which pouches form along the intestine in weak areas of the intestinal muscles. The pouches are caused by high pressure inside the intestine: excessive contractions which force the lining of the intestine through the muscle layer—rather like the ballooning out of a segment of an inner tube. People with diverticulosis often have no symptoms and so are unaware of the fact. However, sometimes fecal material becomes trapped in the pouches, or diverticula, causing inflammation and infection. When this happens, the person is said to have diverticulitis. People with this condition may have cramps, alternating periods of diarrhea and constipation, flatulence, abdominal distension, and dyspepsia. Sometimes the diverticula burst, which can be life threatening.

Patients with diverticulosis should gradually increase the fiber in their diet. At first, this treatment can cause bloating, flatulence, and sometimes heartburn. However, these symptoms soon subside. The high-fiber diet increases the fecal mass, which physically prevents the opposite walls of the intestine from contacting each other and causing excessive intraintestinal pressure, which causes the diverticulosis. (See FIBER.)

Constipation can also be caused by other serious medical conditions such as tumors and irritable bowel syndrome and should always be reported to a physician to rule out anything serious.

IN CONCLUSION

Disorders of the gastrointestinal tract can have a significant effect on nutritional status because they alter food intake, absorption, and nutrient needs. It is difficult for people with disorders that affect their ability to chew and swallow to eat. Similarly, food intake can be altered when a person suffers from nausea, vomiting, or any other abdominal disorder.

Many disorders impair absorption of nutrients, such as a reduced availability of digestive enzymes or a decreased surface area for absorption. When diarrhea is present, both vitamins and minerals are likely to be lost, increasing the likelihood of deficiencies.

With the advent of new drug therapies, dietary regimens for gastrointestinal disorders have become less restricted, especially for ulcers. However, a poor diet can be the underlying cause of many gastrointestinal problems and can exacerbate others. It is difficult to draw up general rules for different disorders as there is a wide spectrum of different reactions to a given food and so each case must be treated individually. (See also HYDROCHLORIC ACID.)

GLUTAMIC ACID

Glutamic acid is an amino acid (building block of protein) that is made in the body from other food-stuffs in sufficient quantities to satisfy its needs. It is used by the body to help make new tissues and replace those that are worn out and is one of the key neurotransmitters (chemical messengers in the brain). In addition, glutamic acid plays a key role in the metabolism of many of the other amino acids. (See AMINO ACIDS.)

GLUTATHIONE PEROXIDASE

Glutathione peroxidase protects the body's cell membranes against damage by free radicals, which are believed to be a causal factor in the development of cancer. Glutathione peroxidase activity in human blood increases with increasing selenium intake, but it reaches a plateau at intakes far below those customarily found in the American diet (200 to 300 micrograms). Thus taking selenium supplements for this purpose is ineffective.

GLYCINE

Glycine is an amino acid which is not essential for the human because it can be manufactured by the body from other compounds. Glycine is found in abundance in most animal and plant proteins. Some people have attributed certain curative or disease preventing properties to glycine. There is no evidence for these properties. Taking glycine in pill form has no rationale, is expensive, and might even be dangerous in large amounts over a long period of time. (See also AMINO ACIDS.)

HAIR ANALYSIS

Hair analysis is a test done on hair to assess the mineral and sometimes the vitamin status of a person. Those using the test claim that there is a good correlation between the level of a given nutrient in the hair and the level in the body. A clump of hair is either pulled from the scalp or cut very close to the scalp, washed, and analyzed for minerals and/or vitamins. *All responsible health professionals would agree that the test is totally invalid for vitamin status assessments.* Most would also agree that its validity for minerals is extremely limited, with the exception of lead and cadmium. If the analyzed hair is cropped from very close to the scalp and includes the root, there is a significant correlation between hair and body levels of each of these minerals.

HERBAL MEDICINES

Many consumers today are put off by the prevalence of pill-popping in our society. As a reaction, many have sought to achieve pharmacological results with concoctions derived from herbs, seeds, roots, etc. In fact, many of the generic compounds in common medications were isolated from plant products; for instance, salicylate in aspirin was derived from willow bark, and we wouldn't have penicillin without bread mold.

The problem with using herbal medications and home remedies is twofold. First, the preparation may be ineffective and a disease may progress untreated. For example, self-administration of watermelon seeds (containing the diuretic cucurbocitrin) by a person with high blood

SOME HERBAL PREPARATIONS—USES AND SAFETY

Preparation Category	Unsafe	Safety Unknown	No Toxicity Reported
Diuretics	horsetail watermelon seeds	corn silk	teas (buchu, quack grass, dandelion, juniper, shave grass)
Cathartics	buckthorn bark senna leaves dock roots aloe licorice root		
Stimulants	(in high amounts) caffeine ginseng		
Weight control	capsicum	chickweed echinacea bladder wrack	hawthorne berries kelp
Miscellaneous	peppermint oil apricot kernel nutmeg Indian tobacco foxglove sassafras root	fennel	bee pollen

pressure is unwise. Not only is a correct dosage undetermined, but excess fluid loss may be accompanied by other problems.

Second, there is the general problem that herbal preparations take on the notion of a panacea and are therefore used inappropriately. Furthermore, herbs are just as prone to abuse and mistaken ingestion as are commercial therapeutic agents.

Though their effectiveness can be contested, many herbs are used for a wide variety of functions. The table on page 173 summarizes the safety of some common herbal preparations.

Everyone appreciates the time-honored preparations of our ancestors. Fortunately, we can now appreciate the advances made in pharmacology. If you feel that medications are not in your best interest, consult your physician before you seek questionable alternatives.

HISTIDINE

Histidine is an amino acid (a building block of protein). It is an essential nutrient for growing infants and children and must be supplied in their diet for normal growth and development. Infants between four and six months of age require 33 miligrams per kilogram of body weight. Humans have the ability to make histidine slowly from other nutrients, and adults can make a sufficient amount to satisfy their needs for short periods of time.

This amino acid is especially important in the growth of muscle proteins. It is also required in the manufacture of histamine—an important neurotransmitter (chemical messenger) in the brain and nervous system. Although histidine supplements may raise histamine levels in the body it is doubtful if this is in any way beneficial. (See AMINO ACIDS.)

HYDROCHLORIC ACID

Hydrochloric acid is a very strong inorganic acid composed of one atom of hydrogen and one of chloride (HC1). It is important in nutrition because certain cells in the stomach manufacture this acid. The hydrochloric acid in the stomach aids in the breakdown of food and there is some evidence that older people cannot produce hydrochloric acid so well as they could at a younger age.

Too much hydrochloric acid production can cause "heartburn" and gas pains and a large number of antacid compounds are on the market which essentially neutralize hydrochloric acid in the stomach. The occasional use of these compounds is justified to relieve the discomfort of excess acid secretion. Chronic use is not recommended. The antacids themselves can cause problems (for example, some are very high in sodium) and the heartburn may be a sign of more serious problems (such as an ulcer).

There used to be a practice of giving some people (particularly the elderly) hydrochloric acid drops in dilute form with meals. This has been widely discontinued because the risks far outweigh the possible benefits. (See also GASTROINTESTINAL DISEASE.)

HYPERTENSION (HIGH BLOOD PRESSURE)

Blood pressure is simply the pressure exerted by the blood on the walls of the blood vessels as it flows through. It is measured by a simple, painless procedure and the results tell us a great deal about the health and circulatory system.

As you probably know, blood pressures are reported by two numbers such as 120/80. This is because while the heart is beating the pressure it exerts is uneven: the 120 refers to the maximum and the 80 refers to the minimum pressure exerted by the heart as it pumps blood. It is generally agreed that blood pressures greater than 140/90 fall into the hypertension category. It must be remembered, however, that factors such as stress and excitement, anxiety, and physical activity can temporarily elevate blood pressure, thus a single blood pressure measurement in excess of 140/90 is not sufficient to diagnose hypertension. To confirm this condition, several such measurements must be made. Once high blood pressure is confirmed, it should be dealt with immediately, since its presence greatly increases the probability of a heart attack or a stroke.

How serious is the problem? Currently, an American male has a 20 percent probability of having a heart attack before he is sixty years old. In a large number of cases, the first attack is fatal. Of those who recover, the chances of dying within the next five years are five times higher than they are for those without any heart disease. In addition, it has been estimated that approximately two million Americans are stroke victims. Stroke patients occupy more hospital and nursing beds and make more use of social welfare services than the total number of cancer and accident victims combined.

It is a mistake to assume that strokes and heart attacks are problems only of the old. If we consider the death rates among the population aged twenty-five to sixty-four (the years we think of as productive working years), it must be appreciated that 25 percent of all stroke and heart attack deaths occurred in this age group. Even among those aged twenty-five to twenty-nine, coronary heart disease ranks among the ten leading causes of death. By age forty to forty-four, it becomes the number one cause of death and it remains so for older groups.

A number of factors have been identified as being responsible for the high incidence of stroke and heart attacks. These include: high levels of cholesterol in the blood, cigarette smoking, too little exercise and physical activity, stress, heredity, hypertension, and diabetes. Although hypertension is the last factor on this list, it may well be the most important. In fact, hypertension is considered the most significant risk factor for developing atherosclerosis (hardening of the arteries), stroke, congestive heart failure, kidney failure, coronary heart attack, and angina pectoris (crippling chest pain due to poor circulation to the heart muscle). Hypertension has been shown to increase the deadliness of a heart attack when it does occur. About 50 percent of all hypertension victims have been shown to have enlarged hearts, and it has been identified as a significant causative factor in kidney disease and eventual kidney failure. Hypertension has also been identified as an important cause of loss of vision and may play a significant role in the memory loss and senility phenomena associated with aging.

The important thing to remember is that today we can treat virtually every single case of hypertension. The task is to identify people suffering from hypertension and to ensure that those who have it receive adequate care. If the condition is neglected, irreversible damage can take place. Too often people fail to get regular checkups, and their condition is left undetected until it is too late. Another problem is that ele-

vated blood pressure does not usually produce unpleasant symptoms, so people feel that the condition can be ignored. Don't be fooled into thinking that you are in good health just because you don't notice any specific ailment.

There are several different kinds of hypertension. Malignant hypertension is a relatively rare disease. In the past, death could be expected to follow within one year after the diagnosis of this condition was made. It occurs more often in the young than in the old and is marked by extreme elevations of blood pressure. Vision is often affected and the condition is usually accompanied by breathlessness, dizziness, and kidney malfunction. Today, malignant hypertension is treatable and people with this disease can usually look forward to leading useful lives. Nonmalignant, or so-called essential hypertension, is accompanied by virtually no symptoms but should not be considered benign. If neglected, mild elevations of blood pressure that are characteristic of nonmalignant hypertension can lead to a constellation of other problems—clogging of arteries, stroke, heart attack, congestive heart failure, kidney failure. Clearly, it is not benign. Fortunately, it too is controllable.

In the majority of cases, the physical cause of hypertension has not been identified. There is currently a controversy within the medical community concerning the cause(s) of hypertension. There are those who believe it is caused by a defective gene. If neither parent has the gene, the chances of the children having hypertension are low. If one parent has the defective gene, the chances of developing hypertension will be higher. Finally, if both parents carry the gene, the chances will be higher still and the hypertension will be more severe.

Some believe that factors in the environment are responsible for the development of hypertension, while others feel that it is a combination of both heredity and environment that is responsible—people who are genetically predisposed to developing hypertension are simply more sensitive to those environmental factors which tend to promote the condition. Some people have argued that the normal aging process is marked by elevations of blood pressure as the years go by. This does seem to hold true in the United States but there are many cultures in which this phenomenon does not occur. There is evidence that increasing pressure with age is influenced by heredity since the blood pressure in the relatives of patients with hypertension is higher than it is in the relatives of others whose blood pressure is normal.

In any case, it has been observed that hypertension is more common among men than women although the statistics for each sex vary according to age. Women taking oral contraceptives may be more likely to develop hypertension, but this may be reversible if the use of the contraceptive is discontinued. Hypertension occurs to a significantly greater extent among blacks than among whites, and for unknown reasons it usually strikes earlier and is more severe in the black population. Blood pressures tend to be lower in active people than in sedentary people. Lastly, there may be a distinct personality type who is subject to developing hypertension. Some studies indicate that hypertensives tend to be tense, anxious, irritable, and restless. In general, these people have been found to have higher levels of emotional arousal and their blood pressures are correspondingly elevated.

ROLE OF NUTRITION IN HYPERTENSION

Nutrition plays an important role in two areas: one is in the prevention of the condition, the other is in the treatment. The correct approach to prevention is not to easy to identify since the cause of hypertension is not clear. But we shall attempt to present several lines of evidence on this important issue.

OBESITY

It is clear that obesity and hypertension are two conditions often found together. They are related, in that hypertensives tend to be more obese than people with normal blood pressure. Also, regardless of age, the higher the relative weight, the higher the prevalence of hypertension. Finally, those people with high blood pressure who were originally lean show a greater tendency to become obese than lean people with normal blood pressure.

Since hypertension is associated with a progressive hardening of the arteries, it would be wise to limit your intake of foods high in cholesterol and saturated fats, because doing so may be beneficial for the prevention of atherosclerosis and hypertension, and can assist you in your weight reduction efforts, as well.

EXERCISE

Unless your physician indicates otherwise, a moderate level of exercise on a regular basis is of value in the treatment of hypertension for a number of reasons. To begin with, it is useful in your efforts to control weight. Exercise has also been shown to be helpful in keeping blood cholesterol levels down. Exercise helps promote improved circulation, especially in the muscles of the heart, and helps the heart to function more efficiently by reducing the heart rate. Also, exercise may help to relieve tension, which has been associated with elevated blood pressure. This may explain why athletically-active individuals tend to have lower blood pressure than more sedentary individuals of the same age and life-style.

SALT/SODIUM

More than two thousand years ago, in a Chinese treatise on internal medicine, the relationship between the amount of salt in the diet and elevated blood pressure was noted: "If too much salt is used in food, the pulse hardens, tears make their appearance, and the complexion changes." (From L. Galton, *The Silent Disease: Hypertension* [New York: Crown Publishers, 1973], p. 16.)

Before the discovery of anti-hypertensive drugs, little could be done to help hypertensives, aside from placing them on a low-salt diet. But it was the effectiveness of this very diet that led some workers to examine the relationship between salt and hypertension. More than twenty years ago, it was suggested that excess salt in the diet may cause hypertension in some individuals. By "salt" we mean ordinary table salt which is added when food is processed by the manufacturer, cooked in the home, or consumed at the table. Table salt is composed of sodium chloride, and it is sodium that may lead to the development of hypertension. In their natural state, most foods are very low in sodium, but as they are processed, so much salt is added that it requires careful planning to reduce one's intake of salt.

A complicating factor is that once you are accustomed to salt in your diet, food tastes bland without it. In other words, a sort of addiction develops. In fact, some people have claimed that we have a salt "appetite" and that we must eat a certain amount of salt in order to remain healthy. This is almost certainly not true. There is good evidence that the amount of salt that exists in food in its natural state is entirely sufficient to sustain us. There may be a need for additional salt in extraordinary circumstances: for instance, when heavy physical labor is undertaken in a very warm environment so that salt losses in sweat are high. But for the vast majority of the US population, this would not apply.

When you compare the amount of salt consumed by the average American with the amount actually needed to stay healthy, we consume anywhere from ten to thirty-five times more salt than we need! This has been true for most of our lives since salt was even added to our baby food. Fortunately, baby food manufacturers recently stopped adding salt to their products.

Is all of this excess salt doing us harm? It is well known that the body regulates its water content mainly by controlling its balance of sodium.

Thus, an excess of sodium obviously implies water excess. It is also known that salt and water retention can increase blood pressure although how this happens is not known.

This may mean that salt and water retention may be intimately involved in the development of hypertension. It should be pointed out, however, that salt and water retention can occur in some individuals who never develop hypertension. Also, several studies have found that some patients with hypertension can have their blood pressure reduced to normal by restricting the amount of salt in their diet, whereas no amount of salt restriction is helpful in controlling the disease in other patients. This could indicate that salt and water retention play a role somewhere in the disease process, but it cannot explain the entire phenomenon.

When salt consumption is compared with the incidence of hypertension, it has been found that the incidence of hypertension in cultures where very little salt is eaten in the diet is extremely low. Moreover, the more salt consumed by a given population, the higher the incidence of the disease in that population. It should be pointed out, however, that this cannot be considered proof that salt causes hypertension.

In order to study the problem in the laboratory, it was necessary to develop a strain of animals capable of developing hypertension. This was difficult since animals usually do not suffer from this particular disease. Such a strain was developed by feeding rats a high-salt diet for several generations. This high-salt diet induced hypertension in these rats, but some animals were found to be more susceptible than others. Thus, it would appear that some animals are resistant to the effects of a high salt intake whereas others exhibit a range of sensitivities to salt. This would suggest that there are genetic differences among the animals. The same may very well be true among people. In other words, some of us seem to inherit a tendency to become hypertensive. A high-salt diet may provide enough of a stress to trigger that hypertension under certain circumstances whereas the same high-salt diet would have no effect on those of us who have no genetic predisposition for hypertension.

Heredity would explain the different incidence of hypertension in the black population. It is estimated that 20 percent of the adult population in the US has elevated blood pressure. Among blacks, this number may be as high as 50 percent. But in countries where the intake of salt is low, even susceptible populations such as blacks show a much lower incidence of hypertension.

What all of this suggests is that those of us with a family history of hypertension might do well to limit salt intake. Unfortunately, a certain number of us may have such a strong genetic predisposition to develop the disease that no amount of preventive measures will help. This is not likely to be true for most of us, however. It is clear that having your blood pressure checked at least twice a year is a wise idea. Whether you should restrict the amoung of salt in your diet is not so clear-cut. There is no evidence that doing so will be harmful and there is at least some evidence that doing so will be beneficial.

There was a time when the only treatment used for hypertension was to place the patient on a low-salt diet. Today, such a diet is sometimes still used to treat hypertension, because if salt is almost completely removed from the diet, blood pressure will almost certainly drop. However, it is more common to use drugs to bring hypertension under control since such drugs can control salt without the patient having to make major dietary changes. A combination of drug therapy and moderate dietary salt restriction is often used.

CALCIUM

In the last few years, evidence has been accumulating linking diets low in calcium with hypertension. The mechanism involved is not understood, but because of the role of calcium in maintaining muscle and nerve activity it has been postulated that the muscular walls of blood vessels may become more rigid, leading to increased pressure within. Since the American diet is relatively low in calcium people at risk for hypertension have an added reason to emphasize calcium rich foods in their diet. (See CALCIUM for a list of foods rich in calcium.)

THE SODIUM RESTRICTED DIET

Sodium is one of the many mineral nutrients that is found in almost all the plants and animals we consume as food. The average level of consumption of sodium in the US diet is estimated to be 6 to 8 grams a day. That amount is equivalent to 3 to 8 teaspoons of table salt (sodium chloride). Even people who do not habitually add salt to food take in a great deal of sodium from commercially processed foods, moderate amounts from what is present naturally in plant and animal products, and small amounts in drinking water.

From our present knowledge of the function of sodium in the body, it is suggested that an adult requires approximately ½ gram of sodium, or less than ¼ teaspoon of salt, per day. Clearly, the desire for and use of salt is not to meet a physical or nutritional requirement, but to satisfy an acquired taste. Adding salt may seem to be only a habit, but it may actually reflect a higher taste threshold: for habitual salt users, more salt is needed

to register the same level of "saltiness" on the palate over a period of time. Those who have become accustomed to unsalted food find their "old favorites" unbearably salty.

Sodium restricted diets fall into three main categories:

- mild, or 2 grams per day
- moderate, or 1 gram per day
- strict, or .5 gram per day

For *mild* restrictions, one simply reduces the amount of table salt used. No salt should be added at the table, but up to one teaspoon can be added per day during cooking. In addition, pickled foods (such as sauerkraut) and extremely salty foods (such as luncheon meats, snack chips, and processed cheeses) should be eliminated.

On a *moderate* restriction one is allowed ¼ teaspoon of salt per day. It is important to learn when foods are salted and when they are not. In some foods salt serves as a necessary preservative, but in others it tempts us so we can't eat just one!

To sharpen your awareness of the sodium content of a food product read the list of ingredients that appears on the label of all packaged foods. Sodium will be in a food if it contains either salt or a sodium compound (such as monosodium glutamate). The food or condiment will be salty if salt (or a sodium compound) appears as one of the first three ingredients. If, on the other hand, it appears very near the end of the list (as in bread) then the food need not be eliminated.

The moderate restriction limits the form of a food eaten rather than eliminating any foods altogether. Corn, for example, is permitted if eaten fresh, frozen unsalted, or canned unsalted. The same is true for all other vegetables, fruits, meats, fish, poultry, fats, and grains. One should consume "unsalted" or "low sodium" dairy products, breads, and cereals. However, to allow flexibility in the diet, up to three servings per day are allowed from restricted foods. This means that a salad bar that offers an array of fresh vegetables along with several dishes of canned beets or canned chick peas is still a welcome stop for someone on the moderate sodium-restricted diet.

The *strict* restriction is the least flexible of the three diets as there are no exceptions permitted. Even though this diet is seldom advised, it is important that it be followed earnestly.

At any level of sodium restriction, the Foods with Insignificant Amounts of Sodium (Later in this section) are allowed without limit.

PLANNING A DIET

In general, a guide to ensure a diet balanced in the essential nutrients for an adult includes at least the following daily servings.

Dairy foods (milk, yogurt, unsalted cheese)	2
Protein foods (meat, poultry, fish, eggs, beans)	2
Fruits	4
Vegetables	3
Breads, cereals, pastas, rice	4

The following meal suggestions apply to a moderate sodium restriction. When prepared at home remember to limit salt to ¼ teaspoon per day and select the appropriate foods as indicated in the following tables.

Gourmet favorites such as stuffed mushrooms, pastry puffs, escargots (snails), steamed seafood, meatballs, and aspics can still be served but should be prepared without salt. Dabble with such spices as coriander, cumin, fennel, ginger, and others you never dared try. When serving dinner for a fancy occasion convert your favorite recipes to a salt-free version. Vegetables tend not to taste "flat" when prepared without salt and therefore should be incorporated more into menus.

When dining out try to patronize restaurants that cook to order and prepare fresh vegetables. This way you will have more control over the amount of sodium that is in your food. Oriental restaurants use soy sauce, monosodium glutamate, and other pickled items; as a result the meals are inescapably high in sodium. Seafood and steak houses may offer some

Breakfast	juice or grapefruit
	egg or unsalted cottage cheese
	toast
	unsalted butter or margarine
	cooked cereal (prepared without salt)
	milk (whole or skim)
	tea or coffee
A Brown Bag Lunch	sliced chicken, lettuce, tomato, alfalfa sprouts on whole wheat bread
	raisins and dry-roasted nuts (unsalted)
	apple
	canned fruit juice, coffee, tea, or milk
A Coffee Shop/ Short-Order Lunch	hamburger on bun with lettuce and tomato
	tossed salad
	vinegar and/or oil (not salad dressing)
	soda pop or flavored milk
	fruit gelatin
A Dieter's Lunch	unsalted wafers or sandwich bread
	hearty tossed salad (with everything except diced cheese and assorted canned vegetables such as those served at salad bars) with vinegar and/or oil
	melon half with unsalted cottage cheese
	fruit juice, coffee, tea, skimmed milk (limit use of sodium-based artificial sweeteners to 2 packets per day)
Evening Meal	broiled cod fish
	broccoli with lemon sauce
	saffron rice (homemade without salt)
	dinner roll
	unsalted butter or margarine
	tossed salad
	fruit compote
	coffee, tea, or milk

advantage if you can ensure that salt is not added during the preparation of your order. Salads and baked potatoes, which usually accompany such entrees, are pretty safe if you forego the dressings and sauces. Fast-food chains and other deep-fried food selections have a lot of added salt; here again a boiled or broiled version of the same food is a better choice.

Your best rule of thumb for sodium restricted diets is to follow the old adage, "Take it with a grain of salt" . . . literally. (See also ARTERIO-SCLEROSIS; CHOLESTEROL; EXERCISE; OBESITY; SALT; SODIUM.)

VEGETABLES NATURALLY HIGH IN SODIUM

Artichokes	Celery flakes	Whole hominy	Parsley flakes
Beet greens	Chard	Kale	Spinach
Carrots	Dandelion greens	Mustard greens	White turnip
Celery			

FOODS WITH INSIGNIFICANT AMOUNTS OF SODIUM (PERMITTED FOR ALL DIETS)

Grains	wheat, oats, rye, rice, barley, and their products (e.g. pasta, breads, flours, uncooked cereals)
Vegetables	all those not listed above in the table Vegetables Naturally High in Sodium or canned/frozen salt-free
Fruits	all fresh/canned fruits and all juices
Meats	all fresh or frozen/canned without salt beef, lamb, pork, veal, poultry, fish, shellfish, and game meats
Eggs	all fresh
Fats	all vegetable oils and shortenings, lard, and unsalted butter and margarine
Condiments	vinegar, all spices, mustard powder, flavorings that do not contain salt
Sweeteners	sugar, honey, syrup, jellies, molasses
Beverages	alcoholic beverages, coffee, teas, soft drinks

HYPOGLYCEMIA (LOW BLOOD SUGAR)

Hypoglycemia, or low blood sugar, may be caused by a number of diseases such as early diabetes or by certain drugs or alcohol. If the blood sugar drops to low enough levels a group of symptoms develop, including, sweating, palpitations, anxiety, dizziness, weakness, and sometimes fainting. The symptoms themselves are not specific, and, therefore, in order to diagnose true hypoglycemia a blood test must show a low blood sugar at the time the symptoms appear and not simply during the course of a show glucose test—a test that is rarely used by knowledgeable specialists. True hypoglycemia, if untreated, can be extremely serious. As the blood sugar falls to very low levels signs of central nervous system impairment may occur. These can include: confusion, blurred vision, loss of memory, bizarre behavior, and depressed intellectual function. If the hypoglycemia gets too severe convulsions and coma may result.

Hypoglycemia may occur either following the ingestion of food—reactive or food stimulated hypoglycemia—or as a result of food deprivation—fasting or food deprived hypoglycemia. The former may be due to early diabetes or to abnormalities of the alimentary tract but more usually is due to an excessive reaction in some people to a rise in blood sugar induced by eating certain foods. The latter is always secondary to other often more serious problems. The following table is a classification of the different types of hypoglycemia.

Any person who suspects that he or she is suffering from hypoglycemia should seek medical advice. If the characteristic symptoms appear between meals, particularly

---

CLASSIFICATION OF HYPOGLYCEMIA

Reactive (food stimulated)	Alimentary
	Early diabetes
	Unknown causes
Fasting (food deprived)	Drugs
	Alcohol
	Hormone deficiency
	Liver disease
	Congenital defects
	Pancreatic tumor

if a meal is skipped, the cause must be carefully sought. Sometimes a drug that you are taking or a heavy bout of alcohol consumption may be involved. A change in life-style may be all that is necessary. Sometimes one of the other problems noted in the table might be present and specific treatment may be necessary.

If the symptoms appear shortly after a meal your physician will wish to determine if you suffer from early diabetes or have certain abnormalities of the gastrointestinal tract. Once these have been eliminated as a possible cause of reactive hypoglycemia, the most probable reason for your hypoglycemia is that you fall into the group which overreacts to the increase in blood sugar which can accompany a meal. Normally when we digest a meal the carbohydrate component is broken down to simple sugars which are rapidly absorbed into the bloodstream. The blood sugar level, therefore, increases after a meal. In response to the elevated blood sugar the specialized cells within the pancreas secrete the hormone insulin which, in turn, brings the blood sugar down. In some people with reactive hypoglycemia the response of the pancreas may be too vigorous and the blood sugar may fall significantly below normal. If symptoms occur accompanying this, low blood sugar hypoglycemia may become a problem.

The treatment of this type of hypoglycemia, which is relatively uncommon, is to consume small frequent meals and frequent snacks and to avoid simple sugars, which are rapidly absorbed into the bloodstream. Foods that are high in protein are useful because they are not broken down to glucose and, therefore, do not significantly affect the level of blood sugar. Dietary fiber should be increased because fiber traps sugars and releases them more slowly, thus reducing the strain on the pancreas. Many people with reactive hypoglycemia find that certain foods precipitate an attack more than others. These foods should be avoided. If an attack is felt coming on a protein snack may abort the symptoms. If an attack is already in progress it can temporarily be aborted using a carbohydrate snack. This can be a simple glass of juice or sweetened tea. It is important, however, to try to avoid this situation because the high blood sugar which is induced can cause a "rebound" and another attack in a relatively short period of time.

Thus a person with true reactive hypoglycemia must establish an eating pattern which works for him or her. Small, frequent high protein meals and snacks rich in protein and fiber are generally helpful, but each person will have to determine what works in his or her individual case and structure eating patterns accordingly. (See also DIABETES.)

IMMUNITY

Nutrition has a tremendous impact on our resistance to infection and ability to cope with disease. In third world countries severe malnutrition seriously compromises the immune systems of millions of severely undernourished people and leads to death from diseases which are not normally life threatening. In America obesity is probably the more prevalent threat to the immune system with over twenty million Americans suffering from this disorder. Severe deficiencies of vitamins or minerals are not common in America, but many people have marginal deficiencies of a single nutrient. The evidence available seems to indicate that even marginal deficiencies of essential nutrients can significantly impair the immune system, although data from humans is sparse.

Megadoses of critical nutrients do not seem to boost the immune system and may even depress it. Hence, at the moment it would appear that a balanced diet containing the recommended daily allowances for all the essential nutrients is the right one for maximum protection against infection. (See also INFECTION.)

INFANT FEEDING

One of the earliest decisions a new mother must make is how to feed her newborn infant. Perhaps the most important decision is whether to breast-feed or to use an infant formula. In this section we will discuss the sequence of infant feeding regardless of whether breast milk or infant formula is used.

For the first four months of life breast milk or infant formula is the only food that the infant needs. Introducing solid food before this is not sensible since the infant has not yet coordinated the swallowing mechanism independent of sucking. Too early introduction of solid foods will either cause a reduction in breast milk or formula consumption or will add unnecessary calories. Neither of these results is desirable. With the former a much poorer food is being substituted, with the latter the infant may gain weight too rapidly. After four months of age solid foods can be introduced. Cereal, fruits, and vegetables are introduced before meat and dairy, otherwise the order is less important than the use of one food at a time. By doing this any food which does not agree with the infant can be rapidly identified and eliminated from the diet. Either commercially prepared baby food or table food ground to the proper consistency in a blender can be used. If the latter course is chosen remember that commercial baby foods no longer add sugar or salt. Many table foods, particularly processed ones, have added salt. It is important, therefore, to be sure that the foods used for a young infant are either fresh or have been processed without added salt or sugar.

Whole cow milk should not be started before about one year of age because of its high protein content. The immature infant kidney may be strained if whole milk is introduced too soon. Skim milk is usually not used until the infant is eighteen months of age.

Certain foods, such as chocolate, are often avoided until the infant is beyond one year of age. Some pediatricians avoid eggs until the infant is almost one year old. Of course, any food which has produced an untoward reaction in your infant should be omitted from the diet and not reintroduced until after a year of age. (See also BREAST-FEEDING; CHILDREN; INFANT FORMULA.)

INFANT FORMULA

In our society infant formula is used in two ways: as a supplement to breast-feeding by mothers who breast-feed their infants, but who for various reasons cannot be available at all times and do not wish to pump their breasts to provide the interim feedings; and instead of breast milk for mothers who cannot or will not breast-feed for various reasons.

The preferable way to feed a young infant is from the mother's breast. However, an infant can be successfully reared using an infant formula either together with breast-feedings or exclusively.

Infant formulas are usually made with a cow milk base. That is, they use cow milk as the source of the protein. Cow milk contains three times the protein of human milk and hence to simulate human milk the protein content of infant formula must be adjusted to that of breast milk. Most commercial infant formulas have done this. However, cow milk protein is different from human milk protein. It contains a different complement of amino acids and a different proportion of the two major proteins found in all milks; whey protein (lactalbumin) and casein. Cow milk is 70 percent casein and 30 percent whey protein; human milk is the reverse. Recognizing this difference, producers of some commercial infant formulas have now changed the proportions of casein to whey protein to simulate breast milk. Even this change, however, leaves the infant formula using a different protein source and hence a different complement of amino acids than human milk. This difference is important since the protein of human milk is easier to digest than that of infant formula and infants consuming formula will have harder curds and firmer stools than infants who breast-feed. In addition, because the infant gut is "leaky" in the sense that it will pass whole protein molecules through, infant formula is more likely to promote allergic responses in some infants than breast milk does.

The carbohydrate used in most commercial infant formulas is lactose and is identical to the carbohydrate found in breast milk. The fat, however, is usually quite different. Breast milk contains a mixture of saturated and unsaturated fat and is rich in cholesterol. (See CHOLESTEROL.) Most infant formulas contain mostly unsaturated fatty acids and are devoid of cholesterol. Whether these differences are important is currently unclear.

In spite of these differences cow milk–based infant formulas are an acceptable way to feed a newborn infant. Almost half of America's new mothers choose to feed their infants in this manner. These formulas have all of the vitamins and minerals necessary to promote proper growth of the infant and hence they, like breast milk, constitute complete infant nutrition for the first three to four months of age.

The only supplements which may be necessary for the infant receiving a commercial formula are iron (if the formula is not fortified with iron) and fluoride. If a ready-to-use infant formula is used it will not contain fluoride. If a powdered formula is used and the local water supply is not fluoridated it, too, will be devoid of fluoride. In both these instances a fluoride supplement should be supplied. If a powdered formula is used and the local water supply is fluoridated then supplementation is unnecessary.

Many mothers who breast-feed choose to stop when the infant is around five to six months of age. Under these circumstances it is better to switch to a commercial infant formula than to whole cow milk. The reason for this is that the high protein content of whole cow milk may put an unnecessary strain on the infant's kidney, which is still immature at this age. By one year of age whole cow milk can be introduced. Skim milk, because of its high protein content per calorie, should be avoided in large amounts until the infant is about eighteen months of age.

There are some commercial infant formulas which do not use cow milk as their base. The most common of these are the formulas which use soybean protein (one of the few complete plant proteins) as their base. These formulas are generally used only if for one reason or another the infant cannot tolerate cow milk–based infant formula. You should consult your physician before beginning one of these formulas.

In some places in the United States "homemade" formulas are still being prepared from whole cow milk or evaporated milk. This is usually done by diluting the milk and then adding carbohydrate, usually in the form of dextromaltose. This practice is not recommended. The final product is too different from human milk.

The use of infant formula in developing countries is a special problem. The water supplies are often contaminated, proper refrigeration may not exist, and to make a little go a longer way, the mother often overdilutes the formula. The result is often infection, diarrhea, and malnutrition, a combination that is the major killer of infants in the world. For this reason, the safest form of infant feeding under these conditions is from the mother's breast for as long as possible. (See also BREAST-FEEDING; CHILDREN; INFANT FEEDING.)

INFECTION

Our ability to fight an infection depends on how well our immune system functions. Any nutritional deficiencies, as well as many excesses and/or imbalances, can seriously impair the various components of the body's immune system. This system has been shown to be compromised in this way not only in developing countries where severe and generalized undernutrition occurs, but also in America, where individual deficiencies may take place, especially in certain high-risk groups, including, hospitalized patients, alcoholics, infants, food faddists, and the elderly.

The body's defense against infectious microorganisms consists of several component parts. The first includes the skin, the lining of the lungs and the gastrointestinal tract, and the various body secretions. Should a foreign organism gain entry to the body, the second system, which includes two types of white blood cells called granulocytes and macrophages are brought into play. At the same time, a third system, consisting of two more types of white blood cells called T cells and B cells, is activated. Both of these cell types are called lymphocytes. All of these systems work together to protect us from viruses and bacteria.

BODY SURFACE DEFENSES

These defenses constitute all surfaces that are exposed to the external environment. The skin prevents microorganisms from getting into the body, and sweat, tears, and the oily secretions of the sebaceous glands in the skin all contain chemicals that kill bacteria. Mucus from the linings of the lungs and body organs sticks to bacteria and contains a chemical that can kill them. Mucus from the lungs can either be coughed up and eliminated or swallowed. The acid in the stomach and digestive juices can kill the bacteria which are swallowed. If bacteria survive these various forms of detoxification and enter the body then the immune system is brought into play.

THE IMMUNE SYSTEM

The cells of the immune system are distributed throughout the body in the bloodstream as granulocytes, monocytes, and lymphocytes and in the lymph tissues which include the thymus, the lymph nodes, the spleen, the bone marrow, and areas lining the gastrointestinal tract. But the most important cells are the granulocytes, monocytes, and lymphocytes. Whenever the body is damaged or invaded by microorganisms, the granulocytes travel to the injured area and ingest and destroy invading organisms. The monocytes also travel to the area, where they mature into macrophages which engulf the foreign microorganisms.

The T cells pass from the bone marrow, where they are made, to the thymus, where they are activated. They then travel directly to wherever the invading substances have gained entry to the body. On making contact with the microorganisms, they become sensitized to them. If these sensitized cells encounter the same type of microorganism a second time they release a chemical that kills it. Further, once the T cells have been sensitized against a particular infectious organism they will be able to act more quickly if the organism attacks the body again in the future. T cells can only be sensitized to one type of microorganism. They are most effective against fungi, viruses, and parasites, but will destroy a few types of bacteria. They can also destroy cancer cells and help the body reject newly transplanted tissues.

The B cells are important in the production of antibodies. When an invading microorganism encounters a B cell it rapidly divides and produces antibodies which kill the invader. The antibodies produced by a given B cell are specific for a single type of organism. If antibodies for a specific organism have been produced once, the body retains the ability to produce them again if the same organism reinfects it. Hence, the B cells will then be able to respond more quickly. Overall, B cells have the most important role to play in the resistance to infection.

THE IMPORTANCE OF NUTRITION

Severe malnutrition, as seen in the present famine in Ethiopia, is definitely associated with an increased susceptibility to infection and a seriously impaired ability to cope with infection due to an impaired immune system. Consistently reduced numbers of T and B cells are found and there is a wasting away of the lymph tissues. On the other hand, the effects of marginal intake of one or more nutrients, as found in some people in this country, are largely unknown, although prolonged mild or moderate deficiencies of any essential nutrient seems to compromise immunity in animals.

Added to the effects of malnutrition are problems associated with age. Both the elderly and infants are more susceptible to nutritional insults than are young adults. In addition, in all people, the extent of immunological impairment depends, not only on the severity of malnutrition, but also on the presence of other metabolic stresses, including, infection, trauma, surgery, cancer, and metabolic disorders, all of which decrease the effectiveness of the immune system. Nevertheless, nutritional repletion usually improves the immune system and decreases the risk of infection in most hospitalized patients.

AGE FACTORS

Both infants and the elderly have less than optimal immune systems and increased susceptibility to infection. If they are also malnourished this further decreases their resistance to disease. Premature infants have a reduced immune function, as do those infants who are growth retarded as a result of maternal undernutrition or infection. Such children may show reduced numbers of T and B cells for several years after birth, despite nutritional rehabilitation. In contrast, correction of nutritional deficits occurring after birth in infants can usually reverse immunological deficits. Undernutrition will also reduce the effectiveness of immunizations against serious diseases in young children.

In the elderly, there is an increased incidence of infection and cancer. This is partly due to a normal progressive decline in immune function with advancing age but is also due to malnutrition resulting from factors which decrease food intake, such as emotional, motivational, dental problems, and altered taste acuity.

OBESITY

Although undernutrition is the most common dietary problem that influences resistance to infection, obesity also affects the immune response. Obese people are very susceptible to infections, especially postoperatively. The obese have a less than optimal immune system with a reduced ability to fight off an infection. Whether these abnormalities are due to obesity itself or to metabolic, hormonal, or other nutritional changes is unknown. (See OBESITY.)

DIETARY PROTEIN

The ability of the body's cells to make new proteins is a necessity for developing and maintaining the immune system at its optimal state. This depends upon the availability of free amino acids to all the immune cells. Even a mild protein deficiency causes defects in all aspects of the immune system. As well as the quantity of protein, the quality also affects how well the immune system works. Infants fed soy protein–based formulas are more susceptible to infection than those receiving formulas based on cow milk protein. Similarly, adults receiving low quality protein diets have been shown to have less effective im-

mune systems and a greater susceptibility to infections, especially ones
of the upper respiratory tract, such
as bronchitis.

DIETARY FAT

In recent years, a good deal of interest has been focused on the effects
of dietary fats on immune function.
Most studies have been concerned
with high intakes rather than low intakes of either saturated fats or polyunsaturated fats. While adequate
quantities of the essential fatty acid
linoleic acid, which is a polyunsaturated fat, are crucial to the normal
functioning of the immune system,
excess polyunsaturated fat suppresses immunity. But this impedi-
ment to immunocompetence is
reversible as soon as dietary polyunsaturated fat intake is reduced. The
mechanism by which polyunsaturated fat suppresses the immune system is not known, but could be due
to the changes in the fat composition
of cell membranes, making them
more readily invaded by microorganisms, or to changes in the hormonal state of the body.

The alleged effects of high intakes of polyunsaturated fat in promoting tumor growth in the breast,
colon, and prostate have been ex-
plained by the fat's suppression of
the body's immune defense, which
might otherwise protect against cancer. Although this idea has not been

proven, it raises some concern because of the increased consumption
of polyunsaturated fat by the American public as a defense against cardiovascular disease.

High blood cholesterol levels
and abnormally high triglyceride levels also seem to increase susceptibility to infection, possibly by altering
the structure of cell membranes.

VITAMINS

Individual vitamins exert widespread effects on the immune system. Of the fat soluble vitamins,
vitamins A and E influence the immune system, whereas vitamins D and
K have little effect.

Vitamin A. Quite a lot of people in
America have marginal intakes of vitamin A. Deficiency of this vitamin
is associated with an increased incidence of infection. This is due in part
to the role of vitamin A in maintaining the functional integrity of the skin
and the lining of the body's organs
(mucosal surfaces) and the production of the mucus secretions that protect and lubricate such surfaces.
Vitamin A is also required for the
production of tears, saliva, and sweat,
all of which contain substances which
have bactericidal properties. In addition, low intakes of this vitamin lead
to reduced numbers of T cells and a
suppressed production of antibodies
by B cells. Animal data also indi-

cates an increased susceptibility to cancer in the presence of vitamin A deficiency. (See VITAMIN A.)

Vitamin E. There is very little information available about the effects of vitamin E on the immune system in humans. However, in animals, low intakes of this vitamin increase susceptibility to infection and up to six times the minimal intake enhances immune function (this would be equivalent to 90 milligrams in humans). Megadoses (150 milligrams or more), on the other hand, have been shown to inhibit several immune functions in humans. (See VITAMIN E.)

B Vitamins. Many individual B vitamins have widespread effects on the immune system, especially vitamin B_6, pantothenic acid, riboflavin (B_2), folacin (folic acid), and vitamin B_{12}. The others seem to have much less influence. Deficiencies in any of the B vitamins will decrease the effectiveness of the immune system, but there is no evidence to show that megadoses of any of them are beneficial.

Vitamin B_6 is needed for cell multiplication and it is not surprising that a deficiency of this vitamin has the biggest effect on the immune system. Such deficiencies lead to dry scaly skin on the face, neck, arms, and legs, a sore mouth and tongue, and cracks in the corners of the mouth and in the lips. All of these lesions

are open to infection by bacteria and fungi. Vitamin B_6 deficiency also leads to a reduced production of antibodies and virtually no production at all if combined with pantothenic acid deficiency. T cells also do not function normally. All of these changes from the norm are reversed upon repletion with the vitamin.

Both pantothenic acid and riboflavin deficiency lead to a reduced production of antibodies. Deficiencies of folacin lead to a reduced resistance to infection and depressed immunocompetence. People with anemia due to folacin deficiency show a reduced production of antibodies and reduced numbers of T cells (with impaired immune functions). When one realizes that up to one-third of all premenopausal women in America have less than optimal intakes of folacin, these effects could actually be widespread.

Folacin and vitamin B_{12} are closely associated in their metabolic effects and it has been difficult to differentiate the effects on the immune system of one from the other. However, vitamin B_{12} deficiency seems to specifically depress T cell function. (See entries for specific B vitamins.)

Vitamin C. Of all the essential nutrients, vitamin C has generated the most public interest. Most of this was begun by Linus Pauling's assertions that adult humans should maintain an intake of more than 1 gram of vitamin C per day. (Although there is no doubt that a deficiency of vitamin C will increase the susceptibility of people to infection, the alleged benefits of taking supplements are in tremendous dispute.) Many studies have tested this hypothesis. Perhaps the biggest effort has gone into examining the questions of whether or not megadoses of vitamin C will cure the common cold. These studies show that a supplement of 80 milligrams a day will reduce the symptoms of a respiratory infection and their duration, and perhaps even the number of episodes of infection experienced by a given person in any specific period to a minor extent. The vitamin seems to do this by enhancing the ability of the granulocytes and macrophages to engulf and destroy bacteria but does not have any direct effect on viruses. Supplements larger than 80 milligrams do not seem to be associated with any additional benefit and megadoses may even suppress immune system activity.

Recent studies have also shown that vitamin C has no value in the treatment of cancer. The use of vitamin C for this purpose was first proposed by Pauling and Ewan Cameron who claimed that they had been able to extend the lives of cancer patients by 160 to 255 days by giving them 10 grams of vitamin C daily. In addition, they claimed they were able to reduce tumor size in several patients.

The Mayo Clinic recently completed a study which followed the same design as that of Pauling in giving 10 grams of vitamin C per day to patients with cancer of the colon and/or rectum. The investigators could find absolutely no benefit associated with the supplement. Patients neither lived longer than a placebo group given sugar pills nor did the vitamin appear to reduce the size of the tumors, or prevent them from spreading in any of the patients.

Pauling had severely criticized a previous study carried out at the Mayo Clinic that had also shown no benefits associated with the use of vitamin C supplements, because the patients had been given chemotherapy prior to trying the supplements. Such drugs, he claims, interfere with the beneficial action of the vitamin. However, none of the patients in the more recent study had been given chemotherapy prior to inclusion in the study.

Pauling's own studies have been universally criticized by accepted authorities as being improperly designed. His results, therefore, would seem to have no validity. In light of the new evidence, it must be concluded that megadoses of vitamin C will not cure or help in the treatment of cancer. (See VITAMIN C.)

MINERALS

Many minerals are necessary for the normal functioning of the immune system. Iron and zinc are especially important to a patient's resistance to infection and ability to destroy invading microorganisms. Deficiencies of cobalt, manganese, copper, calcium, chromium, magnesium, selenium, and iodine depress the immune system. Excesses of lead, mercury, and cadmium compromise the system.

Iron. Over one-third of premenopausal women in America have less than optimal body stores of iron. Many people of both sexes and all ages experience some degree of iron deficiency at one time or another in their lives. It is perhaps the most likely form of a single nutrient deficiency to occur in the absence of any other accompanying form of malnutrition. Iron is also one of the most important nutrients in terms of its effects on the immune system.

Both deficiencies and excesses of iron will increase susceptibility to infection. Iron deficiency, whether serious enough to cause anemia or not, will impair most functions of the immune system. However, iron is needed for the growth and multiplication of bacteria. Hence, any supplemental program to replete a deficient person must be approached with caution. Such supplements can promote bacteria growth and cause infection in a person who is generally poorly nourished, but this should not

be a problem in a well-nourished individual. (See IRON.)

Zinc. As with iron, zinc deficiency can compromise a variety of immune functions and a person's resistance to infection. It is a key factor in cell division. The developing immune system is especially vulnerable to a deficiency. A zinc deficiency during pregnancy or the first few weeks of life slows down the normal development of the immune system and makes the infant more susceptible to infection at this critical time of life. There are also reports of impaired immune function in some elderly people due to zinc deficiency. When zinc supplements are given to these people their immune function appears to return to normal. However, it should be noted that megadoses of zinc (150 milligrams or more) have a detrimental effect on the immune system. (See ZINC.)

NUTRITION AND THE IMMUNE SYSTEM: AN OVERVIEW

Obviously, nutrition has a tremendous impact on our resistance to infection and ability to cope with disease. In third world countries severe malnutrition seriously compromises the immune systems of millions of severely undernourished people and leads to death from diseases which are not normally life-threatening. In America obesity is probably the most prevalent threat to the immune system with over twenty million Americans suffering from this disorder. Severe deficiencies of vitamins or minerals are not common in America, but many people have marginal deficiencies of a single nutrient. The evidence available seems to indicate that even marginal deficiencies of essential nutrients can significantly impair the immune system, although data from humans is sparse.

Megadoses of critical nutrients do not seem to boost the immune system and may even depress it. Hence, at the moment it would appear that a balanced diet containing the recommended daily allowances for all the essential nutrients is the right one for maximum protection against disease.

WHO SHOULD TAKE VITAMIN AND MINERAL SUPPLEMENTS TO AID IN RESISTANCE TO INFECTION?

In the adult population, the question of whether or not one should routinely take vitamin supplements is not an easy one to answer. Heavy alcohol consumption can deplete the body of thiamine and folacin, and heavy smoking can reduce vitamin C levels. When these types of habits are added to the constant struggle for weight maintenance and the consumption of highly processed foods the natural intake of certain vitamins and min-

---

Food Sources of Nutrients Critical To An Optimal Immune System

Nutrient	Food Sources
Vitamin A	Liver, butter, cream, egg yolks, leafy green vegetables, deep yellow and orange fruits and vegetables.
Vitamin E	Vegetable oils.
Vitamin B_6	Wheat germ, meat, liver, whole grains, peanuts, soy beans, and corn.
Vitamin B_{12}	Liver, eggs, meat, milk, and cheese.
Folic Acid	Liver, yeast, leafy green vegetables, legumes, whole grains, fruits and other vegetables.
Vitamin C	Citrus fruits, strawberries, tomatoes, cantaloupes, broccoli, cabbage, green peppers, leafy greens, and potatoes.
Iron	Liver, meat, oysters, leafy green vegetables, dried apricots, prunes, peaches, raisins, legumes, nuts, and whole grains.
Zinc	Oysters, liver, wheat germ, yeast, and seafood.

erals through our diet becomes lower than it should be. In spite of this, however, there is little evidence to show that the average adult male has any signs of lowered vitamin or mineral levels, and so routine supplementation for adult males is not necessary. However, supplementation for heavy drinkers or smokers is beneficial.

In women, the situation is different, as many women have less than optimal levels of one or more nutrients in their bodies. In addition to heavy consumption of alcohol and heavy smoking, there is the problem of iron loss through menstruation, vitamin depletion during pregnancy and lactation (if supplementation has not been given), and the use of oral contraceptives (which can interfere with folacin and vitamin B_6 metabolism). The American woman is also very weight-conscious and so millions of women follow "fad" diets for weight loss, which invariably fall short in the area of essential nutrients. Women who fit into any of these categories can often benefit from taking a vitamin and mineral supplement containing the RDA. All women whose calcium intake is less than 1000 milligrams—the majority of women in the US—should take a supplement of 1000 milligrams of calcium. The average American woman's diet contains only about 400 milligrams of calcium and the high phosphorus and protein nature of the diet causes her to absorb very little of it.

Older Americans form yet another special population group. They often eat convenience foods which may be low in certain vitamins and minerals. In addition, the elderly often have to exist on low incomes and hence try to save money by cutting out more expensive foods. Finally, they may have specific health problems which affect vitamin and mineral metabolism. Many older people also have difficulty chewing their food properly and so must eat softer foods. Many have problems with iron and vitamin B_{12} absorption. A lot take medications for one or more nutrients. As a result, all elderly people with a history of dietary inadequacies should at least take supplements of iron and vitamin B_{12} as recommended by their physicians. (See also IMMUNITY.)

INTOLERANCE

Unlike food allergy, food intolerance is a very imprecise term. It means simply what it says—that a particular food is, for some reason, not tolerated well. Many foods fit this definition. No doubt you have a particular food that makes you sick to your stomach or causes gas pains or even diarrhea. Such foods are usually easy to recognize and can be quickly removed from the diet.

Certain food intolerances are not recognized so easily and will produce very severe symptoms. Lactose, or milk, intolerance is the most prevalent food intolerance, since, as we shall see, it is present in one form or another in most of the people in the world.

GLUTEN INTOLERANCE

The classic food intolerance in children is called celiac disease. It is characterized by poor growth, loss of appetite, a potbellied appearance, and a persistent, foul-smelling, fatty diarrhea. The disease usually occurs during the first three years of life and is caused by an intolerance to a single substance, gluten, found mostly in wheat but present in some other grains, such as rye, as well. Unfortunately, even minute amounts of gluten are enough to cause severe symptoms.

If your child has true celiac disease, your doctor will place her or him on a careful diet. It is very important that the diet be followed, since even small indiscretions can lead to recurrence of most or all of the symptoms. The principle of the diet is simple—avoidance of all foods containing gluten. In practice this is no simple task. The table on page 202 is an abbreviated list of foods which must be avoided and foods which can be used on a gluten-free diet.

As soon as he or she is able, your child will have to be taught about the diet, for celiac disease is a long-term problem (sometimes lifelong). A child who has been suffering from symptoms for any length of time will probably also have anemia as a result of microscopic losses of blood in the diarrheal stool. The anemia can be easily corrected with iron supplementation at the same time as the gluten-free diet is instituted.

In some children this diet may be necessary for the rest of their lives; in others some tolerance to gluten may develop. Therefore, after successful dietary therapy for five years, your doctor will probably slowly introduce small amounts of gluten-containing foods. If they are tolerated, the child can begin to eat a regular or nearly normal diet.

Any illness that lasts for a lifetime is a difficult thing for a parent to accept and can seem like a tragedy of insurmountable proportions. If your child has celiac disease, remember that before the discovery of its cause it was a chronic, debilitating, and sometimes even fatal disease. Today, however, if your child sticks to the diet, she or he can live a perfectly normal life in every way.

Celiac disease, or gluten sensitivity, can sometimes occur in adults. The symptoms are similar to celiac disease in children except for the characteristic potbelly and of course the growth failure. Usually it is the chronic fatty diarrhea that brings an adult to the doctor. The treatment is the same as in children with careful attention to a gluten-free diet. Remember that the bowel, in anyone suffering from celiac disease, is sensitive to gluten, and so even one drink of rye whiskey can set off an adverse response.

GLUTEN PRESENCE IN FOODS

	Present	Absent
Grains	wheat, rye, oats, barley, products made from the above	corn, gluten-free wheat starch, rice, soybean flour, millet, buckwheat (Kasha), products made from the above
Vegetables, fruits	cream soups	all types, juices, fruit ices
Nuts, beans	bean soups thickened with flour	all types, nut butters
Dairy	some ice cream, cheese spread, malted milk	milk, cheese
Meats, fish, poultry	breaded, made with filler, canned (read label)	all fresh and frozen unprocessed
Fats, Oils	salad dressing thickened with wheat starch	oils, margarine, butter, salad dressing
Miscellaneous	wheat starch, Postum, gravies and sauces	tapioca, hard candies, coffee, tea, arrowroot, jellies, jams, syrup, honey

MILK INTOLERANCE

The carbohydrate in all milk is called lactose (milk sugar). Lactose is actually two simple sugars (glucose and galactose) joined together in a tight chemical bond. All newborns and young infants have an enzyme, lactase, in their gastrointestinal tracts that is capable of breaking this bond and releasing the free glucose and galactose. These simple sugars are then absorbed and used by the body.

In certain races, lactase remains very active throughout life; in others, the activity of this enzyme slowly diminishes, so that at about age eight or nine, the lactose in milk is no longer split efficiently. The majority of the people in the world fall into this latter category. Only Europeans, particularly western Europeans and their descendants, seem to maintain high levels of lactase into adult life. In Asians, Africans, Polynesians, and their descendants, the activity of the enzyme slowly diminishes. Consequently, schoolchildren and adults from these populations do not tolerate large quantities of milk very well.

If you come from a non-European background, it is very likely that you will have some degree of difficulty in digesting lactose. The extent of the difficulty, however, varies widely. For example, neither you nor your husband may have noticed any trouble, since neither of you consumes large quantities of milk at one time, and yet, your older child could be very sensitive. Conversely, one glass of milk might make you very uncomfortable while your child might easily tolerate larger quantities.

The problem is the undigested lactose. As it gets into the lower gastrointestinal tract it is fermented by bacteria, releasing products that are gaseous and cause bloating and abdominal discomfort. Lactic acid is also produced, which irritates the intestine and can cause diarrhea. These symptoms come on within minutes after the ingestion of lactose and are called lactose intolerance. If you or one of your children suffer from this, the amount of milk consumed should be controlled. Usually, small amounts in cereal or added to a dessert cause no problems. Often, half a glass or even a full glass can be consumed without problems. Observe your children carefully; don't force them to take more milk than they can tolerate. This is not an allergy but a normal physiologic state in most of the older children in the world.

It would appear that consumption of large quantities of milk was designed for infants and very young children. Only certain older children and adults can tolerate large quantities. In our society, where milk has taken on a special role in the feeding of young children, care must be taken not to force children who cannot tolerate large quantities to consume more than is comfortable for them. Fortunately, there are many dairy products, lower in lactose, which will supply most of the nutrients in milk. See the following table for the foods that fall into this category. Remember, it is not the fat but the lactose which is the culprit. Skimmed or low-fat milk will not solve the problem. The only solution is moderation. Lactose-sensitive people will soon learn how much they can take and what consititutes too much. Respect their wishes.

All people, even those who have adequate levels of lactase and can easily tolerate large quantities of milk, can become lactase-deficient with certain illnesses that are accompanied by diarrhea. Therefore, when a person has diarrhea or is recovering from diarrhea, milk should be avoided. (See also ALLERGY; GASTROINTESTINAL DISEASE.)

DIETARY GUIDELINES

It has long been recognized that some foods present problems to some people. The old saying "One man's medicine is another man's poison" is an indication of the instances of food intolerance from many generations ago. Although it is important to recognize the possible link between physical symptoms and inges-

---

LACTOSE IN COMMON FOODS

	High Amount	**Low Amount**	**Absent**
Milk	fluid milk, evaporated milk, powdered milk	yogurt, buttermilk	soybean milk, Nutramigen, Pregestimil (milk substitute or formula)
Milk products	ice cream, sherbert, some non-dairy milks	cheese	
Meat, fish, poultry, eggs	creamed items	some cold cuts	all fresh forms
Vegetables, fruits		creamed items	all fresh or plain forms
Baked products, grains	baked with milk	baked with cheese	French and Italian bread, "Parve" goods, pasta, rice, cereals, crackers

Read the label to check for the presence of milk.

tion of some foods, it is more important not to incriminate and thus eliminate categories of foods because of a hunch that they may be causing problems. Any suspected problem should be carefully investigated through an elimination diet and medical screening.

Elimination Diet. Certain categories of foods rarely produce severe reactions following their ingestion. These include most vegetables, some fruits, meats, beans, and rice. An elimination diet should concentrate on these foods for a period of time. An example of an elimination diet is given below. Portion sizes in this and all other sample menus should be adjusted to suit individual appetites.

It is best not to stay on a diet restricted in variety for an extended period of time. If a food allergy is suspected, add other foods to the elimination diet—one at a time, with two to three days between adding each new food—until symptoms appear or until symptoms can be attributed to some other factor.

If a sensitivity has been clearly identified as triggered by milk or wheat, the following menus will illustrate how to plan balanced diets without the offending foods.

Breakfast
hominy grits
margarine (containing no milk solids)
ham
apricot juice
peach slices

Lunch
lemonade
rice
pink beans
carrot & raisin salad (made with egg-free, corn oil salad dressing)
pear halves

Snack
apple

Dinner
apricot nectar
kale
yellow squash
lamb
lettuce (with corn oil & vinegar)
fruited gelatin

Milk-Free Diet. Milk-free diets result in the elimination of a very good source of calcium. Include other calcium rich foods often if milk and milk products are eliminated. (See CALCIUM for list of other calcium sources.)

Milk-Free Menu

Breakfast
orange juice
toast
margarine (without milk solids)
melon slice
poached egg
coffee or tea (with lemon, sugar optional)

Lunch
noodle soup
salmon salad
tossed salad
French bread
angel food cake

Snack
dried fruit & nuts

Dinner
baked potato
margarine (without milk solids)
broccoli
broiled chicken
tomato slices
Applesauce Gingerbread (see p. 207)

Wheat and Gluten-Free Menu

Breakfast
orange juice
puffed rice
milk
blueberries
ham
hash brown potatoes

Snack
rice cakes
grapes

Lunch
chicken-rice soup
broiled fish (not breaded)
coleslaw
green peas
fruited gelatin

Dinner
kernel corn
brussels sprouts
sliced turkey
cranberry sauce
tossed salad
vinegar & oil
rice pudding

Snack
popcorn
fruit juice

Wheat-Free Diet. Wheat-free diets require particular attention to labels when you shop. As noted in the table on page 202, wheat is widely dispersed in the food supply. When eating out, try to select plain, uncomplicated items. Consider the foods suggested in the following menu.

Modifying Recipes. Rice can be used in a manner similar to macaroni and other pasta products in baked cheese or cold salad recipes. Rice cakes and tortilla chips, once found only in specialty stores, are now available in supermarkets. These make excellent side snacks for soups and fish or egg salads.

When recipes call for an egg or 2 tablespoons of flour as a thickener use 1 tablespoon of cornstarch instead. Carob powder can substitute for the flavor of cocoa in cooked products. Use cornflake crumbs for breading. Almost all pastries are forbidden on wheat-free diets. In their place consult a basic cookbook for cornflake macaroons and meringue cookies. Tofu in milk-free diets can be made to spread, whip or pour like any dairy product.

It may seem like a nuisance to have to avoid certain categories of foods. But, for many, it trains the eye and the palate to be more discriminating. Instead of being repetitive, a restricted diet can feature a great deal of variety through creativity.

Applesauce Gingerbread

2 cups unbleached flour
1½ tsp baking soda
2 tsp ground ginger
1 cup molasses
⅓ cup corn oil
1 cup applesauce
1 egg

1. Sift together the flour, baking soda, and ginger.
2. Heat together the molasses, corn oil, and applesauce just until the mixture pours easily and is well blended.
3. Add a beaten egg to the molasses mixture.
4. Combine all ingredients and stir until the batter is smooth.
5. Pour into a greased and floured 8-inch square pan and bake at 325 degrees F for 30 to 40 minutes.

IODINE

Iodine is necessary for the normal function of the thyroid gland. You need a daily intake of 150 micrograms which can be obtained from iodized salt, seafood, milk, and kelp. Certain other foods contain substances called goitrogens, which prevent the thyroid gland from utilizing the iodine to produce thyroid hormone. These include brussels sprouts, cabbage, carrots, cauliflower, kale, peaches, pears, soybeans, spinach, and turnips. If eaten in large quantities regularly, these can cause iodine deficiency. This is characterized by an enlarged thyroid gland (goiter) and sluggish metabolism tending to cause weight gain. A deficiency during pregnancy can cause fetal growth retardation and mental retardation and deficiency during childhood can cause growth stunting. Cooking goitrogen-containing foods inactivates these toxic substances to a great degree.

An overdose of iodine, which is extremely rare, causes skin lesions. This cannot occur by dietary means as you need to consume more than 2 milligrams daily. (See also KELP.)

IRON

The amount of iron in the body is proportional to the weight and gender of a person. The adult male has about 50 milligrams of iron per kilogram of body weight, or 4 grams of iron for a 175 pound man. The adult female has about 35 milligrams of iron per kilogram of body weight, or about 2 grams of iron for a 125 pound woman. About 70 percent of the total body iron is in a functional pool, 85 percent of which is in the form of hemoglobin which carries oxygen from the lungs to other tissues of the body via the bloodstream. The remaining 15 percent of the functional pool is found in metabolic enzymes, most of which are involved in energy production from fuels such as carbohydrates and fats. The other 30 percent of the total body iron is in a storage pool distributed mostly in the blood cell–forming organs (spleen and bone marrow) and stored in the liver where blood cells are destroyed after their normal lifespan and their contents, including iron, recycled for use in the rest of the body.

Iron deficiency is not readily detected in the clinical situation, because the symptoms are similar to those of other diseases. Iron deficiency is marked by fatigue, headache, pallor (paleness), and shortness of breath during mild exertion. The latter condition arises from a decreased ability of the blood to transport oxygen to the tissues. Blood tests can confirm an iron deficiency, which can be treated by iron supplements, and in more severe cases by intramuscular iron injections. Iron deficiency causes anemia, but anemias can arise from deficiencies of other nutrients, such as folacin, vitamin B_{12}, and in severe cases of vitamin B_6 (pyridoxine) and protein deficiencies. (See ANEMIAS.) Iron deficiency can arise from several factors, including decreased dietary intake, malabsorption, excessive loss due to bleeding or blood donation and with the added burden of pregnancy.

Iron is widely distributed in foods and fortification of cereals and flour has had a very positive impact on alleviating iron deficiencies in the United States and other developed countries. Liver is a rich source of iron, as are most red meats and the dark meats of poultry. Many vegetables contain iron, but the iron is not absorbed well from these sources because of phytates in the leaves of many vegetables that inhibit iron absorption. Eggs also contain iron, but they too contain substances that inhibit iron absorption. Antacids and digestive disorders which decrease stomach acid also lead to poor iron absorption. Iron deficiency seems to be on the increase in the US in recent years, because of a trend away from the cast-iron cookware toward aluminum, stainless steel, and Teflon coated utensils. Cooking foods in cast-iron cookware increases the amount of iron in the foods. Fruits and vegetables that are rich in vitamin C will aid in the absorption of iron. However, large doses of vitamin C should not be taken with iron supplements because this combination can act as a prooxidant, leading to free radical generation and tissue damage in the digestive tract.

The recommended dietary allowance (RDA) for iron varies with age and sex. Infants and children have a high demand for iron because it is an essential component of all body tissues and blood, which are ever expanding in the growing process. The RDA for infants and children is 15 milligrams from six months to three years of age, and 10 milligrams at other times through age ten. The RDA is 18 milligrams for males and females ages eleven through eighteen. The RDA for adult males is 10 milligrams and for adult females is 18 milligrams. The increased requirement for iron during pregnancy cannot be met by the iron content of most American diets, and the Food and Nutrition Board recommends the

IRON SOURCES

(each portion provides approximately 6 mg iron)

Food	Weight	Serving
Beans, kidney, cooked	240 g	1¼ cup
Beans, lima, cooked	238 g	1⅓ cup
Beef (lean only)	168 g	6 oz
Beef liver	70 g	2½ oz
Calves' liver	42 g	1½ oz
Chicken (fresh only)	364 g	13 oz
Chicken liver	70 g	2½ oz
Pork, loin (lean only)	170 g	6 oz
Sardines, Atlantic	168 g	6 oz
Tofu (soybean curd)	360 g	2½ pcs
White bread (firm crumb)	243 g	9 sl
White bread (soft crumb)	280 g	10 sl
Whole wheat bread (soft and firm crumb)	196 g	7 sl

(See VEGETARIAN DIETS for additional iron sources.)

use of a 30 to 60 milligram daily supplement for preganat and lactating women. Although iron needs during lactation are not substantially greater than those of non-pregnant females, the supplement is recommended after parturition to replenish stores that were depleted during pregnancy.

A copper-sufficient status is essential for the absorption and metabolism of iron, and several nutrient interactions that can lead to a copper deficiency may also contribute to iron deficiency. (See COPPER.) Dietary vitamin C is also essential for iron absorption, but it is recommended that large doses of these two nutrients in the form of supplements not be taken together because of undesirable effects these may have on the digestive tract. Amino acids derived from the digestion of dietary protein aid in the absorption of most minerals. For this reason, iron supplements should be taken at meal time, preferably with meals containing sufficient protein and vitamin C. Dietary fiber impedes absorption of most minerals and for this reason iron supplements, when needed, should be taken with a low-fiber meal. (See also MANGANESE.)

JUNK FOOD

In many ways the labeling of a food as "junk food" is unfortunate. It imparts a sense that the food is not good for you but does not give any indication of why. Even with this broad definition, many foods have been labeled as junk foods which when taken in moderation provide excellent nutrition. In general, junk food has been used to describe foods that are high in calories but low in, or sometimes devoid of, other nutrients. These include highly sugared foods and drinks containing little more than the sugar. A second category of foods often classified as junk food are certain fast foods which are often high in fat, calories, and salt. These foods may contain generous amounts of other nutrients and therefore may have a place in the overall diet if used in moderation and in conjunction with other foods which are low in these substances. Thus, a burger is high in fat and relatively high in calories, but it is rich in iron and zinc and certain vitamins. If you balance this with lower calorie foods rich in other nutrients and low in fat, your overall diet may be perfectly acceptable. The rule of moderation in your choices of food applies particularly well with so called junk foods. Some of them, when taken in moderation and complemented by other kinds of foods, can be a source of good nutrition. Others, while providing empty calories, can be used in small amounts without ruining your overall diet.

KELP

Kelp is a kind of seaweed used by the Japanese as a foodstuff. It is a rich source of iodine, which is needed by the thyroid gland to enable it to produce thyroid hormone to regulate the rate at which the body's various processes work. Kelp tablets, which are made from the dehydrated seaweed, are widely available and are sold in health food stores as a putative aid to dieting. Unfortunately large amounts of kelp taken over long periods (several months) can cause an underactive thyroid. This means that the body's metabolic reaction will be slowed down and a person would tend to gain weight rather than lose it. In fact iodine is sometimes used to treat hyperthyroidism (overactive thyroid) because of its slowing effect on the gland. This should only be done under strict medical supervision and you should not medicate yourself with kelp as this could permanently damage the thyroid. (See also IODINE.)

KIDNEY DISEASE

One of the major functions of the kidney is to excrete the products (usually nitrogenous products) of protein metabolism. If the kidney is badly diseased this process becomes impaired and these nitrogenous products build up in the person's blood. This can be extremely dangerous and if severe enough must be treated by kidney dialysis. The buildup of these nitrogenous products can be slowed if only very small amounts of protein are consumed. Hence, the best diet for a person suffering from chronic kidney disease is a very low protein diet in which the protein consumed is of extremely high biologic value (i.e., rich in essential amino acids). Thus the diet is essentially one in which carbohydrate and fat are consumed in large amounts and small amounts of egg white or milk proteins are used to provide the essential amino acids. (See also PROTEIN.)

KIDNEY STONES

Ninety percent of all kidney stones contain calcium. Many people produce kidney stones as a manifestation of disease elsewhere in the body. For this reason anyone who has kidney stones should be under the care of a physician. Some kidney stones occur in people who are otherwise healthy. If these stones contain calcium they may be due to the fact that too much calcium is being excreted in the urine. This can be determined, and if so, a diet which is restricted in calcium can be very effective. Such a diet, of course, avoids milk and dairy products, certain greens such as collards and turnips and certain nuts such as almonds. (See CALCIUM for a list of foods rich in calcium.)

Some kidney stones are a combination of calcium and oxalate. Certain vegetables (rhubarb, spinach, Swiss chard, and beet roots), chocolate, and tea are rich in oxalate and should be restricted for anyone who has formed calcium oxalate stones.

There are several rare types of kidney stones which require specialized fluids which can be prescribed by a physician.

LEAD

Lead is a trace element widely present in industrial societies. Ingestion of lead (by eating paint chips, chewing on batteries, etc.) can lead to lead poisoning. This serious intoxication is prevalent among disadvantaged children living under poor environmental conditions. In its most severe form it may lead to brain damage and even death. There is some evidence that a craving for eating abnormal substances (pica) is the major cause of lead poisoning. This abnormal craving has been associated with iron deficiency and some nutritionists feel that iron deficiency in some children may actually cause pica and directly contribute to lead poisoning. (See ANEMIAS and IRON.)

Lead can also be taken into the

body by breathing fumes containing this element. The use of leaded gasoline has raised lead levels in many urban areas. There is some evidence that high lead levels in the environmental air may be associated with poor pregnancy outcome.

Lead poisoning is a treatable disease and if caught in time can be cured. It is important, therefore, for any person who has been exposed to high amounts of lead to be seen by a physician. (See also CHEMICAL CONTAMINANTS IN FOODS.)

LECITHIN

Lecithin is a phospholipid, or phosphorus-containing fat, found in animal tissues. It was originally isolated from egg yolk. Lecithin and other phospholipids play a key role in the structure of all cell membranes, where they help transport fat and fat-soluble nutrients to and fro across the walls of the cells. Good food sources of lecithin include meat, fish, oatmeal, soybeans, wheat, wheat germ, wheat bran, peanuts, rice, ham, and Canadian bacon. It is also made by the liver in sufficient quantities to satisfy the body's needs. Hence it is not an essential nutrient.

Many people take large supplements of lecithin for a number of disorders. They claim that it reduces blood cholesterol levels and prevents fat from depositing on the inside of arteries and causing hardening of the arteries. No evidence has been found to corroborate this claim. It is also taken to improve memory. Acetylcholine, the neurotransmitter, or brain-chemical messenger, responsible for coding new information in the brain is made from choline, which is an integral part of lecithin. Clinical trials have failed to show any benefit from taking lecithin supplements in the vast majority of people with Alzheimer's disease.

LEUCINE

Leucine is an essential amino acid widely present in proteins from both animal and plant sources. There are no known reasons for taking leucine as a supplement since dietary leucine deficiency does not occur. The use of leucine in high doses to cure or prevent disease is unwarranted. There is no evidence that it has any use in this regard. As with any other single amino acid very high doses may cause an amino acid imbalance and therefore have the potential of being toxic. (See also AMINO ACIDS.)

LINOLEIC ACID

Fat is carried and stored within our bodies in a number of forms. One of the major forms in which fat is found is as small organic molecules known as fatty acids. Fatty acids are not only part of our fat tissue but are also structural components of all cells. Thus, fatty acids are necessary for our bodies to function and without them we could not survive. Most fatty acids can be synthesized from other compounds and therefore need not be taken directly in the diet. At least one fatty acid cannot be synthesized and must therefore be supplied in the diet. This is linoleic acid. Linoleic acid, therefore, is an essential dietary component and is sometimes called essential fatty acid, or EFA.

Only small amounts of linoleic acid are necessary to provide for the body's needs: about 1 percent of the fat that a person takes in. Even in a very low fat diet there is more than enough linoleic acid. Young infants are much more prone to a deficiency of this fatty acid than older children or adults. Breast milk and commercial infant formulas have plenty of linoleic acid. Too early use of skim milk, however, in a young infant can lead to a deficiency.

There is no evidence that quantities above the required amount offer any health benefit. Supplementation with linoleic acid in the form of pills or capsules is not necessary.

LYSINE

Lysine is one of the eight essential amino acids. Amino acids are the constituent molecules, or building blocks, of protein. The body cannot make the eight essential ones which means that they must be supplied by the diet. Cereals contain very little lysine but meats, fish, dairy products, eggs, beans, lentils, peas, soy products, and nuts are good sources of the nutrient. Every day our body is continuously replacing worn out tissues which have a high content of protein. For instance, the cells lining the digestive tract are replaced every three days. Hence it is important that foods rich in lysine be included in the diet every day. Some people advocate the use of lysine supplements in the treatment of herpes. However there is no scientific evidence available at present to support this practice. (See also AMINO ACIDS.)

MACROBIOTIC DIETS

These diets are vegetarian in nature and become progressively more and more restrictive in the kinds of vegetables and fruits which can be consumed. In their least restrictive form they will often provide all of the needed nutrients (with the exception of vitamin B_{12}) if care is taken to complement protein sources. (See VEGETARIAN DIETS.) In their most restrictive forms, when they allow only herb teas and rice, they are deficient in many nutrients and if such diets are consumed for a long period of time they can be extremely dangerous. The forms of the macrobiotic diet between these two extremes will vary as to which nutrient or nutrients may be deficient. In general, nutrients in the shortest supply are protein, iron, calcium, and vitamin B_{12}. Children consuming certain macrobiotic diets and not exposed to sunlight may develop rickets. Sometimes a simple modification of the diet can be of great benefit. For example, the person who is consuming only fruits and rice could benefit by the introduction of nuts, certain pulses, and other whole grains. Sometimes the diet is so rigid that no changes are allowed. Under these circumstances a vitamin and mineral supplement should be taken if possible. During pregnancy and lactation a rigid form of macrobiotic diet should not be practiced since it can endanger the health of the infant and the mother.

MAGNESIUM

Magnesium is used by enzymes in the body responsible for storing and releasing energy from our foods. It also plays an important role in muscle contraction and in maintaining the blood's calcium levels.

A deficiency of this mineral is rarely found in the American population because all cereals and vegetables provide a good supply. However, deficiency is sometimes seen in alcoholics, people with prolonged diarrhea, those taking diuretics, and kidney disease sufferers. Alcohol impairs magnesium absorption and the others are at risk due to excessive losses of the nutrient in the urine or stool. Symptoms associated with magnesium deficiency are depression, instability, muscle weakness, tremors, irrational behavior, and leg cramps.

The recommended dietary allowance (RDA) for magnesium is 400 milligrams. A toxic intake would be 6000 milligrams, which is unlikely unless a person takes megadose supplements or excessive amounts of magnesium-based antacids. Toxicity causes phosphorus and calcium depletion from the body and leads to drowsiness, lethargy, profuse sweating, slurring of speech, unsteadiness, diarrhea, and, rarely, paralysis. (See also CALCIUM; PHOSPHORUS.)

MANGANESE

Manganese is needed for the growth of bones and tendons. Weak bones could theoretically occur with inadequate dietary manganese, but no case has yet been reported in the medical literature. However, iron supplements decrease manganese absorption. (See IRON.) Although a recommended dietary allowance (RDA) for this element does not exist, most experts would agree that your daily intake should be about 5 milligrams. This is easily obtained from peas, beans, nuts, tea, bran, and coffee. Industrial workers have been known to inhale excessive amounts of manganese. Such workers showed a reduced ability to produce the proteins necessary for blood clotting (that is, they bled for prolonged periods whenever they cut themselves), weight loss, and slow growth of hair and nails.

MERCURY

Mercury is a heavy metal which is often found in toxic waste produced as a by-product of certain processes used in various industries. Mercury, when ingested in even small amounts, is a poison and can cause severe toxic reactions, often leading to death. The contamination of fishing areas in the ocean around areas of Japan some years ago, lead to a number of deaths of individuals consuming fish which had ingested mercury. It is, therefore, very important that any toxic jwaste material containing mercury be kept from getting into any part of our food supply. (See also CHEMICAL CONTAMINANTS IN FOODS.)

METHIONINE

Methionine is an essential amino acid belonging to a class of amino acids which contain sulfur as one of the atoms in their structural make-up. Methionine is widely distributed among proteins of animal origin but may be absent or present in only small amounts in certain plant proteins, for example, some beans. Hence, pure vegetarians must be careful to choose foods which contain methionine. There are other essential amino acids, for instance lysine, which may also be missing from certain plant foods. A simple procedure has evolved to ensure that people subsisting mainly on plant foods get adequate amounts of all of the essential amino acids. The use of corn (which is low in lysine but adequate in methionine) and beans (which are low in methionine but adequate in lysine) in the same meal is an example of complementing plant proteins to supply all of the necessary amino acids. It is no accident that Mexicans eat corn tortillas and beans or that Asian countries use rice and various beans as the staple of their diets. Without these combinations they would not survive.

Like many amino acids, methionine is thought to have special healing properties by some people and has been advocated in pill form to prevent or cure certain diseases. There is no evidence that this works; it is potentially dangerous. Methionine should be supplied by the diet. A certain amount is necessary. More is not better. (See also AMINO ACIDS; VEGETARIAN DIETS.)

MILK

The secretion of the mammary glands (milk) of a number of animals—cow, buffalo, goat, ass, mare, ewe—is used as a food in different parts of the world. The milk of each of these animals differs considerably in nutrient content. Cow milk is the most widely used and contains 3.3 percent protein, 3.6 percent fat, 4.7 percent carbohydrate; 150 calories, 8 grams protein, 11 grams fat, 291 milligrams calcium, 1 milligram iron, 7 milligrams zinc, 94 retinol equivalents vitamin A, .09 milligram thiamine, .4 milligram riboflavin, 2 milligrams niacin, 12 micrograms folacin, 2 milligrams vitamin C, 226 milligrams phosphorus, and 50 International Units vitamin D per cup. Milk is possibly the best source of dietary calcium. (See also CALCIUM.)

MINERALS

See CALCIUM, CHLORIDE, CHROMIUM, COPPER, FLUORIDE, IODINE, IRON, MAGNESIUM, MANGANESE, MOLYBDENUM, PHOSPHORUS, POTASSIUM, SELENIUM, SODIUM, SULFUR, and ZINC.

MOLYBDENUM

Molybdenum is an integral part of the enzyme xanthine oxidase which helps you metabolize xanthines found in coffee, tea, meat, and fish. No recommended dietary allowance exists for this nutrient, but experts agree that you need between .06 and .5 milligram per day. A deficiency has never been reported in people possibly because it is found in so many foodstuffs. Beans, peas, nuts, organ meats including liver, cereals, and dark green vegetables are all rich sources of this substance. Occasionally industrial accidents have led to an excessive intake of molybdenum causing sharp pains in the joints similar to those experienced in gout. Molybdenum impairs copper absorption and high intakes can lead to copper deficiency. (See COPPER.)

NIGHTSHADES

Infusions or preparations of the leaves and dried tops of nightshades are sometimes used as an aid to preventing stomach upsets. This is an extremely dangerous procedure. The nightshades, in particular belladonna, contain a substance called atropine, which is a very potent drug. Although it will reduce acid secretion in the stomach it also can cause glaucoma, reflux of the food in the stomach into the esophagus (the tube conveying food from the mouth to the stomach), an inability to urinate, prevention of stomach contractions, severe dryness of the mouth, and loss of memory.

NUTRITION AND EXERCISE

A well-balanced diet is the best diet for an athlete, and emphasizing protein to "strengthen or increase muscle" does not improve performance. In fact, an athlete only needs more energy to meet greater expenditure, which is more available in the form of carbohydrate and fat and not protein. More than 1½ to 2 grams of protein per kilogram of body weight confers no extra benefits. Taking vitamin supplements does not improve performance either.

Athletes trying to increase muscle mass, such as weight lifters or wrestlers, need to exercise the muscle more and do not need to adjust the diet, as the average American diet contains more than enough protein to provide the building material for the new muscle. Obviously, any increased energy intake will enable a person to gain weight. Fat is more calorie dense than carbohydrate and protein and so less bulk needs to be consumed to take in the same number of calories. However, a high fat intake increases the risk of heart disease and so this is not a good idea. Any form of rapid weight gain means an increase in body fat and not muscle and so it is not going to add to an athlete's strength. Patient exercising with a balanced diet is the best way to achieve the desired weight gain.

The athlete must remember to cut down on calorie intake between and after training periods. As he or she is using less energy at this time, any extra calories will simply be laid down as fat. This is why people who are active in sports in their youth, and who continue to eat the same amount when they cease to participate, become flabby in later life. Their calorie intake far exceeds their energy needs now that they are not training heavily.

Many athletes try to lose weight to achieve the ideal ratio of muscle strength to body mass. To do this they must only lose body fat. However, the quick weight loss methods often used, such as sauna baths, sweat suits, diuretics, and laxatives, simply achieve weight loss at the expense of body water. Such dehydration impairs athletic performance, as do fad diets which lead to loss of muscle, glycogen (used by the muscles for energy), bone mass, and water, all of which are necessary for optimal athletic performance. The best way for an athlete to lose weight is to cut down on calories enough to lose 2 to 3 pounds a week. Even then, if such a regime is followed for an extended period and is combined with a heavy training schedule, it can be hazardous. Hence it should not be followed for more than a few weeks at a time. Women athletes can experience menstrual irregularities and even loss of menstrual periods if they lose too much body fat. Anemia is a danger in weight-losing athletes and so iron supplements may be necessary. (See ANEMIAS.)

Muscles use carbohydrate and fat for energy. During intensive exercise they mainly use glucose which they store as glycogen. Glycogen is made up of hundreds of glucose molecules joined together in chains. When the muscles exercise this is broken down to supply glucose. The first few steps in the breakdown of glucose do not need the presence of oxygen to liberate energy. However, the partially broken down glucose accumulates as lactic acid in the muscle and causes pain and fatigue. Hence the aim of the athlete is to provide the muscle with enough oxygen to break down the glucose completely and prevent the accumulation of lactic acid. This is done by doing training exercises that condition the heart and lungs and so supply the muscles with blood that is saturated with oxygen in the most rapid and efficient way. Training exercises like running speed up breathing and heart rate and so are conditioning. Exercises like weight lifting do not help in this respect but merely strengthen the muscles.

However, no matter what the conditioning, during heavy physical exertion the heart cannot pump enough blood to the muscles to supply them with all the oxygen they need and lactic acid accumulates. There are several tricks employed by athletes to limit the accumulation of the lactic acid and the fluid that accumulates with it which help to drain it away to the liver, where it is degraded after the bout of exercise when more oxygen is available. Every opportunity is taken to relax the muscles during the event which reduces the lactic acid buildup. After an event, shaking and moving the muscles shifts the lactic acid and fluid out of the muscles and prevents the usual stiffness caused by them. After an event, breathing is more rapid, as is the heart rate which helps to get rid of these accumulated substances.

Fat can only be used during moderate exercise as it can only be broken down when there is a good supply of oxygen. This is why moderately intense activity, such as long brisk walks, is effective in burning up excess fat and acts as a useful addition to any weight loss regimen. The physically fit athlete does, however, use fat more efficiently than the "out of shape" individual. Conditioned muscles burn fat easier, which means that the muscles will go for longer before depleting their glycogen stores for energy. This confers a tremendous advantage as glycogen stores are limited. During an endurance event this means that the athlete starts using up glycogen stores further into the event and the "wall," when performance drops off, which signifies when the glycogen stores are used up, is reached at a later stage.

Once depleted, it takes forty-eight hours to restore the muscle glycogen stores to normal. If an athlete trains every day over an extended period the glycogen stores become depleted and performance falls off. Hence it is a good idea to have rest days during training. Similarly, an athlete should rest for a day or two before an event and eat a carbohydrate-rich diet.

Carbohydrate loading is a way of tricking the muscles into storing more glycogen than normal. This process involves reducing carbohydrate intake for several days by eating a diet high in protein and fat and simultaneously exercising heavily to deplete muscle glycogen. Then exercise intensity is reduced and the athlete is abruptly switched to a diet high in carbohydrate. The result is that muscle glycogen stores rebound to about two to four times the normal level and so provide a store of energy to last for a longer period than would otherwise prevail. (See The Carbohydrate-Loading Diet in EX-ERCISE.)

Recently this practice has been questioned. Glycogen is stored with considerable amounts of water. As a result, so much weight may be gained by this storage that the athlete suffers from a feeling of heaviness and stiffness. The increased weight is also believed to decrease the athlete's ability to take up oxygen. It may also impose a strain on the heart. In view of these problems, most experts agree that glycogen loading should not be used more than three times a year.

Athletes should be sure to stay in good water balance during an event. The loss of 5 percent of body water impairs performance by 20 to 30 percent. Water lost during an event should be replaced by drinking small amounts of plain water or orange juice diluted four to one with water. No more than 1 liter per hour can be absorbed by the stomach, and so no matter how much is lost, taking more than this is pointless. Although salt is lost in the perspiration during an event this need not be replaced until after the event. Even then salt tablets are unnecessary and the better way to replace the salt is by simply following the regular diet, which contains excess salt. (See also EXER-CISE.)

OBESITY

OBESITY AS A PUBLIC HEALTH PROBLEM

Obesity may be the most serious health problem in America today, 10 to 13 percent of children are overweight and 80 percent of all overweight children become overweight adults. Obesity is associated with an increased risk of heart disease by increasing the chances of an individual's being hyperlipidemic or hypertensive. The higher prevalence of hypertension, in turn, increases the risk of cerebrovascular accidents. Obesity is also associated with an increased incidence of adult-onset diabetes and with all the complications that may follow. Thus, obesity kills through its complications. It should be noted that people who are obese but who develop none of these complications do not have a reduced life expectancy. In fact, some data suggests that such people may actually live longer.

This concept that obesity kills through its complications is an important one when the public health consequences of this disease are examined. Obesity is more common in women than in men. It is particularly prevalent among poor black women. However, since the mortality from cardiovascular disease is much higher in men than in women, obesity may be a more serious disease in men. What is needed is the establishment of criteria for populations and individuals who are at risk not only for obesity but for the complications of obesity.

In addition to an increased mortality and morbidity due to its complications, obesity itself leads to considerable inconvenience within our society. The obese person leads a more difficult life. Thin is the image that Americans have adopted as chic. The fat person is afflicted with many social problems even though 20 percent of the population is overweight. It has been said that the obese may be one of the oppressed minorities in America.

Thus for both medical and social reasons, obesity represents a challenge to the health professional, a challenge that until recently has not been seriously accepted.

DEFINITION

Obesity can be defined as a relative increase in total body fat. Thus, at any given weight an individual can be obese if body fat makes up too much of the total body mass. In adults, we have used weight for height as a reasonable estimate of total body fat. In children, weight for height corrected for age has been used. The following table gives the "ideal" weight for height for adult men and women. It should be remembered that while these are good approximations for average people, there are certain important exceptions. For example,

MEN			
Height	Small Frame	Medium Frame	Large Frame
5'2"	128-134	131-141	138-150
5'3"	130-136	133-143	140-153
5'4"	132-138	135-145	142-156
5'5"	134-140	137-148	144-160
5'6"	136-142	139-151	146-164
5'7"	138-145	142-154	149-168
5'8"	140-148	145-157	152-172
5'9"	142-151	148-160	155-176
5'10"	144-154	151-163	158-180
5'11"	146-157	154-166	161-184
6'	149-160	157-170	164-188
6'1"	152-164	160-174	168-192
6'2"	155-168	164-178	172-197
6'3"	158-172	167-182	176-202
6'4"	162-176	171-187	181-207

WOMEN			
Height	Small Frame	Medium Frame	Large Frame
4'10"	102-111	109-121	118-131
4'11"	103-113	111-123	120-134
5'	104-115	113-126	122-137
5'1"	106-118	115-129	125-140
5'2"	108-121	118-132	128-143
5'3"	111-124	121-135	131-147
5'4"	114-127	124-138	134-151
5'5"	117-130	127-141	137-155
5'6"	120-133	130-144	140-159
5'7"	123-136	133-147	143-163
5'8"	126-139	136-150	146-167
5'9"	129-142	139-153	149-170
5'10"	132-145	142-156	152-173
5'11"	135-148	145-159	155-176
6'	138-151	148-162	158-179

*In indoor clothing weighing 5 lbs. for men and 3 lbs. for women; shoes with 1" heels.

Courtesy of Metropolitan Life, Health and Safety Division, New York, NY.

the athlete who weighs 240 pounds and is 6 feet 1 inch may not be obese. Much of the increased weight is due to an increase in lean body mass.

Recently, obesity has been defined at the cellular level, and by using this definition, we can distinguish at least two distinct forms of obesity. Many individuals, often those with mild or moderate obesity beginning in middle age, have an adipose tissue depot that is made up of a *normal* number of adipocytes (fat cells) each containing a very large fat droplet (type I, or hypertrophic obesity). Other individuals, often those with marked obesity and a history dating to early childhood, have an adipose tissue depot made up of *too many* adipocytes each containing a fat droplet reasonably normal in size (type II, or hyperplastic obesity).

During weight reduction, only the size of the fat cell is reduced; the number of fat cells is not affected. Hence, an obese person whose fat cells are just too large can reduce the size of each fat cell to normal and will then have adipose tissue identical in every respect to that in thin persons (type I). By contrast, an obese individual who has too many fat cells that are normal in size will have to reduce the size of those fat cells to below normal in order to maintain a normal quantity of adipose tissue. This person will still have too many fat cells (type II) and will now be in the doubly abnormal state of having too many too small fat cells. These people have a particularly difficult time maintaining the reduced body weight.

The significance of the discovery of type II (hyperplastic) obesity is that preventive measures must be taken early in life if this type of obesity is to be avoided. The evidence suggests that there are two critical periods in life when too many fat cells may develop—infancy and adolescence. Overfeeding during these critical periods may lead to a permanent abnormality with which a person must struggle throughout life—excessive numbers of fat cells.

ETIOLOGY

Recent evidence implies that obesity is a disease with multiple causes. Both genetics and environment contribute in determining the amount of body fat and the cellular make-up of the adipose depot. Animal experiments suggest that the rate of cell division within the adipose depot is to some extent under genetic control. Moreover, the cells within the adipose depot in certain genetically obese strains of rodents continue to divide long past the time when cell division has ceased in the adipose depot of lean littermates. Observations of identical human twins raised in completely different environments suggest that their body types, whether lean or fat, tend to be the same. By contrast, fraternal twins raised in different environments will tend to have different body types. Thus, a certain amount of obesity has a genetic basis, and no doubt this kind of obesity is more difficult to control. The precise incidence of this type of obesity, its cellular make-up, and just how purely it occurs is still unknown.

By far the most common type of obesity is environmentally induced; that is, more calories are consumed than expended over a variable period of time. This type of obesity may begin in mid-life when eating patterns have been established and exercise is replaced by martinis, or it may begin in early life when parents struggle to stuff their children in a well-meaning but misguided attempt to keep them healthy. The average American six-month-old is consuming 135 percent of the recommended daily amount of calories. From whatever the original food source, excess calories will be converted to fat and deposited into the adipose depot. What makes the problem much more difficult, however, is that because of individual metabolic differences what is a slight excess for one person may not be an excess for another. Minute differences in metabolic rate, in the energy used to digest food, in "activity" at rest, and in energy expenditure during exercise, when sustained over a long period of time, can account for large differences in weight be-

tween two individuals who are consuming similar amounts of calories and expending what appear to be similar amounts of energy. The observation that one person will gain weight although he or she consumes fewer calories than another who gains none is no doubt valid.

DIAGNOSIS

The diagnosis of obesity can be made with different degrees of accuracy. Is the distribution of adipose tissue and lean body mass such that there is a relatively larger proportion of fat tissue? In most adults, simply comparing weight for height is enough. In children, weight for height corrected for age is often used. As pointed out above, this method is not always correct and is most inaccurate for individuals who are only slightly obese, the very individual in whom the diagnosis may be most difficult to make. Recently, the use of skinfold calipers has become more prevalent in the diagnosis of obesity. With proper use of these instruments a precise diagnosis can usually be made. Recent evidence suggests that in experienced hands, measurement of triceps and subscapular fatfold thickness is as accurate a method for determining total body fat as the methods of determining total body water or potassium.

Once obesity has been diagnosed, the type of obesity can be ascertained. While precise diagnosis of type I or type II obesity requires an adipose tissue biopsy, a good approximation can be obtained from the history. Although not all childhood obesity is hyperplastic, most individuals with hyperplastic obesity will have a history of obesity since childhood. Although not all severe obesity is hyperplastic, most individuals with hyperplastic obesity are severely obese. Hence, a severely obese individual with a clear history of obesity since childhood is potentially an individual with hyperplastic obesity.

The diagnosis of genetic obesity is at best very difficult and may not be possible except in extraordinary situations. We know that if one parent is obese there is a 40 percent chance that the child will be obese. If both parents are obese, the chance increases to 80 percent. We know that fat women are more likely to marry fat men and vice versa. Although this might suggest genetic influences that can be historically traced, environmental explanations may be equally applicable. Simply stated, obese parents may overfeed their children and this tendency to overfeed may be greater if both parents are obese. There is strong evidence that such environmental pressures do occur in these types of families. Hence, whether a strong family history implies a genetic etiology remains an open question. Re-

gardless of the cause, however, a family history of obesity must immediately alert the parents to the fact that their child is particularly at risk. Since there is little that can be done about the genetic problem, attempts to control the "energy environment" should be made.

CONTROL OF OBESITY

Prevention. Obesity often begins subtly with very slight increases in weight over relatively long periods of time. There are certain signs which should alert an individual to the possibility of becoming obese. Below is a list of several signs that are helpful in determining the likelihood that obesity may develop.

Risk Factors for Obesity

Family history of obesity
Obesity present in childhood
Change in life-style, such as, a more sedentary occupation, increased consumption of alcohol, change in patterns of meal consumption
Major family or personal crisis

The prevention of childhood and adolescent obesity may be the key to controlling its most malignant form—hyperplastic obesity. Since fat cell number is determined during these periods, any tendency to obesity at these times of life should be vigorously resisted. Parents should be alert to the dangers to their children and should feed their children a balanced diet, restricted in calories, which maintains growth but prevents obesity. During adolescence the problem is more difficult because the eating patterns of adolescents are sometimes unconventional and often difficult to change. Parents should work with the adolescent to develop an acceptable diet that fits within the adolescent life-style and controls calories sufficiently to control weight gain and still permit the adolescent growth spurt. Although this sounds complicated, it is really quite simple. It requires a moderate restriction of calories—70 to 80 percent of the recommended daily allowance for an adolescent of that sex and height—and meticulous attention to providing adequate amounts of such essential nutrients as iron. If caloric restriction cannot be achieved without compromising other nutrients, then supplements should be given during this period of life.

Obesity often begins to develop in early middle age; in men after they settle into a job (often in an office) and begin to raise a family, in women often after the birth of the first or second child. People who have a family history of obesity or who have been obese during childhood are especially at risk. Changes in life-style, such as the acquisition of a more sedentary job, an increase in the con-

sumption of alcohol, eating more in restaurants—especially fast-food chains—and major family crises are also danger signs.

Women should try to revert to their prepregnancy weight after childbirth. There is evidence that, besides its advantages to the infant, breast-feeding can help a mother resume her prepregnancy weight more efficiently than bottle-feeding. If the mother has a tendency to obesity or is not losing weight after her delivery, mild caloric restriction that provides adequate amounts of essential nutrients will often be effective. If the problem of postpartum obesity in women and "middle-age spread" in men can be prevented, many people might be spared a life of constant dieting.

Treatment of Obesity. The moderately obese person has a potentially serious problem and should try to lose weight. The person who is grossly obese is suffering from a disease that may lead to life-threatening complications. Such an individual should be under the care of a physician. Both the physician and the patient must understand that losing weight and keeping it off is at best a difficult task; the patient must know what to expect and must understand that there will be periods of disappointment. But she or he must also realize how important it is that the weight loss be maintained. The physician should help the patient set realistic goals. These goals depend in part on the nature and severity of the obesity and whether complications are present. Hence the goal will vary with the individual and the exact nature of the problem. The 350 pound person who has been obese from childhood is unlikely to be able to attain a weight of 150 to 175 pounds and to maintain that weight for life. Such a person is likely to have a hyperplastic adipose depot and therefore will never be able to achieve normal weight with adipocytes of normal size and number. Therefore a more moderate goal should be set. It may be better for this person to get down to 250 pounds and remain at that weight.

Almost every mode of therapy employed in medical practice, and many not usually employed, have been tried in treating obesity. Controlling caloric intake and expenditure has always been, and still remains, the mainstay of therapy.

All of the various diet plans, when they work, owe their success to the establishment of an overall negative caloric balance. The success of one diet plan over another depends entirely on the motivation of the person to try and to maintain one type of regimen rather than another. Regardless of its claims, there is no evidence that any diet that works does so by any mechanism other than caloric reduction. However, since millions of people are constantly experimenting with one diet or another, the next section will be devoted to an evaluation of the various types of diets currently in use.

Recently, it has been recognized that since obesity often results from a change in life-style, redirecting the individual's life-style by behavior modification in such a way as to reduce caloric intake and increase energy expenditure often results in lasting weight reduction. Behavior modification, especially in a group setting, has been very effective. This approach, in an abridged fashion, is probably the major reason for the success of Weight Watchers. There are a number of competent psychiatrists and psychologists employing these techniques, and clinics are being established using the same principles. Fundamentally what is done is that people are made aware of those habits peculiar to themselves which lead to overeating. Often participants do this by keeping a diary, which is then examined in detail by themselves, their peers, and the therapist. A plan is evolved by which behavior patterns are changed gradually in a manner acceptable to the person and consistent with the goal of reducing caloric intake. For example, if the person watches the Monday night football game and consumes 2 pounds of peanuts and 4 bottles of beer, the substitution of a bowl of fruit and light beer or iced tea or coffee can save hundreds of calories. The person may not have realized what he or she was doing and the change might be readily accepted. Several distinct changes such as this can result in reduction in caloric intake in excess of 1000 calories per day and over time may establish a pattern of living that is compatible with a stable reduced weight.

Exercise has been receiving more and more attention as a method of weight reduction. While increasing exercise as a way of expending calories is an excellent adjunct to dietary management, it is in itself not a definitive treatment. Exercise is much more important in prevention and maintenance than in weight reduction. The type of exercise is very important. Dynamic exercises, such as swimming, cycling, walking, and jogging are much better than static exercises, such as weight lifting, pushups, situps, etc. (See EXERCISE for table of the caloric expenditure of various forms of exercise.)

Almost every type of drug has been tried in the treatment of obesity. Appetite depressants, metabolic stimulants, amphetamines, and hormones each has had its vogue. Some still have their advocates. None works in the long run; all have side effects, some serious. For this reason, they should not be used in the management of obesity.

Surgical therapy has also been used. The current surgical procedure is intestinal bypass. This procedure produces severe side effects. Long-term follow-up experience has for the most part been poor. In our judgment, there is almost no indication for this operation. Other operations, such as wiring the mouth or teeth, have been used in the past; none has had any good long-term results.

Thus, there is not an easy approach to the treatment of obesity. Dietary therapy is still the best approach. Unfortunately, there is no easy way to diet. The reason fad diets come and go is that although they are easy for some patients to use in initial weight loss, they cannot be indefinitely maintained, and hence they ultimately fail. The best diet is one that will allow the person to eat as normally as possible and yet reduce his or her caloric intake. A number of these are available.

DIETARY MANAGEMENT OF OBESITY

The cornerstone of any obesity regimen is the diet. Any successful diet must ultimately result in a reduced intake of calories. The reduction can be achieved either by limiting the quantity of food or by altering the quality of the overall diet so that the individual foods are lower in calories. Since all three macronutrients, fat, carbohydrate, and protein, can be burned as energy or converted to adipose tissue, any calorie, regardless of its source, is potentially fat tissue. When caloric intake is reduced to a level below caloric expenditure, body fat begins to break down to make up the deficit. Fat is never burned exclusively; carbohydrate stores (in the form of glycogen) and tissue protein (lean body mass) are also consumed. The premise under which many of the unusual diets operate is that one can increase the rate of adipose tissue breakdown while decreasing or sparing the loss of lean body mass. If this were true, certainly the diet that accomplished it would be useful. However, there is no evidence that there is any significant difference between high-carbohydrate and low-carbohydrate, high-fat and low-fat, high-protein and low-protein diets when compared on a calorie for calorie basis. And yet, each week a new diet becomes the rage. Atkins or Stillman, high carbohydrate or low carbohydrate, high protein, protein powder, or hydrolyzed protein, high alcohol, and Scarsdale. Many of these diets will result in weight loss, sometimes even rapid weight loss. The reason, however, is that the intake of calories is reduced, sometimes because the diet itself limits calories (Scarsdale) and sometimes because the very nature of the diet results in a reduction of food intake (Atkins or "grapefruit"). Some of these diets can be dangerous, especially if sustained for a long time. In addition, all of these diets suffer from the same

primary problem—the weight lost is usually rapidly regained when the individual is finished dieting and returns to previous eating habits.

Unusual or "fad" diets can be separated into two major groups—those which limit calories and those which allow unlimited calories. The first group cuts out all foods high in calories but permits the person to eat as much as he or she wants of whatever is left. If the permissible foods supply adequate amounts of the essential nutrients, these diets are all usable and, depending on palatability, variety, and personal preferences, will have varied success. Many of these diets, however, are so constructed that the "forbidden lists" prevent the person from consuming adequate amounts of both macronutrients and micronutrients.

The popular Scarsdale diet is an example of the low calorie approach. The menu is rigidly set forth. It is calculated to provide 1200 to 1500 calories per day. Almost all carbohydrate and significant amounts of fat are forbidden. Hence, it is a relatively high protein diet. The diet is such that iron, unless consumed in fortified foods, is at best marginal. Calcium requirements are also not adequately met on this diet. Hence the diet, though effective and reasonably safe over a short period, must be monitored.

The second group of diets is represented by the Stillman diet, which consists almost solely of protein, or the Atkins diet, which consists of both protein and fat. Both restrict carbohydrates severely. Stillman tells you to "eat as much of the protein food as you want without stuffing yourself." Atkins presents his diet as a revolution and markets it as the "high calorie way to stay thin forever." Both of these diets are unbalanced and extremely high in protein, presenting a heavy nitrogen load to the kidney. In addition, the Atkins diet encourages the consumption of large amounts of saturated fat and cholesterol. A diet high in saturated fat should be avoided in general and should be avoided particularly by people with high blood lipid levels or with a history of cardiovascular disease. Moreover this high fat intake, combined with the reduced intake of carbohydrate, inevitably leads to the formation of certain chemicals in the blood called ketones (ketosis). Ketosis in itself can be troublesome in many people, producing headache, nausea, and vomiting. In certain people, ketosis may be extremely dangerous. For example, ketosis during early pregnancy may result in fetal damage.

Some people lose weight on these diets. Despite the fact that one is allowed to eat unlimited amounts of the permitted foods, many find they simply cannot tolerate large quantities of such foods. Hence, in reality, they are limiting their calories. In the long run, people find that they cannot maintain such an unbalanced diet for long and sooner or later they return to previous eating patterns and inevitably regain weight.

The dietary approach that is likely to produce the greatest long-term success is one which sets attainable goals, restricts calories, is nutritionally sound, and supplies the greatest variety of choices. Such a regimen requires patience and determination. The person should learn

---

FOOD CATEGORIES FOR CONSTRUCTING A LOW-CALORIE DIET

1.	Free foods	lettuce, parsley, pickles, coffee, tea, bouillon
2.	Vegetables	almost all green and yellow vegetables
3.	Fruits	almost all fruits, dried fruits, berries, melons in prescribed amounts
4.	Starch	breads, rolls, crackers, starch, vegetables, cereals, alcohol
5.	Meat	beef, veal, lamb, pork, cheese, poultry, fish, seafood
6.	Milk	buttermilk, yogurt, skim milk
7.	Fats	creams, butter, certain meats, dressings

the caloric content of foods and how calories are converted to fat. For example, 1 pound of fat represents 3500 calories. Therefore, a reduction of 500 calories per day should result in weight loss of approximately 1 pound per week. Most adults will lose weight on a calorie intake ranging from 1000 to 1800 calories per day. This can be started immediately and will provide good nutrition and adequate variety. An abbreviated list of Food Categories for Constructing a Low-Calorie Diet is on page 235. (See the Exchange Lists in DIABETES for more complete lists of foods in various categories.) Pick a number of foods from each category depending on the number of calories prescribed. The Sample Menu on page 122 shows how this might be done for a person consuming 1500 calories.

The following rules may help reducers avoid some of the common problems of dieting.

1. Do not be discouraged when the rapid initial weight loss begins to taper off as dieting proceeds.
2. Eat smaller portions five times a day instead of larger ones three times a day.
3. Use a smaller plate so smaller portions do not look too small.
4. Allow yourself a treat once a day.
5. Do not be fooled by high-calorie "health food" snacks. Some of these snacks are just as high in calories as a chocolate bar.

6. Avoid cold cuts, since these are usually very high in fat.

Keep in mind that dieting and weight maintenance are lifelong processes. Other factors, such as regular exercise, play a part in weight maintenance, but for the moderately and severely obese, long-term dietary regulation is mandatory. Evidence shows that the body resists changes in weight. This phenomenon is known as the set point. If you have been fifty pounds overweight for a few months, the initial rate of weight loss when you go on a diet may be slow. Your body uses food more efficiently and needs up to 30% less energy to stay at the same weight. Conversely, if you have been underweight you have to eat more than the calories needed to gain the weight you want, because the body uses food inefficiently and burns it to produce heat.

Studies show that people who repeatedly go on and off diets find it increasingly difficult to lose weight. This may be because the body becomes more efficient each time and eventually remains at peak efficiency. This could mean that after repeated diets a dieter who experienced weight loss on 1200 calories a day may need to restrict caloric intake to 800 to have the same weight loss. (See also ARTERIOSCLEROSIS; DIABETES; HYPERTENSION; REDUCING DIETS.)

OSTEOPOROSIS

Each year more than 500,000 American women progress to a state which can be called osteoporosis; 200,000 osteoporotic women over the age of forty-five fracture one or more bones; 40,000 die of complications which follow their injuries; and thousands of others are disabled, many seriously, for the rest of their lives. Osteoporosis and its complications is the twelfth most common cause of death in the United States and in women it must be considered a major killer disease. The disease has no single course and is associated with a number of risk factors. Some of these factors are easy to control and so the risk can be modified. Proper diet and certain types of exercise are two major ways in which the risk may be reduced.

THE NATURE OF OSTEOPOROSIS

The hard substance of bone is made mostly from calcium and phosphorus. This substance is called hydroxyapatite and is constantly remodeling. Calcium and phosphorus move freely from the blood into the bone and from the bone into the blood. When new bone is being made, more of these minerals pass into the bone. When bone tissue is being destroyed, more of these minerals move out of the bone.

Maintaining the structural integrity of bone is only one of the important functions of calcium. This mineral is essential for the proper working of every cell in the body. For instance, without calcium nerve cells cannot conduct impulses and muscle cells cannot contract. Ninety-nine percent of body calcium is found in bone and the remaining 1 percent circulates in the blood or is present in the other tissues. If insufficient calcium is available for the tissues from the diet it will slowly be withdrawn from the bones. The more calcium that is withdrawn, the thinner the bones will become. Eventually, they become so thin that they fracture easily. When the bones get into this state a person is said to be suffering from osteoporosis, or brittle bones.

The amount of calcium absorbed by the body is rigidly controlled by dihydroxy-vitamin D, a hormone made in the kidneys from the vitamin D in the diet. If the level of calcium should fall below a critical point parathyroid hormone is secreted by the four parathyroid glands at the base of the thyroid gland, which raises the level of calcium in the blood. It does this by signaling the kidneys to convert vitamin D to its active form, thereby increasing calcium absorption and stimulating the breakdown of bone to release its calcium into the bloodstream. To protect against too much calcium being withdrawn from bone the body uses another hormone, calcitonin, which is made in the thyroid gland. This inhibits the action of osteoclasts, which are the bone cells that break bone down. By the use of these three hormones to regulate calcium metabolism, the calcium level in the blood never gets too high or too low.

Other hormones within the body play an important role in determining whether bone loss will occur. These hormones are not directly involved in the regulation of blood calcium but still have a major effect on the body's calcium status. The most important of these is the female sex hormone estrogen. Estrogen is a bone-protecting hormone, and yet, it does not have any activity on bone itself. Estrogen works indirectly by blocking the action of parathyroid hormone. Thus, when estrogen is present greater amounts of parathyroid hormone are necessary in order to cause bone resorption and the release of calcium from bone to the blood. If estrogen is not present, the brake is released and even small amounts of parathyroid hormone will release large quantities of calcium from the bones. When the fine tuning of the calcium-regulating mech-

anism is upset, more calcium gets into the blood than is needed and the excess spills out into the urine and is lost to the body. In addition, estrogen stimulates the secretion of calcitonin and so when estrogen levels are low, calcitonin levels tend to be low and bone resorption tends to increase.

Finally, recent evidence suggests that high levels of estrogen (like those occurring during pregnancy) stimulate the conversion of vitamin D to its active form in the kidneys, thereby increasing the amount of calcium absorbed and available for deposition into the bones. Thus, the absence of estrogen will produce an imbalance between the bone-resorbing parathyroid hormone and the bone-protecting calcitonin hormone, favoring the former. As a result, calcium will be lost from the bones and excreted in the urine. In addition, the one hormone which might reverse this situation, dihydroxy-vitamin D, may not be so efficiently made in the absence of estrogen. It is no wonder, then, that the state of menopause, where estrogen levels fall sharply, is a key event in the development of osteoporosis in women.

Another group of hormones affecting bone metabolism are the adrenocortical hormones. These hormones directly affect bone tissue, causing resorption. Both estrogen and progesterone prevent the action of adrenal hormones on bone tissue.

Thus menopause, when both of these sex hormones decline, allows the adrenal hormones free license to cause a breakdown of bone. Two other hormones also affect bone. Growth hormone from the pituitary gland promotes the growth of all tissues including bone, while thyroid hormone promotes bone resorption.

So, as you can see, bone tissue is under a variety of hormonal influences within the body. When these groups of hormones are in balance bone growth and bone loss are equal. You are then said to be in calcium balance and your bone mass does not change. If those hormones involved in bone growth predominate, bone mass will increase. If those hormones involved in bone loss predominate, bone mass will decrease. Anything which promotes the action or maximizes the effect of the first group of hormones will lower your risk of developing osteoporosis. Anything which promotes the activity or maximizes the effect of the second group of hormones will raise your risk for developing osteoporosis.

During infancy and early childhood the bone growth hormones predominate and calcium is deposited into the growing bones. When puberty occurs estrogen and progesterone levels increase sharply, further promoting bone growth. During pregnancy, levels of estrogen and progesterone again rise promoting bone growth in the mother and fetus.

In addition, more dihydroxy-vitamin D is made during pregnancy by the placenta, further promoting bone growth. If the mother nurses her infant, the levels of estrogen remain high and bone growth is stable. A few years prior to menopause, progesterone levels begin to fall and the balance tips in favor of the bone-loss hormones. At menopause estrogen levels fall dramatically and the bone-loss hormones become even more dominant. The result is that bone is rapidly resorbed. At around age sixty-five adrenal-cortical activity lessens and the levels of adrenal steroids like cortisone drop. This reduces the imbalance and bone loss slows down.

The best way to minimize the risk for developing osteoporosis is to take advantage of the periods when the hormonal balance favors bone growth. Thus, a woman should do whatever is possible during her childhood and childbearing years to promote maximum bone growth. In this regard both diet and exercise can be wisely used to increase bone mass.

If a woman has been confined in bed for long periods of time or has spent a significant amount of time in a wheelchair, she is at increased risk for osteoporosis. Leading a sedentary life also increases the risk for osteoporosis. Exercise which emphasizes weight-bearing on the bones is beneficial for several reasons. First, exercise will place actual physical stress on the bones. As a result, the bones respond by becoming bigger and stronger. Second, exercise will increase the flow of blood to the bones thereby increasing the availability of bone-building nutrients. Third, exercise generates mini–electrical currents within the bones which stimulate bone growth. And fourth, exercise alters the hormonal balance favoring those hormones which protect the bones. It is important to note that the type of exercise which produces these results consists of maneuvers which put stress on the bones. Walk-

---

OSTEOPOROSIS—WHO IS AT RISK?

Risk Factor

Sex	Women are ten times more likely to suffer from severe osteoporosis than men.
Menopause	The earlier menopause occurs the greater the risk. Twenty-five percent of women undergoing natural menopause exhibit osteoporosis in later life; 50 percent of women having their ovaries removed before natural menopause develop osteoporosis.
Family history	The greater the history of fractures among elderly relatives, especially of the hip and vertebrae, the greater the risk.
Ethnic background	Those of British, Northern European, Chinese, or Japanese extraction are at the highest risk. Jewish women are at moderate risk and black women are at low risk.
Body build	The smaller the build, the greater the risk.
Body weight	The thinner the person, the higher the risk.
Oral contraceptives	Lower the risk.
Pregnancy	Women who have never been pregnant have an increased risk.
Smoking	Increases the risk.
Alcoholism	Increases the risk.
Cortisone	Increases the risk.
Anticonvulsants	Increases the risk.
Antacids	Antacids containing aluminum increase the risk.
Illness	Hyperparathyroidism, hyperthyroidism, Cushing's syndrome, diabetes, rheumatoid arthritis, kidney disease, and gastrointestinal problems that impair absorption all increase the risk.

ing, jogging, cycling, gymnastics, basketball, and tennis all fit the bill. Swimming, an excellent exercise for cardiovascular fitness, is a poor exercise for lowering the risk of osteoporosis.

But even more important than undertaking a specific exercise program is maintaining an active lifestyle. Walking rather than driving, climbing stairs instead of taking elevators, standing rather than sitting; these simple adjustments in life-style can significantly lower the chance of developing osteoporosis.

As shown in the Dietary Guidelines in this section, a diet which is deficient in calcium will promote bone loss. Not only is the amount of calcium in the diet important but so is the amount that can actually be absorbed from the gastrointestinal tract. Certain elements in the diet promote calcium absorption and therefore indirectly promote bone growth. Other elements in the diet inhibit calcium absorption and therefore promote bone loss. Other external factors influencing calcium balance and hence the risk for osteoporosis are listed in the table opposite.

DIETARY GUIDELINES

There are a number of dietary factors which can contribute to the development of osteoporosis. First, and most important, is a deficiency of calcium.

There are periods in life when calcium deficiency is more dangerous than at other times. The early growing years, particularly during infancy, are very important. Bone is being produced at a rapid rate and the hormonal balance is favoring bone growth. The reserves are already being built up for later life. If the diet is deficient in calcium at this time or if calcium cannot be absorbed properly the impaired bone growth which may result can never be made up. This is one reason why breast milk is the best food for a young infant. The calcium found in breast milk is much better absorbed by the human infant than the calcium found in cow milk. For mothers who do not or cannot breast-feed, an infant formula which simulates breast milk as closely as possible is preferred for the greater part of the first year of life, to ensure maximum calcium absorption.

Adolescence is another time when an inadequate calcium intake can be very dangerous from the standpoint of developing osteoporosis in later life. The adolescent is undergoing the most rapid rate of bone growth that will occur during any period of life. Unfortunately, many adolescents have eating habits which tend to promote calcium deficiency. Some just eat foods that are low in calcium or high in phosphorus (which interferes with calcium absorption). Others are dieting so rigidly they are simply not taking in enough food to supply their calcium needs, and an ever-increasing number are carrying this to such extremes they can be classified as suffering from anorexia nervosa. Obviously, any adolescent girl suffering from this disease has significantly increased her risk for osteoporosis.

Pregnancy is another period when insufficient intake of calcium can lead to a reduction in bone mass. The fetal skeleton is rapidly consuming calcium and, although the mother's body is in a hormonal state which favors bone growth, adequate calcium must be available or the maternal bones will be the fetus' only source of this mineral. If forced, fetal bone growth will take place at the expense of maternal bone mass. The saying "for every child a tooth" is equally applicable to your bones if during pregnancy you do not get enough calcium. However, it need not be that way. A diet which is adequate in calcium will not only supply enough for your fetus but will also allow your own bones to increase their mass.

If you nurse your infant, your milk will have to supply large amounts of calcium. If dietary calcium is inadequate during this period your bones will supply the calcium. Thus, lactation is a critical period when a lack of calcium in your diet can erode your bones. But, as with pregnancy,

the opposite will occur if enough calcium is available. Your body's hormones now favor bone growth and even with the calcium drain produced by your hungry infant you can finish nursing with an increase in bone mass.

Even at other times of life, severe calcium deficiency can result in significant bone loss. Several constituents of your diet besides calcium itself will affect the amount of calcium you absorb. The principles of a diet designed to lower your risk for osteoporosis include:

- adequate calories to attain and/or maintain ideal weight
- a calcium intake of 1 gram (1000 milligrams) per day (1500 milligrams during periods of high calcium need such as adolescence, pregnancy, and lactation)
- a relatively low phosphorus intake
- a relatively low protein intake
- avoidance of excess dietary sodium
- adequate but not excessive amounts of vitamin D (not over 400 IU)

Calories. Calories are important for two reasons. If a person is too thin the risk of osteoporosis is increased and, in addition, if a woman is consuming very few calories she is unlikely to be able to fulfill her calcium requirement.

Women who are constantly consuming under 1500 calories per

day to maintain their cosmetic appearance, which often means they are 10 or 20 percent below their ideal weight, are endangering their bones. We often hear about the problems of being overweight and assume that the thinner we are the better. Clearly this is not true if a person is at high risk for osteoporosis. Too thin may be just as much of a health risk as too fat.

A person who is truly obese and at the same time at increased risk for osteoporosis should avoid crash dieting or the use of fad diets—they are often very low in calcium. Foods should be emphasized that are of a high nutrient density with specific attention to calcium. Foods should be chosen with a low calorie and high calcium content. For example, skim milk is much better than whole milk; low-fat yogurt is better than sour cream; cottage cheese is preferable to cream cheese. Finally, attainable goals should be set which can be met and maintained without constantly restricting calories to unrealistically low amounts. (See OBESITY.) A woman who is overweight but out of the danger zone will have reduced her risk for the complications of obesity and at the same time will reap at least one benefit of being slightly overweight. Her risk of developing osteoporosis will be reduced, as it seems that the fat tissue in postmenopausal women can make small amounts of estrogen. The added

weight also exerts more stress on the bones and so reduces calcium resorption.

Dietary Calcium. The recommended dietary allowance for calcium is 800 milligrams per day for an adult woman and 1200 milligrams per day during periods of increased calcium demand. We have set the amounts slightly higher because women who are at risk for osteoporosis are often beginning with a deficit. These levels, however, are attainable by eating a proper diet. (See CALCIUM for a list of foods rich in calcium.)

Most of the high calcium foods fall into the category of dairy products—Americans normally get about 80 percent of their calcium from dairy products. However, by making careful choices, it is possible to get the required amount of calcium with a much lower percentage coming from milk and milk products. For example, a daily menu which includes single portions of any two of the following will supply more than half of the calcium requirement: almonds, broccoli, canned fish (with bones), kelp, tofu, tortillas, kale, turnips or collard greens, macaroni and cheese, pizza, beef tacos, and cheese or meat enchiladas. Although the rest of the diet will supply some calcium it will still be necessary to include some dairy foods to reach the requirement. If dairy foods are not tolerated a calcium supplement should be taken. (See CALCIUM.)

Dietary Phosphorus. A diet high in phosphorus will inhibit adequate calcium absorption and thereby effectively reduce the amount of calcium getting into the body. For optimal calcium absorption one should strive for a dietary pattern that supplies twice as much calcium as phosphorus. The major sources of phosphorus in the diet are particularly red meats, and for some people carbonated soft drinks. In addition, these foods contain little calcium. Thus, the calcium/phosphorus ratio, which should be 2:1, is very low. Foods such as beef liver, bologna, fried chicken, corn on the cob, frankfurters, ground beef, ham, lamb chops, and pork chops have a calcium/phosphorus ratio from 1:15 to 1:45 which is very bad for calcium intake. Some of the phosphorylated soft drinks contain almost no calcium at all. By contrast, many of the green leafy vegetables such as spinach and lettuce have more calcium than phosphorus and hence favor calcium absorption. Dairy products which are high in calcium also contain significant amounts of phosphorus and so the calcium absorption from these foods is not so good as from some of the plant foods. From a practical standpoint what this means is that a diet designed to lower your risk for osteoporosis should not only be high in calcium but should also be low in phosphorus.

In addition to the overall content of calcium and phosphorus in the diet, the time in which these two nutrients are consumed in relation to each other is very important. Because these nutrients compete with each other for absorption, the more the intake of these two minerals is separated the better. (Those meals which emphasize calcium-rich foods are better if they avoid phosphorus-rich foods). Thus, calcium from the sour cream in the baked-potato-and-steak meal is not absorbed so well as from the late-evening-ice-cream snack. A good idea is to emphasize calcium in snack foods, which are often taken by themselves. (See PHOSPHORUS.)

Protein. The very high protein diet consumed by most Americans will result in more calcium being excreted in the urine than occurs in people who consume less protein. Like phosphorus, the main source of dietary protein is meat. The more meat a person eats the more calcium will be lost, and so the greater the risk for osteoporosis. This does not mean that meat must be eliminated from a diet designed to lower the risk for osteoporosis. However, meat consumption should be limited to one meal a day; portion size should also be reduced. Remember—if dairy products are being used to supply dietary calcium they also contain significant amounts of protein and hence there is no need to worry about protein deficiency.

Vegetarians, particularly ovo-lacto vegetarians, have a lower incidence of osteoporosis than meat-eaters. This is probably because of the lower protein and phosphorus content of their diets. A well-balanced vegetarian diet that allows milk and milk products is probably the best diet for the prevention of osteoporosis. The closer we all come to eating such a diet, the better. A pure vegetarian or vegan diet can prove to be a problem unless attention is paid to the nondairy sources of calcium. Such a diet has the advantage of good calcium absorption and low calcium excretion and hence the actual calcium requirement on such a diet is generally less than on the typical American diet. However, even with these factors in the favor of calcium absorption, if a woman's risk for osteoporosis is high, she must pay special attention to her calcium intake. Diets which claim to be variations of vegetarianism but which are much more restrictive, for instance, macrobiotic diets, will increase the risk of osteoporosis. They will be too low in calcium to supply the body's needs. (See PROTEIN.)

Sodium. A very high sodium intake will force the kidneys to excrete more sodium. In the process of excreting this excess sodium the kidneys will also excrete calcium. A low sodium diet need not be followed to protect the bones from osteoporosis, but a "salt-aholic" should cut back. A mild sodium-restricted diet is a good place to start. This is where one simply reduces the amount of table salt used. No salt is added at the table, but up to one teaspoon can be added per day during cooking. In addition, pickled foods and extremely salty foods should be eliminated. (See SALT; SODIUM.)

Vitamin D. Most American diets, particularly those which are adequate in calcium, will be adequate in vitamin D. Thus, a diet for preventing osteoporosis should always be adequate in this important vitamin. However, we get most of our dietary vitamin D from dairy products made from milk which has been fortified. In the case of milk intolerance, other foods which have been fortified must be emphasized in the diet, or a supplement taken. Remember—vitamin D in excess amounts can be very dangerous and since it is stored in the body its effects can be cumulative. Supplements should never contain more than the recommended dietary allowance (400 IU). (See VITAMIN D.)

(See also AGING; CALCIUM; PREGNANCY; WOMEN.)

PANTOTHENIC ACID

Pantothenic acid is one of the B vitamins. It is an essential part of coenzyme A which plays a critical role in our ability to derive energy from the food we eat and helps us make fats which are an integral part of all cell membranes. The vitamin was discovered by Dr. Roger Williams in 1933. A daily intake of 5 to 10 milligrams satisfies the needs of adults and 10 milligrams is ideal for pregnant and nursing mothers. Good food sources of the vitamin include beans, meat, broccoli, dairy products, eggs, cereals, mushrooms, fish, oranges, brewer's yeast, and nuts. Less good sources are all cuts of chicken, lamb, dried beans, lentils, and beans.

Because of the large variety of foods containing the vitamin, pantothenic acid deficiency is rare. Chronic alcoholics who often have a multiple B vitamin deficiency state are the highest risk group for this deficiency. Deficiency symptoms include malaise, stomach ache, vomiting, leg cramps, nausea, reduced resistance to disease, fatigue, sleeplessness, pins and needles, and numbness in the hands. No human toxicity has been reported in people taking as much as 7 grams a day. However, there is absolutely no discernible benefit to taking pantothenic acid supplements. The vitamin will not prevent graying of the hair or prevent or cure diseases. (See also VITAMINS.)

PAPAIN

Papain is a protein-digesting enzyme extracted from papaya. It is used in medical research to break down proteins in test tubes under controlled conditions. However, when taken by humans as an aid to digestion it serves no purpose whatsoever. This is because the enzyme is broken down and inactivated in the stomach before it has a chance to work. (See also ENZYMES.)

PARENTERAL NUTRITION

In the past the only way for a person to be nourished was through the gastrointestinal tract. Thus if severe disease was present or if a large segment of the gastrointestinal tract had to be removed, the patient could not be fed and death from starvation ensued. In the middle 1960s a method became available for providing complete nutrition directly into the bloodstream. Today carbohydrate in the form of glucose, protein in the form of amino acids, and fat in a special emulsion can all be delivered in sufficient amounts to keep a person in energy balance and to supply the necessary building blocks for protein metabolism. In addition, all of the known vitamins and minerals can be administered in pure form directly into the bloodstream.

The availability of total parenteral nutrition has radically changed many aspects of medical practice. Patients can be kept in a well nourished condition prior to and after surgery without using the gastrointestinal tract. Patients with severe disease of the gastrointestinal tract have been maintained on total parenteral nutrition for years. They are able to live relatively normal lives at home and to administer the necessary solutions themselves (usually before and during sleep at night).

Obviously total parenteral nutrition must be initiated by, and constantly managed by, a team of physicians and other professionals specially trained in this technique. (See also ENTERAL NUTRITION.)

PHENYLALANINE

Phenylalanine is an essential amino acid and as such is present in all complete proteins. Phenylalanine is converted by the body into another amino acid, tyrosine. Both of these amino acids are necessary for proper body function and for adequate growth and development. There is a serious and, fortunately, rare condition called phenylketonuria (PKU) in which the body cannot make this conversion. The result is an accumulation of large amounts of phenylalanine in the blood and a deficiency of tyrosine. The high levels of phenylalanine can be toxic to the developing brain. Hence, children with this genetic disease must be maintained on diets very low in phenylalanine. Such diets are very difficult to construct and maintain and therefore should be consumed under the careful supervision of a physician. Phenylalanine has been advocated by some as a useful supplement for preventing or treating a variety of diseases. There is no evidence for these claims. Phenylalanine is also found in the artificial sweetener aspartame. Therefore, any person with PKU would not use any products containing aspartame. (See also AMINO ACIDS; ASPARTAME.)

PHOSPHORUS

Phosphorus combined with calcium helps build strong bones and teeth. In addition, it is also needed by many enzymes (catalysts) in the body that liberate the energy from our food and store it in the body as glycogen or fat.

As the American diet tends to be very high in phosphorus, deficiencies are rare. However, people who take large quantities of antacids containing aluminum and magnesium compounds can develop a deficiency. The aluminum and magnesium combine with phosphorus in the gastrointestinal tract to form aluminum and magnesium phosphates which cannot be absorbed and so pass out of the body in the stool. In order to maintain blood phosphorus levels the body liberates the nutrient from the bone, leading to demineralization and weakening of the bones. This causes bone pain and a feeling of weakness. It also increases the risk of osteoporosis—a bone weakening disease which is a fairly common disorder among the elderly.

A toxic level of phosphorus would be 12,000 milligrams, which is unlikely to be consumed in the normal course of events. However, most Americans consume more than the recommended dietary allowance of 1000 milligrams. An excess of phosphorus over calcium in the diet impairs the absorption of calcium, which can lead to a calcium deficiency. The National Academy of Sciences recommends a dietary calcium to phosphorus ratio of 1.5 to 1 for optimal calcium absorption. Liver, red meats, nuts, beans, peas, whole grains, cereals, and many soft drinks are all good sources of phosphorus. (See also CALCIUM; ENZYMES; OSTEOPOROSIS.)

POTASSIUM

Potassium with sodium regulates the amount of water in the cells of the body and is essential for the proper functioning of the kidneys, the heart and other muscles, the secretion of stomach juices, and the transmission of nerve impulses. Although there is no recommended dietary allowance (RDA) for this nutrient you require between 755 and 5625 milligrams a day to be consumed in your daily diet. Dried apricots, avocados, bananas, lima beans, brussels sprouts, carrots, flounder, spinach, tomatoes, and yogurt are all rich sources of potassium.

People who suffer from severe diarrhea or kidney disease and those taking certain diuretics can lose sufficient potassium from their bodies to cause a deficiency state. If a deficiency does occur the patient will exhibit one or more of the following symptoms: weakness, a loss of appetite, nausea, vomiting, dryness of the mouth, increased thirst, listlessness, apprehension, diffuse pain throughout the body, and an irreg-

Good Sources of Potassium	
Food	**Potassium Content**
Milk, skim, 1 cup	406 mg
Dates, 10 pitted	518 mg
Banana, 1 small	440 mg
Apricots, dried, 1 cup	1273 mg
Prunes, dried, 5 large pitted	298 mg
Yogurt, plain, container	531 mg
Baked potato, 1 medium	782 mg
Chopped spinach, cooked, 1 cup	688 mg
Tomato, raw, 1 medium	300 mg
Avocado, 1 Florida avocado	1836 mg
Chicken, broiled, 6.2 oz	483 mg
Orange juice, 1 cup	496 mg
Lima beans, 1 cup	724 mg
Brussels sprouts, cooked from fresh, 1 cup	423 mg
Carrots, cooked, 1 cup	344 mg

ular heartbeat. It is impossible to develop a potassium deficiency in a normal diet unless you fall into one of the above risk groups.

Patients in the risk groups are often given potassium supplements, but nobody should take such supplements without the guidance of a physician. Not only does potassium in high doses impair the absorption of vitamin B_{12} (a B_{12} deficiency causes anemia) but it can be life threatening by causing an irregular heart rate and eventually death from heart failure. (See also SALT; SODIUM; VITAMIN B_{12}.)

PREGNANCY

WEIGHT GAIN

Pregnancy is a time when a woman undergoes a series of adaptations that create an environment optimal for fetal growth and that prepare her for a period of lactation which is to follow. These adaptations involve a certain amount of weight gain independent of the gain resulting from the weight of the developing fetus. For example, early in pregnancy, while the placenta and fetus are still quite small, the woman begins to increase the size of her uterus, develop her breast tissue, expand the volume of circulating blood and deposit "storage" fat deep within her body. The expanded uterine size is to accommodate the anticipated products of conception. The increased blood volume facilitates the flow of oxygen and nutrients across the placenta into the fetus as well as the removal of carbon dioxide and water products. Breast enlargement and fat deposition prepare the woman for lactation, a period that will immediately follow delivery. Before the introduction of infant formulas, this particular adaptation of pregnancy was crucial to the survival of the infant.

As pregnancy proceeds, the products of conception begin to enlarge; first the placenta and then the fetus and its surrounding amniotic fluid. These changes account for a certain amount of the weight gain during pregnancy. The total weight gain during a normal pregnancy to allow for proper maternal adaptation and for adequate fetal growth should be around 25 pounds (between 11 and 12 kilograms).

In order to gain sufficient weight, the woman must increase the number of calories she consumes. This is not difficult, since as part of the maternal adaptation, she will experience an increased appetite. The extra 300 to 500 calories per day required for a normal pregnancy are readily consumed by most women.

What happens if the diet is inadequate because insufficient food is available, unwise food choices have been made, or because dietary restrictions have been imposed by well-meaning friends and relatives and sometimes even by well-meaning physicians, midwives, and nurses? Fetal growth is impaired and the birth weight of the infant is reduced. Thus, the fetus is unable to extract the necessary nutrients to maintain optimal growth. This might seem unlikely in view of the relatively large size of the woman when compared to the fetus. One might expect her to tap her own stores to supply the fetus. But, in fact, this does not occur, and until recently, science had no explanation for this inability of the pregnant woman to adequately mobilize her own reserves and transfer them to the fetus. In the last few years, we have begun to understand this apparent paradox.

As previously mentioned, in order for the fetus to grow optimally the woman must undergo a series of adaptations to pregnancy. Recent evidence, both in animals and in humans, suggests that inadequate nutrition, especially in consumption of insufficient calories, will result in an incomplete adaptation to pregnancy. Thus, the expected increase in the pregnant female's blood volume will not take place in undernourished animals and humans. This, in turn, leads to a reduction in the amount of blood flowing to the uterus and placenta. As a result, the placenta itself will not grow properly and will not transfer nutrients adequately. Thus, the process by which nutrients are actually passed to the fetus is impaired and even though these nutrients are available from maternal reserves they cannot reach the fetus in normal quantities.

It is interesting to speculate as to why such a state of affairs should exist—why would fetal growth be sacrificed and maternal reserves be protected? The present view is that these reserves are essential so that they may be called upon during lactation. Inability to lactate once meant certain death to the infant and therefore the woman had to be prepared. Even if the fetus grew more slowly and was smaller at birth, its chances of survival would be better if the woman could supply it with adequate amounts of milk. It is only when we view pregnancy and lactation as a continuum that we can see the body's logic in protecting the woman at the expense of the fetal growth. These adaptations of pregnancy developed well before infant formulas were invented, and the adaptation for lactation represented nature's way of ensuring that the woman's breasts would be prepared for infant feeding.

Since we know today that optimal fetal growth and development increase the infant's chances of survival and for subsequent normal development, proper nutrition during pregnancy leading to an increase of 25 pounds above prepregnancy weight in the nonobese woman is strongly recommended. Pregnancy is no time to diet and no time to lose weight even if the mother is obese! Pregnancy is a time to consume adequate nutrients, to gain enough weight so that the baby will develop properly in utero and will therefore emerge into the world with the best chance to survive and prosper.

SPECIFIC NUTRIENT REQUIREMENTS

To gain approximately 25 pounds during pregnancy a woman should increase her caloric intake by about 300 to 500 calories per day. While the source of those calories is not important from the standpoint of adaptation to pregnancy and subsequent fetal growth, it is very important in terms of providing specific nutrients which may be in short supply and which are particularly needed by the growing fetus. These nutrients include: protein, which is required for the building of fetal tissues; calcium, which is necessary for ensuring adequate development of the bones; iron, for making hemoglobin, the molecule within the red blood cells that carries the oxygen; zinc, which is needed for proper cell division; and folacin and pyridoxine, two of the B vitamins particularly important in fetal development.

As part of the overall adaptation to pregnancy, certain changes occur in the woman which favor absorption and retention of these nutrients. For example, both calcium and iron are more efficiently absorbed by the gastrointestinal tract of the pregnant woman. In spite of this, we recommend a diet rich in these nutrients. Such a diet is outlined below. It would be fine if this were the only dietary advice necessary for the pregnant woman. Unfortunately, the very nutrients in greatest demand during pregnancy are in the shortest supply. For example, iron is present in marginal amounts in many diets and many women tend to be iron deficient even before pregnancy begins. Calcium, while abundant in milk and milk products as well as in certain green leafy vegetables, is not taken into the body efficiently when large amounts of phosphorus are consumed at the same time. Because so many foods are highly processed, the American diet is far too rich in phosphorus. For example, much of it is supplied by red meat and soft drinks. Hence calcium, while abundant in the food supply, may not be readily available for use by the body.

Folacin (folic acid) is the most scarce vitamin in our diet, and in women who were previously on contraceptive pills, body reserves of both folacin and pyridoxine (vitamin B_6) may already be depleted. Thus, many women enter pregnancy in a nutritional state which is marginal for these nutrients. For this reason, we would recommend supplementation either through fortified foods or directly in tablets of iron, folacin, and vitamin B_6. In addition, if a woman is unable or unwilling to increase her calcium intake by consuming more milk or milk products, then calcium supplementation is also advised. The following table outlines the recommended requirements for selected

---

NUTRIENT REQUIREMENTS DURING PREGNANCY

Nutrient	RDA	Best Sources
Calories	2300–2400	meat, fish, poultry, fats, fruits, grain, legumes, nuts
Protein	76 g	meat, fish, poultry, eggs, milk, milk products, legumes, grains
Calcium	1200 mg	milk (all forms), yogurt, cheese, leafy green vegetables, clams, oysters, almonds
Iron	18 mg*	liver, meats, fish, poultry, whole grain and enriched cereals and breads, legumes, foods cooked in an iron pan, leafy green vegetables, dried prunes, apricots, raisins
Folacin	800 mcg*	liver, yeast, leafy green vegetables, legumes, whole grains, fruits, assorted vegetables
Pyridoxine (B$_6$)	2.5 mg*	wheat germ, meat, liver, whole grains, peanuts, soybeans, corn
Zinc		same as iron plus oysters, clams, and other shellfish

*Supplementation with these nutrients is recommended as follows: iron, 30–60 mg per day; folacin, 400–800 mcg per day; pyridoxine, 3–6 mg per day.

---

nutrients during pregnancy and the most important sources of these nutrients.

PROPER DIET DURING PREGNANCY

"Eat for two," and other time-honored hints abound in the discussion of the proper diet during pregnancy. Despite modern awareness, food-related superstitions—such as losing a filling with every pregnancy or causing a birthmark on the child which resembles a food frequently consumed by the mother—still stick in the minds of many. While some "old wives' tales" are harmless or even support sound nutritional practices, others which restrict foods that are beneficial should be discontinued. All these practices illustrate the long-held recognition that the diet during pregnancy is critically related to the ensuing health of both the mother and the infant.

As already mentioned, a woman must consume significantly more food (for additional calories and nutrients) than what she was accustomed to eating before conceiving. Unless your appetite is poor, this "open season" for eating comes as a special bonus of pregnancy! Some discretion is necessary, however. Judge your calories by the company they keep. Foods that are excessively fatty or sweet offer very little other than calories and may be replacing foods that could be enhancing the nutritional status of you and your baby. A good example is made by comparing 5 marshmallows to 1½ ounces of raisins. While nearly equal in calories (approximately 120 each), the raisins contain more than twice the amount of protein, five times as much calcium, three times as much iron, and significant amounts of vitamins A and B—of which the marshmallows have none. Clearly, benefits can be gained by making the right choices.

A guide for daily food selections for pregnant and lactating women is listed below.

No matter what your particular food preferences are, this guide will help you select foods which will provide almost all the nutrients needed in increased amounts (see the table on page 255 for more specific details). As noted earlier, calories are also needed in increased amounts. The use of spreads, cooking fats, salad dressings, sweeteners, etc., as well as additional servings from the food groups listed above, will help achieve

FOOD SELECTIONS FOR PREGNANT AND LACTATING WOMEN

Main Nutrients	Food Group	Minimum Number of Servings
Protein and iron	meat, fish, poultry, eggs, legumes/grains, nuts	4
Calcium and protein	milk (all forms), yogurt, cheese	4
Vitamins A and C (fiber)	citrus and other fruits, leafy, red/orange and green vegetables, potatoes and other tubers	5
B Vitamins, iron (fiber)	whole grain, enriched grain products (such as whole wheat products, enriched and fortified cereals)	4
Water (fluid)	juices, fruits, vegetables, beverages, water	6

the recommended calorie intake.

SPECIFIC NUTRITIONAL PROBLEMS

In the first three to four months of pregnancy some women experience nausea and vomiting. The discomfort occurs at different times and in differing degrees of severity. Nevertheless, it is possible to prevent or lessen the symptoms in the following ways.

• Make sure you are relaxed, comfortable and have fresh, odor-free air.
• If nausea is felt soon after getting up in the morning, keep crackers beside your bed and eat a few before getting on your feet.
• Meals should be smaller (even only a bite or two) and taken more often.
• Liquids should be sipped and taken between meals.
• Have dry foods (such as breads). In general, eat foods that you know are not unsettling. Foods well tolerated by some women are upsetting to others, so there is no set list of foods to eat or avoid.

Symptoms common in the latter months of pregnancy, such as heartburn or fullness (even after eating only a small amount), can also be lessened by controlling meal size and frequency.

Constipation may occur at any time during pregnancy but may be a particular problem during the last months, when the fetus presses against the large intestine and decreases intestinal movement. This is a time when it is very important to consume five or more servings a day of raw fruits or vegetables, dried fruits, whole grain products, and ample fluids. One or 2 tablespoons of bran or bran cereal may also help.

Pica, a craving for unnatural or nonfoods, is very common in pregnancy. In different parts of the world, pregnant women seek chalk, ashes, clay (earthen), or laundry starch. This practice may permit ingestion of harmful bacteria, reduce the amount of dietary zinc and iron absorbed from the intestinal tract, and take the place of nutritious foods. For these reasons, pica is discouraged at all times—and particularly during pregnancy.

Cravings for unusual combinations of food (such as the classic pickles and ice cream) are occasionally experienced and seem to be harmless. The worst that might come of satisfying a craving is the repeated consumption of a food—nutritious or not—with a resulting lack of variety in the diet. That is, fortunately, a minor and easily resolved problem.

Though there is an emphasis on the consumption of meat, vegetarian women can easily select a well-balanced diet. Sufficient calories, the most important aspect of the diet during pregnancy, are obtained from a variety of foods that do not conflict with the lack of meat in the diet.

In the absence of meat or eggs, complete proteins can be derived from dairy products and/or from combinations of legumes (beans and peas) and grains (wheat, oats, rice, etc.) eaten at the same meal. If the diet contains no dairy products, generous amounts of leafy green vegetables, nuts, and seeds should be consumed and supplements of 12 grams of calcium and 400 international units of vitamin D taken daily are recommended.

A sample menu, based on the food guide on page 255, is given below. Remember that variety is very important. If you are tired of drinking milk, try combining it with ce-

---

Sample Menu

Breakfast
orange juice
bran flakes with peaches
milk

Morning Snack
peanut butter & jelly on whole wheat toast
glass of milk
pear

Lunch
glass of vegetable juice
egg salad on lettuce
two slices of pumpernickel bread
tomato slices

Afternoon Snack
cup of yogurt
carrot sticks
glass of water or other beverage

Dinner
chicken
carrot-raisin-apple salad
whole baked potato
green peas
glass of apple juice

Evening Snack
crackers with cheese
glass of milk
dried apricots

---

real, in puddings, or in soup. At this time, when you should be so aware of the importance of following a nutritionally sound diet, remember that it is a continuing concern and the good food habits you establish now will take you and yours through a healthier lifetime.

POSTPARTUM OBESITY

Pregnancy and lactation must be considered as a continuum when assessing the effects of maternal nutrition on fetal growth. Recent data suggests that the interruption of this continuum may have long-lasting effects on the mother quite apart from any effects on the infant.

An important part of the maternal adaptation to pregnancy is the deposition of fat deep within the body. Because the pregnant woman deposits fat by filling up previously existing fat cells, she develops a unique type of hypertrophic or type II obesity. (See OBESITY.) This fat is a storage depot which will be used during lactation when energy demands are greater than at any other time in a woman's life. Studies in rats show that if the mother nurses her pups, all this stored fat is "burned up" by the end of the nursing period. By contrast, if the mother is not allowed to nurse her pups, this fat remains. If the animal becomes pregnant shortly thereafter, it is possible that still more fat will be deposited

and the effect will be additive. In humans, there are studies which show that women who nurse their infants revert to their prepregnancy weight more quickly than those who do not nurse. In other words, women who do not nurse remain "fatter" for a longer period of time than those woman who do.

We have often heard the complaint "I started to put on weight only after my first child was born and this got worse with subsequent pregnancies." Could this postpartum obesity be real? And could it be due to repeated pregnancies coupled with a lack of breast-feeding? Wouldn't it be ironic if part of the reason for the so-called maturity onset obesity in women was due to the replacement of breast by bottle? The data at present is still only suggestive, but the importance of this possibility is such that research directed at answering these questions is already in progress. We'll try to keep you up-to-date on these studies as the data becomes available.

SUBSTANCES TO AVOID DURING PREGNANCY

Alcohol. Consumption of large amounts of alcohol during pregnancy can result in severe damage to the developing fetus. The type of damage is so characteristic that it has been given the name "fetal alcohol syndrome." It consists of growth retardation, abnormal facial development, and mental retardation. Although this syndrome occurs only in "heavy" drinkers, the exact amount of alcohol which must be consumed to cause it varies. There is some evidence gathered recently that suggests alcohol consumed in so-called moderate amounts during pregnancy may cause more subtle changes in the fetus. Again the exact quantity of alcohol which must be consumed is unknown. The changes in the fetus include slight growth retardation and transient behavioral abnormalities. Although it appears to be perfectly safe to consume an occasional cocktail or a glass of wine with dinner the inability to know the exact amount of alcohol which for a given mother will damage her fetus makes us recommend abstention from alcoholic beverages during pregnancy.

Tobacco. Smoking during pregnancy will retard fetal growth. The mechanism by which this occurs has been recently uncovered. The nicotine (and perhaps other substances) in the cigarette smoke causes a constriction of the blood vessels leading to the uterus and the placenta. The resultant reduction in blood supply to these organs causes a form of fetal malnutrition. Every time you smoke a cigarette you are reducing the amount of oxygen and nutrients reaching your fetus. The more you smoke the greater the effect. The earlier you stop or at least cut back the better for you and your offspring.

Caffeine. There is evidence in animals that consumption of large amounts of caffeine during pregnancy can retard fetal growth and induce behavioral abnormalities in the offspring. In human populations consumption of large amounts of caffeine (8 to 10 cups of coffee per day) has been associated with an increased incidence of spontaneous abortion. Smaller amounts of caffeine appear to be safe. Therefore we would recommend that any woman who consumes more than 3 to 4 cups of coffee per day or numerous glasses of caffeine-containing soft drinks cut back to more moderate levels. (See CAFFEINE.)

Megadoses of Vitamins and Minerals. Many people, convinced of deriving a multitude of health benefits, consume a variety of vitamins and minerals in doses of ten to one thousand times the recommended dietary allowance. Some of these nutrients in very high doses can be extremely toxic, particularly if taken by a woman who is pregnant. Vitamin A and vitamin D taken in large doses can be directly toxic to the fetus. Vitamin C in large amounts taken by the pregnant woman can create a dependence on large doses in the young infant which may persist for several months. The consequences of very high doses of some of the other vitamins and of most of the minerals are unknown. For a pregnant woman the best advice is to take a prenatal vitamin and mineral preparation. This practice, along with a varied diet, will supply all of the vitamins and minerals which are needed. Higher doses are of no further benefit and could prove to be dangerous.

Drugs. As far as possible, all drugs should be avoided during pregnancy. If symptoms are present which require the use of drug therapy check with your physician before beginning. Narcotics are particularly dangerous and infants of narcotics addicts often suffer from withdrawal symptoms which if not promptly treated can lead to death. Smoking marijuana during pregnancy while not so dangerous as using narcotic drugs can still be harmful to the fetus.

THE PREGNANT ADOLESCENT

The nutritional requirements of a pregnant teenager are much higher than those of a mature woman since the teenager is still growing, herself. Her needs, therefore, will parallel her rate of body growth at the time when pregnancy begins. Thus, dietary recommendations should be carefully adjusted to each individual need and

to the nutritional status of the adolescent at the start of pregnancy. An extremely young teenage mother with an adequate nutritional status should be encouraged to gain her estimated growth increments in weight in addition to the expected weight gains of pregnancy. Thus, an adequate weight gain for a pregnant teenage mother could range fom 27 to 35 pounds. If she was underweight at the start of pregnancy, the estimated weight deficit should be added to the recommended weight gain.

In addition to an adequate caloric and protein intake to achieve these body-weight goals, a teenage mother should receive generous supplements of iron and calcium as well as the vitamin and mineral supplements routinely prescribed to pregnant women. (See ADOLESCENT for a more complete discussion of nutrition during adolescent pregnancy.)

DIABETES

During pregnancy, uncontrolled diabetes can have devastating effects on both the mother and the fetus. By contrast, if the diabetes is carefully controlled both mother and fetus will usually have a smooth course. Thus, any woman who has diabetes should be under constant medical supervision throughout the entire length of her pregnancy. Using a combination of insulin injections and proper diet, blood sugar levels can be kept close to normal. The exact regimen will vary from patient to patient but certain general dietary principles are usually employed. These include: frequent (5 or 6) small meals, reducing fat to 30 percent or less of the total calories consumed, limiting the consumption of refined sugar, increasing complex carbohydrate to 45 or 50 percent of total calories consumed, and increasing dietary fiber. With a little care on the part of the patient and close supervision by her physician, the pregnant woman with diabetes can usually look forward to a normal outcome of pregnancy.

TOXEMIA

Toxemia is one of the most serious complications of pregnancy. It is characterized by a rapid accumulation of fluid in the tissues (edema) and hypertension (high blood pressure). It used to be thought that by limiting salt (sodium) intake during pregnancy toxemia could be prevented. This has not been borne out and routine salt restriction during pregnancy is no longer used. In fact severe salt restriction can be dangerous. Similarly, the use of diuretic drugs to promote salt and water excretion during pregnancy can be dangerous. There is some evidence which suggests that toxemia of pregnancy may be associated with poor nutrition. At present, the best way for a

woman to lower her risk for developing toxemia is to practice good nutrition as outlined above throughout pregnancy.

NUTRITION PRIOR TO PREGNANCY

For a variety of reasons, many women today are carefully planning their pregnancies. Such women should focus on their nutritional status as soon as they plan to become pregnant. As mentioned above, the normal adult woman should gain between 25 and 30 pounds during pregnancy. However, this assumes that she was close to her ideal weight (as defined in the 1983 Metropolitan Life Insurance Company Tables) before becoming pregnant. If she is underweight she will have to make up the difference for her fetus to grow adequately. If she is obese she must still gain about 15 pounds during pregnancy. Thus for different reasons both the overweight and underweight woman should attempt to begin pregnancy as close to her ideal weight as possible. The underweight woman will then need to gain less weight during pregnancy and the overweight woman can gain the desired amount during pregnancy without worrying about increasing her weight problem.

There are two additional reasons why the period prior to actual conception is so important from a nutritional standpoint. First, body stores of particular nutrients which are often in short supply during pregnancy can be built up. Second, by waiting until she knows she is pregnant a woman usually misses the earliest stages of fetal development, a time when her nutrition is particularly important. Thus, as soon as a woman plans to become pregnant she should consult her physician and begin consuming her prenatal vitamin and iron supplement, as well as a calcium supplement if necessary. This is particularly important if she has been using oral contraceptives since many of these agents affect the metabolism of certain vitamins. Finally, the time to stop drinking, smoking, or using drugs is before becoming pregnant. Waiting until pregnancy is diagnosed may be too late. (See also BREAST-FEEDING; WOMEN.)

PROTEIN

Protein is the substance from which all our tissues are made. There are thousands of different protein molecules all made up of long chains of amino acids. The arrangement of the individual amino acids determines the structure of the protein. In addition to being the basic structural molecule of the tissues of our body, protein is necessary for almost every essential body function. Enzymes are specialized protein molecules as are certain hormones. Protein is used for transporting molecules in our blood, for digesting our food, for causing our blood to clot, and for a host of other functions without which life would be impossible.

Protein in our diet can come from either animal or plant sources.

Protein from animal sources is in general of higher quality (higher biological value) than protein from plant sources because it contains all of the essential amino acids. Plant proteins are often missing one or more amino acids and hence must be combined to give a complete protein. (See VEGETARIAN DIETS.) The American diet is relatively high in protein and the recommended daily allowance of 45 grams is easily met by most people. Protein deficiency, however, commonly occurs in developing countries, particularly among children, and can have extremely serious consequences. See also AMINO ACIDS; ENZYMES; PROTEIN-CALORIE MALNUTRITION; SULFUR; VEGETARIAN DIETS.)

PROTEIN-CALORIE MALNUTRITION (PCM)

Protein-calorie malnutrition (PCM) is the single greatest health hazard to children worldwide. In some underdeveloped countries, virtually one-half the children are said to be suffering from primary PCM, and it's estimated that over 300 million people alive today once had the syndrome, with many still bearing permanent sequelae.

Primary PCM is typically found among the poor of developed and developing countries, and in more recent years, even among the not so poor. The victims in more affluent societies are infants whose parents have placed them on "fad" diets, usually at the time of weaning. These diets, often well tolerated by adults, can induce primary protein-calorie malnutrition or severe undernutrition in children.

Regardless of how PCM develops, its effects can be devastating and lifelong in terms of mental and physical development. Protein-calorie malnutrition can be divided into two types; marasmus and kwashiorkor.

MARASMUS

Marasmus usually occurs during the first year of life. The primary form involves infants who aren't being breast-fed and whose bottle-feeding is improper or inadequate owing to a lack of refrigeration or sterilizing facilities, use of contaminated water, or formulas that are too expensive and are therefore overdiluted. An infant fed under such conditions will develop profuse, unremitting diarrhea; the parents, in an effort to help, often make matters worse by further diluting the formula or switching to a liquid starch.

Affected infants quickly and completely exhaust all body reserves. In addition, these children generally develop profuse diarrhea and several mineral imbalances. Such infants are small and underweight, and often look emaciated. Emaciation in some children makes the head appear relatively large, though in fact head circumference is markedly reduced. As for behavior, marasmic infants are both apathetic and hypersensitive: They'll often lie quietly for hours, but will become extremely hyperactive when touched or moved.

KWASHIORKOR

Kwashiorkor generally affects children, one year or older, who are abruptly weaned and placed on a low-calorie diet that is also markedly deficient in protein.

Edema (swelling due to water

retention), skin rash, hair depigmentation, and growth failure characterize the child with kwashiorkor, although all these symptoms may not appear at once. Frequently, kwashiorkor develops: growth slows; the face takes on a moonlike look, with edema beginning around the eyes and gradually spreading downward; and finally a skin rash develops and hair loses its color. In other cases, frank kwashiorkor is precipitated when the chronically malnourished child contracts an infection like measles.

Diarrhea is not always found in kwashiorkor, but edema is. Though edema sometimes masks weight loss, height retardation is always apparent in affected children. Head circumference may also be smaller than normal, but less so than in marasmic infants.

MILDER FORMS OF PCM

Reduced intake of calories and protein in infants does not always lead to distinct marasmus or kwashiorkor.

Children with these milder or less distinct forms of PCM share certain common traits—growth failure, low weight for height, and reduced midarm circumference. Diet therapy generally assures a good outcome, except for those children whose mental development already has been compromised.

MENTAL DEVELOPMENT

The most serious permanent effect of PCM is an impairment of mental development. Recently collected evidence strongly suggests that infants who have recovered from PCM (either marasmus or kwashiorkor) may have severe behavioral abnormalities, poor motor skills, and a reduced capacity to learn. Given the enormous number of children who are affected each year this becomes one of the most serious health and social issues facing modern society. (See also CHILDREN; PROTEIN; VEGETARIAN DIETS.)

REDUCING DIETS

With the growing prevalence of overweight in the United States, interest has been increasing in weight reduction diets. This preoccupation with weight control is occurring because of the social, psychological, and economic rewards that are perceived to be derived from a trim figure. Concern is actually related less to anxiety about health than to cosmetic considerations. Nevertheless, because the concern is so widespread and because losing weight with nutritionally balanced, low-calorie diets is so difficult over extended periods of time, a great many methods or gimmicks for losing weight have been proposed over the years.

REDUCED EFFICIENCY OF UTILIZATION

One strategy for weight loss is to use diets which reduce the efficiency with which the body utilizes the calories consumed. For many years it was thought that proteins in the diet would temporarily increase the amount of energy dissipated in the body as heat. Therefore, fewer of the calories ingested would be available for utilization or deposition as fat. This, in fact, has been shown not to be the case. Carbohydrate and fat contribute essentially as much as protein to this heat loss.

There is some suggestion that a high-fat diet may be more efficient than a high-carbohydrate diet in its ability to deposit fat. The data is not conclusive concerning this concept, but some investigators have been able to induce weight gain much more easily with a high-fat than with a mixed diet. Whether this increased efficiency of fat occurs in low-calorie diets has not been experimentally tested, but if it does, it would tend to militate against diets with a high proportion of fat and in favor of high carbohydrate ones for weight reduction programs.

IMPAIRED ABSORPTION

A second strategy for weight reduction is to add constituents which impair absorption to the diet, so that some of the calories ingested remain in the gut and are excreted rather than utilized. High-fiber diets have been suggested in this regard. To date, however, there is little evidence to demonstrate that high-fiber diets affect intestinal absorption or have a significant impact on weight. Certainly, no evidence exists that high-fiber diets cause intestinal malabsorption of nutrients high in calories.

Nondigestible fat substitutes are beginning to be developed. Sucrose polyester is an example. Virtually the same as corn oil in taste, it can be used as a replacement for up to 900 calories of fat in the diet. Theoretically, it has the potential to reduce the total daily calorie intake significantly, but to this date it has not been tested for such a long-term effect.

Other agents have also been suggested. Perfluoracetyl bromide is an inert substance that coats the gastrointestinal tract and has been reported to be useful in preventing some absorption of calories.

Also being tried are agents which will inhibit the natural breakdown of the macromolecular nutrients in the gut into smaller absorbable molecules, a necessary process for absorption. As a result, malabsorption of these macromolecules occurs and these are partly excreted in the stool unutilized.

The acceptability of all these substances however is likely to be quite low because of the unpleasant side effects of fat and carbohydrate malabsorption, the most significant of which is diarrhea.

EXERCISE

Exercise is a popular addition to the weight-control regimen. Data is accumulating to show that exercise may indeed be quite helpful. A recent study suggests that subjects eating low-calorie diets, whose resting energy consumption would be ex-pected to decrease, maintain this energy consumption with exercise. Thus, exercise as an adjunct to dieting may help in the utilization of energy out of proportion to the actual exercise calories expended. However, long-term studies investigating the effect of exercise by itself on weight reduction have been disappointing. Nevertheless, until new data is obtained, we still feel that exercise may be a good companion to a balanced low-calorie diet in a weight reduction program. (See Exercise.)

UNBALANCED LOW-CALORIE DIETS

The most common strategy is to use diets unbalanced in carbohydrates, protein, and fat and low in calories. These unbalanced diets focus on particular food groups and prohibit or reduce others. Such diets are generally easier for individuals to follow rigorously and, therefore, are quite popular. Numerous fad diets have swept the country, and millions of volumes describing them have been sold, usually for short periods of time, after which new versions displace them. The diets all have in common a marked imbalance of macronutrients (protein, carbohydrate, or fat) which also often creates an imbalance of micronutrients.

One type of hypocaloric unbalanced diet is a low-carbohydrate, high-protein, high-fat diet. Notorious examples of this type are found in *Calories Don't Count, Dr. Atkins' Diet Revolution, The Snack Diet* (or Wisconsin Diet), *The Doctors' Metabolic Diet,* and *The Drinking Man's Diet.* Many of these diet books claim that the presence of ketone bodies (ketogenesis), which are formed when the diet lacks a proper amount of carbohydrates, decreases the appetite. In fact, no inhibitory effect of these substances on food intake in humans has ever been demonstrated.

A second unbalanced diet is high in protein, low in carbohydrate, but also low in fat. The two most common examples are in *The Scarsdale Diet* and *The Stillman Quick Weight Loss Diet.* These diets also induce ketogenesis but, because of the emphasis on low fat as well as low carbohydrate, tend to be lower in calories. Another type of regimen is a high-carbohydrate, low-protein, low-fat diet. Examples are the Macrobiotic diet, and the diets in *The Kempner Rice Diet, The Pritikin Diet,* and *Stillman's Quick Inches Off Diet.* A fourth approach uses a protein-supplemental fast. A popular example of this is the *Last Chance Diet.*

Finally, there is the possibility of total fast, publicized in the *Fasting as a Way of Life Diet.* The hazards of the above-mentioned diets will be enumerated later.

There are also specific focus diets. These diets target on one or a few particular items invested with magical powers for weight reduction. One example is the Human Chorionic Gonadotrophin (HCG) Diet, in which not only is a diet prescribed, but injections of this hormone are given every day. This has been found to be useless but still commands great popularity. In the Mayo Clinic Diet (no relation to the Mayo Clinic) eggs, grapefruit, and tomato juice are invested with certain fat-burning powers which actually do not exist.

In Mary Ann Crenshaw's Lecithin, B_6, Apple Cider Vinegar, and Kelp Diet, kelp (a seaweed) is supposed to provide iodine to stimulate the thyroid gland, the apple cider vinegar to give potassium, the vitamin B_6 to help burn fat, and the lecithin to mix everything up! The Banana and Milk Diet consists of 6 bananas and 3 glasses of milk a day, and causes weight loss because its 1000 calories per day are taken with such boring food that it is easily kept. Because of its imbalance, it is hazardous if extra vitamins and minerals are not conscientiously taken.

We do not have the space here to review in detail all of the diets enumerated above, so instead the focus will be on a few of the most popular unbalanced diets.

The Atkins diet is a typical low-carbohydrate, high-protein, high-fat diet. It recommends an unlimited consumption of proteins and fats and severely limits carbohydrates. It has an unspecified energy level though portion sizes and types of food are suggested. Atkins states that one can eat as much as is desired because the appetite will be diminished by the ketonemia (amount of ketone bodies in the blood) and an inhibition of food intake will occur. This diet tends to be low in vitamin C. Its side effects are nausea, hypotension, and fatigue. Calcium loss can occur. High uric acid levels develop which make it dangerous for people with gout, and it has a very high cholesterol content, dangerous for people with a propensity to hypercholesterolemia.

The Stillman Quick Weight Loss Diet is a low-carbohydrate, high-protein diet in which the fat content varies depending on the meats which are chosen. It designates types of food—lean meat, poultry, fish, eggs, cottage cheese—but not quantities. It stipulates a high water intake and prohibits fruit, vegetables, breads, and cereals. It is very low in carbohydrate, high in saturated fat and cholesterol, and is low in vitamin A, C, thiamine, and iron. This diet has about double to triple the amount of cholesterol found in a regular diet.

The Scarsdale diet is primarily a low-carbohydrate diet but it is also low in fat. It prescribes no set calories, but fluids are limited to black coffee and tea. People like it because it does have a fixed menu. It is low in milk, bread, and cereal groups, and in iron, vitamin A, calcium, and riboflavin. This diet was first introduced as only a two-week regimen. The doctor who popularized it was wise enough to realize that the diet was deficient and that subjects should not follow it for longer than the two-week limit. In actuality, people unfortunately stay on it for much longer periods of time. While fat is lost, there is an associated increase in urinary excretion of water and sodium in the urine, typical of ketogenic diets.

The Pritikin diet is a very high carbohydrate diet in which only an extremely low 10 percent of total calories are fat. It has an unspecified energy level and emphasizes fruits, vegetables, breads, and cereals. Since these carbohydrate foods are bulky, it becomes difficult to eat excessive calories. No sugar, table fats, oils, or dairy products except skim milk are allowed. It is low in salt, iron, essential fatty acids, and the fat soluble vitamins.

PROTEIN SUPPLEMENTED FASTING

While total fasting has been tried for weight reduction, it is hazardous and ethically requires hospitalization, which makes it expensive and impractical. The protein-supplemented fast has been an attempt to obtain the rapid weight loss characteristic of fasting while preserving lean tissue in the body. A popular example of this plan, mentioned earlier, is the Last Chance Diet, in which a protein powder is the sole dietary item.

The Last Chance diet has a specific energy level, while a certain number of grams of protein are recommended for each individual. Many such protein preparations are on the market, some in liquid form and some in powder form. Some include vitamin and mineral supplements, while others simply suggest their use. Many people take the protein supplements and do not take the vitamins and minerals. With or without them, however, real problems may develop. Particular dangers are dehydration, losses of sodium and potassium, and an inadequate intake of vitamin A, riboflavin, iron, and calcium.

Individuals have been enthusiastic about the protein-supplemented fast because the diet is severely limited in calories, allowing only 300 to 500 calories per day, which achieves a great energy deficit and generates a rapid weight loss. The protein which the patients take, if of high quality, has been reported to prevent the loss of body protein that occurs during a standard fast. The protein-supplemented fast can produce several side effects including dehydration, hair loss, cold intolerance, menstrual irregularities, and cardiovascular abnormalities.

Although the conservation of lean tissue seems to be better with these diets than in the case of total starvation, both of these strategies for weight reduction are dangerous and should not be followed without professional advice.

Commercial preparations of liquid protein are available for over-the-counter purchase. Since 1977, when these preparations began to gain popularity, fifty-eight deaths have been associated with the use of these agents. One liquid protein label states: "Hydrolyzed animal collagen, water, sorbitol, citric acid, tryptophan, sodium saccharin, benzoin soda, potassium sorbate, flavor. Calories 72/30 ml, protein 15 grams, fat 0, carbohydrate 3 grams. The protein in this product is predigested and is utilized 100%." "Utilized" here means that it is absorbed.

BALANCED DIETS

Since restricted diets must be followed for long periods of time, the nutritional adequacy of the diet becomes crucial. Acceptable meal patterns, proper food selection, and allowance for individual preferences are necessary prerequisites. Very limited and unbalanced diets are unhealthful because of the loss of macro- and micronutrients which can result from following them. A mixed, balanced diet is a much more sensible and healthful approach to weight reduction.

Diets in the 1100 to 1200 calorie range, in contrast, can be followed for months without serious side effects. While these diets are more difficult to maintain, it is certainly possible to do so. A great many people have lost significant amounts of weight on balanced hypocaloric diets which give all the required nutrients. In addition, these diets can educate patients to a lifelong awareness of high-quality foods and the need for balance in the diet.

If a more restricted diet must be followed, then it seems sensible to offer one that provides about 800 calories of high-quality protein mixed with carbohydrate. In addition, adequate vitamins and minerals should both be given and every effort made to ensure that these are actually taken. Long-term diets providing fewer calories than this do not appear justified at this time.

PLANNING WHAT TO EAT

Planning a balanced weight reduction diet has been simplified by using "exchange lists." (See DIABETES.) The foods in the lists are grouped according to their nutrient similarities: vegetables; fruits and juices; and starchy foods (breads, cereals, beans) are grouped together.

The total number of servings allowed for each calorie level (check how many calories you should be consuming on your diet) is given in the table below. At all levels the protein intake will be adequate and vitamin and mineral supplements

NUMBER OF PORTIONS ALLOWED FOR VARIOUS CALORIE LEVELS

Food Exchanges*	Calories			
	1000	1200	1500	1800
Free Foods	*******UNLIMITED*******			
Vegetables	2	2	2	2
Fruits	3	3	3	3
Starches	3	5	7	9
Protein	6	6	7	7
Milk	2	2	2	3
Fats	2	1	6	7

*See the Exchange Lists in DIABETES (page 120) for specific foods and quantities.

should not be needed if selections are to be made from a variety of foods. It is advisable, if the calorie level chosen is under 1200 calories, to take a low dose multivitamin such as those available in grocery stores and pharmacies.

If you just can't seem to follow a diet, a few things may be responsible. First, you may be trying one of the ineffective, short-term regimens. If so, examine why it hasn't worked for you and let our guidelines steer you to a more suitable plan for yourself. Second, to lose weight in an environment seemingly crazed with food consumption, you must be well motivated. Well motivated means you have realistically decided that this is what you want to do. It means you are willing to change some of your attitudes, such as what's "tasty" and when you're satisfied. Occasional gains or plateaus in weight are normal and should not undermine one's determination. The dilemma between wanting to lose weight and being able to do so is almost erased when one is effectively motivated and ready. (See also EXERCISE; FASTING; OBESITY.)

SALT

Although salt is a necessary constituent of our own body fluids, in many ways the problem of adding salt to our food supply is much more serious than that of adding caffeine. First of all, this is because salt is added to a tremendous variety of processed foods, whereas caffeine is restricted to just a few. Second, salt has been implicated as a causal factor in hypertension (high blood pressure).

Salt is added to food to improve taste and, in some cases, as a preservative. It is added to flour and to most baked goods. Canned peas may contain one hundred times as much sodium as fresh peas. Pickled and smoked foods are soaked in brine until they are saturated with salt. In a society where our diet is laden with processed foods, it is difficult to design a low-salt diet. However, salt consumed in large amounts, over long periods of time, has been associated with hypertension.

Hypertension is a condition in which the pressure exerted by the blood, in the vessels through which it circulates, is greater than it should be. The heart must pump with extra force against this pressure. Prolonged, sustained high blood pressure can therefore lead to heart failure or to diseases of the walls of the arteries, leading to vessel clogging and coronary or other arterial diseases. Finally, a vessel no longer able to resist the increased pressure may burst. If this occurs in the brain, a serious cerebral hemorrhage (or stroke) may occur. As it happens, high blood pressure is often not accompanied by serious symptoms until heart attack or stroke strikes. Therefore, many people have high blood pressure without knowing it.

In populations that consume little sodium, blood pressure does not rise with age and hypertension is rare. By contrast, in populations consuming relatively high amounts of sodium, blood pressure does increase with age and hypertension is quite common. Among the Greenland Eskimos, Australian Aborigines, Polynesians, African Bushmen, and American Indians hypertension is virtually unknown and blood pressure remains constant throughout life. But as these societies begin to become westernized and consume processed foods in bulk, salt intake rises as does the incidence of both hypertension and obesity.

Obesity and a high salt intake seem to be independent risk factors in the development of hypertension. An interesting study was carried out in a group of Samburu tribesmen from northern Kenya. Traditionally, these nomads consume a diet of meat and milk, which is low in salt. A group was followed after being drafted into the Kenyan army, where the ration consisting of maize and meal and other foods increased their salt intake fivefold. During the second year of service, the blood pressure of these men began to increase and continued to increase throughout their six years of duty. By contrast, their weights remained relatively constant during their army term. Thus, increased sodium consumption without an increase in weight resulted in higher blood pressure values in this population.

Hypertension runs in families and is much more common in certain ethnic and racial groups. It is particularly prevalent among American blacks and to a lesser extent, among Eastern European Jews. By contrast, in the black population of Africa, where American blacks had their origins, hypertension, until recently, was very rare. Thus, while there is a genetic component to hypertension, this inborn disposition must be catalyzed by a particular environmental circumstance such as high exposure to salt, or particularly to the sodium, in the diet.

High blood pressure can often be lowered by drastically curtailing the intake of sodium. A strict, sodium-restricted diet contains less than half a gram per day. As most of the common foods eaten in the US contain sodium, it is a very inflexible diet. The following list gives you some idea of common foods which are high in sodium.

FOODS TO OMIT ON A SODIUM-RESTRICTED DIET

- Canned and frozen vegetables, soups, and vegetable juices if processed with salt
- The following fresh vegetables: artichokes, beet greens, carrots, celery, chard, dandelion greens, whole hominy, kale, mustard greens, parsley flakes, spinach, and white turnips
- Meats, fish, poultry, and eggs if canned or frozen with salt
- Bread and grain products if prepared with sodium
- All milk and dairy products except low-sodium products
- Miscellaneous: salt, salted butter or margarine, catsup, mustard, commercial salad preparations, and seasoning salts

Because of the difficulties in following the more strict sodium restriction diets, diuretic drugs, which induce the kidneys to excrete more water and with it more sodium, have been used in treating high blood pressure. The success rate with both strict restriction diets and drugs has been impressive. Thus, if the amount of sodium is drastically reduced or the amount of sodium excreted is significantly increased, blood pressure will usually fall in a person with hypertension (blood pressure higher than 140/90). Many people impose mild restrictions (fewer than 2 grams per day) on their salt intake where the amount of table salt used is reduced. No salt is added at the table, but up to 1 teaspoon per day can be used during cooking. In addition, pickled foods and extremely salty foods are eliminated.

Whether or not mild salt reduction is sufficient to reduce the incidence of hypertension is unknown. This is a very important point to clarify when you consider that 20 percent of the adult population in America has elevated blood pressure. Among blacks it may be as high as 50 percent. However, it does seem advisable to reduce our salt intake, particularly if there is a strong family history of hypertension.

IN CONCLUSION

What can be done to lessen the health risks associated with dietary salt? Foods should be labeled with their sodium content. The public has a right to know what the manufacturer is adding to their food supply. Only then can the average consumer decide whether one product is better than another, if he or she is trying to limit the amount of salt in the diet. Manufacturers should take the responsibility of offering a wide enough variety of foods so that a real choice is available within food categories.

Actually, this is already beginning to happen. Salt-free foods are becoming more available. In addition, added salt has been removed from all baby foods. This is a very positive step, since a liking for salt is an acquired taste. Young infants do not automatically favor salty foods. They develop such preferences only after long-term exposure.

It is crucial for consumers to become aware of the health hazards of too much salt so that this knowledge can be taken into consideration when they are choosing the foods which make up their diets. Food manufacturers do watch these choices and react very rapidly, making available more foods which reflect what is being chosen. Hence, the best way to make sure that we all get a food supply which contains less salt is to restrict our food purchases to those items which are low in this additive. (See also HYPERTENSION; OBESITY; POTASSIUM; SODIUM.)

SEAWEED

A wide variety of seaweeds have been sold in health food stores in recent years, the most popular of these being kelp and spirulina. Claims are made that both aid in weight loss but there is no evidence to support such claims. Kelp is certainly a good source of iodine. It is claimed that spirulina is a rich source of vitamin B_{12} but this is totally false. (See IODINE; KELP.)

SELENIUM

Selenium is a trace element essential for maintaining good health. The requirement for this element is very small and deficiency is very uncommon when the food supply is mixed and when foods come from a variety of growing areas. This is because the selenium content of food depends to a large extent on the selenium content of the soil on which the food is grown. Deficiency symptoms were first noted among livestock, particularly cattle, which grazed exclusively in areas devoid of selenium in the soil. A muscle disease (white muscle disease) involving most of the skeletal muscle and causing progressive weakness and ultimately death in these animals was found to be caused by selenium deficiency.

Recently, selenium deficiency has been found to be the cause of a long known disease found in a large region of China. The disease, known as Keshan disease (named after the city where it was first found), is present in a wide region extending from northeast to southwest China. Its principle victims are children and women of childbearing age. There is degeneration of the heart muscle with heart failure. Keshan disease is a major cause of death in China, affecting several million people. When Chinese investigators noticed that white muscle disease in cattle was very common in the same area as Keshan disease, they suspected that selenium deficiency might be involved. In a series of brilliant studies, they were able to demonstrate a cause and effect relationship between low levels of selenium and Keshan disease. Supplementation of the population and spraying of crops with selenium has largely eradicated the disease in the last two years.

It is estimated that you need between .05 and .2 milligrams of selenium each day to work in conjunction with vitamin E in the body to prevent the breakdown of fats and the formation of free radicals, which are believed by some authorities to be a causative agent in cancer. In fact people with a high selenium intake tend to be at lower risk for cancer. However, selenium supplements have not been successful in curing cancer. Seafood, egg yolks, chicken, garlic, and whole grain cereals all contain significant amounts of this nutrient.

In the western world, selenium deficiency is very rare since there is great diversity in the food supply which is grown in many different regions. Most water supplies also contain sufficient selenium to prevent deficiency.

Large amounts of selenium can be toxic and there is no evidence that selenium supplementation in a non-deficient population has any health benefit. (See also ANTICARCINOGENS; ANTIOXIDANTS.)

SODIUM

Sodium with potassium regulates the amount of water in the cells of the body and is essential for proper transmission of nerve impulses and contraction of muscles. There is no recommended dietary allowance (RDA) for sodium, but you need at least 450 milligrams a day. Up to 3300 milligrams per day is safe for most people. More than this amount may cause high blood pressure in some people. In people with already impaired cardiac function or renal disease, excessive amounts may even result in congestive heart failure and kidney disease. Table salt, processed foods, luncheon meats, meat, fish, pickled foods, bacon, baked beans, salted butter, buttermilk, cheese, canned corn, beets, and certain food additives such as monosodium glutamate (MSG) all have a high sodium content. People with high blood pressure should limit their intake of these foods and limit the salt used in cooking to 1 teaspoon per day. In addition, no salt should be added at the table.

Sodium deficiency is rare as the American diet is very high in salt (sodium chloride). However, certain medications can deplete the body of this nutrient as can excessive sweating. When this occurs the patient experiences a loss of appetite, nausea, vomiting, muscle weakness, and headaches. (See also POTASSIUM; SALT.)

SPROUTS

Sprouts belong to a family of vegetables known as cruciferous vegetables. These include broccoli, cauliflower, cabbage, and certain lesser known varieties. Consumption of these vegetables has been associated with a reduced incidence of certain cancers of the gastrointestinal tract. The agent or agents within cruciferous vegetables which reduces the risk of gastrointestinal cancers has not been identified and is the subject of intensive investigation. At present, the dietary recommendations advise including a generous amount (three servings per week) of cruciferous vegetables as part of a well-balanced diet.

STRESS

Some people suffer deeply from stress, while others thrive on it. Some completely lose their appetite for food, while others eat more. Whatever a person's reactions may be to either severe or mild stress, eating habits are always one of the first things to be affected. Stress can age people and/or take a lot out of their emotional and physical well-being, and so it is important to know exactly how stress affects the body and its nutritional status. In this way, you can learn what to do before, during, and after periods of stress so that your body does not suffer too much from its effects.

WHAT IS STRESS?

Stress can be generally defined as any condition or set of conditions which you experience as a threat to your stability. The types of stress we will be discussing are those which bring about the body's hormonal stress response, which would include any type of major physical or emotional disturbance. Major physical stresses would include pain of any type, illness, wounds, burns, surgery, a very hot or humid climate, infections, toxic compounds, radiation, and pollution. The chief emotional sources of stress are listed on page 281.

The stress response is the body's way of responding to these perceived emotional or physical threats. It is first mediated by the nerves and hormones. It begins with an "alarm reaction," then goes to a stage of "resistance," and then on to a recovery, or, if prolonged, to exhaustion. This three-stage response has also been called the "general adaptation syndrome." The hormones that the stress response involves affect all the tissues of the body.

EFFECTS OF THE STRESS RESPONSE

The stress response makes the body ready to effectively deal with danger. It can also stimulate people to solve problems and overcome great obstacles in order to achieve their dreams. But it can destroy a person's health, as well. This is because the stress response is designed to help the body cope with physical danger, while so much of the stress experienced today is more emotional in nature. This response makes the body ready for the vigorous muscular activity of "fight or flight," and not for the uptight and worried state of a person holding stress-producing problems inside, not being able to respond actively to them.

LEADING TYPES OF EMOTIONAL STRESS*

Event	Stress "Points"
Death of spouse	100
Divorce	73
Marital separation	65
Being sent to jail	63
Death of close family member	63
Personal injury or illness	53
Marriage	50
Losing a job	47
Retirement	45
Change in health of family member	44
Pregnancy	40
Sexual problems	39
Addition of new family member	39
Change in business status	39
Change in financial state	38
Death of close friend	37

*People ranked these events on a scale of 1 to 100 according to how much stress they felt each would produce. Individual people may score these events higher or lower than these averages, according to their own particular reactions to these events.

The reaction begins when a threat to your stability is perceived by the brain. A loud noise exploding near your ear, a strange person chasing you down the street and screaming out threats, the excitement of planning a wedding, or a feeling of sudden pain or illness are all examples of incidents which can serve as alarm signals. What follows is a chain of physical events, acting through both the nerves and hormones, which causes a state of readiness to develop in every part of the body. For ex- ample, the pupils of the eyes widen so that you can see better; the muscles tense so that you can jump, run, or fight with top strength and speed; the heart races to rush more oxygen to the muscles so they can burn the fuel they need for energy; the liver pours forth the needed fuel, glucose, from its stores, and so on. There are few parts of the body which are not called into dramatic action.

The totally-involving reaction to stress provides excellent support to a person should she or he need to take any type of emergency physical action. And anyone can respond in this highly efficient way to stress of a sudden physical nature for a short period of time. But if the stress is prolonged, and especially if a physical action is not a permitted response to it, then it can drain the body of its reserves and leave it weakened, aged, and more susceptible to illness.

BODY RESERVES USED DURING TIMES OF STRESS

All three energy fuels—carbohydrate, fat, and protein—are drawn upon in increased amounts during stress. If the response to the stress requires heavy physical action, and if it involves injury, all three are used. And while the body is occupied by responding and not by eating, internal sources are drained for these fuels.

Conserving bodily water at this time is essential, and the body uses several methods to conserve its water supply. First, it retains sodium. But to retain sodium the kidney exchanges, and loses, potassium. Hence, you can see why you need sufficient stores of potassium to be able to withstand the loss.

For energy, glucose is taken from stored glycogen in the liver and muscles for as long as the supply lasts, but actually, the supply is exhausted within a day. After that, body protein provides the only continuing glucose supply, and this is mainly drawn from the muscles. Some tissues can use fat for energy, and in a person who regularly eats balanced meals, fat stores are sufficient to meet this need for many days. To summarize, the body uses not only dispensable supplies (those which are there to be used up, like fat) but also functional tissue which one doesn't want to lose, like muscle tissue. So first, in preparation for prolonged periods of stress, such as a long illness, you would want to have as much protein in the muscle tissue as possible. Second, you would want to make sure that you minimize the wasting of muscle during stress.

Another nutrient lost from the body during stress is calcium, which is taken from the bones. The evidence tends to show that people lose varying amounts of this essential bone mineral, depending partly on their hormonal state, although the studies are not yet completely clear on this point. Adult bone loss is common anyway, and so the same measures should be taken here as we suggested with protein—one should know how to prepare for these losses and also how to minimize them.

PROPER NUTRITION PRIOR TO PERIODS OF STRESS

A healthy body, which has tissues that contain the optimal amounts of all essential nutrients, is best prepared for stress. Overall, a balanced diet should include a daily intake of the following:

- 2–3 servings of vegetables (raw and cooked)
- 2–3 servings of fruits (raw and cooked)
- 3–4 servings of whole grain products
- 2 servings of milk products
- 1–2 servings of poultry, meat, fish, eggs, beans, or peas

Protein and calcium are among the vital nutrients needed for stress, and you must get ample supplies of both of these. (See CALCIUM for a list of calcium sources.) But you must do two things to get enough of these nutrients into your body. First, you must eat foods which contain them, and then you must exercise to make them as effective as they can be. Muscles cannot grow and retain protein without activity. They don't respond passively to what's in their environment, but rather actively to the demands that are put upon them. Only when they have to do work do they grow and accumulate protein. Hence, being in optimal health in this case implies both nutrition and exercise. It means daily or every-other-day workouts, which are demanding enough to build up that muscle tissue. This can be done easily, by starting with only 20 minutes or so of vigorous exercise every other day at first. (See EXERCISE.) In this way,

when you encounter a stressful situation, even if eating is cut down or out for a short time, the wasting that can occur will have a less severe impact. And by the way, if you increase your muscle mass, you will also add significantly to your supplies of potassium.

Bones, like muscles, also need active work to build up their supplies of calcium. In response to the "good" stress of physical work, your bones store calcium and become denser, stronger, and able to carry more weight. Like the muscles then, when they are confronted with the "bad" stress of anxiety or illness, they can better afford to give up some of their calcium stores without becoming too weak.

So the best way to prepare for stress is to eat a balanced diet every day and to take some form of exercise in order to protect your body from being depleted of its essential nutrients during trying times.

NUTRITION DURING PERIODS OF STRESS

The appetite is normally suppressed during severe stress, because it is an adaptive reaction to a physical threat. Energy at such a time is needed to facilitate the fight or flight response, and is not usually used to look for or to eat food. The blood supply has been redirected to the muscles in order to maximize strength and speed, and so even if you do eat, you may not be able to digest or absorb it efficiently. In fact, during extreme upsets, the stomach and intestines may even reject solid food through processes like vomiting and diarrhea. What this all means is that a person under severe stress should not be forced to eat—they may not even be able to digest and absorb what they have eaten.

On the other hand, fasting is not a good idea either, and the longer one fasts, the harder it will be to start eating normally again. It is sad to watch a person who is under so much stress that they cannot eat, and by not eating become even less able to handle the stress. Hence, it is best not to let stress become so all-consuming that eating stops. Managing stress so that it does not overwhelm you is both a nutritional and a psychological task.

If a person under stress can eat, then he or she definitely should do so. You might eat only a little if that's all you can handle, but you can eat more often in order to meet nutrient and caloric needs. A person in this position should choose a variety of foods, and drink plenty of fluids as well. Although the body conserves fluids during stress, it will excrete what it does not need, and by taking in fluids a person enables the kidneys to excrete the sodium they might otherwise have to retain.

Whenever someone can't eat at all, nutrients will be depleted. Aside from the protein, calcium, and potassium (see POTASSIUM for a list of good potassium sources) we have already mentioned, the other nutrients most likely to be depleted are the vitamins and minerals which are not stored in the body in adequate quantities. Water soluble vitamins like C and the B vitamins fall into this category, as well as approximately two dozen minerals. So, if one is not eating properly during periods of extreme and prolonged stress, it is best to take a vitamin-mineral preparation which supplies a balanced assortment of all the nutrients that might be needed by the body, not in "megadoses" but in amounts comparable to the RDA. Generally, people taking in less than 1200 to 1500 calories per day need such supplements.

EATING TOO MUCH DURING PERIODS OF STRESS

Now that we have discussed the type of people who can't eat when confronted with stress, we should mention the other type—those people who eat more and too much during such times. It is not clear why stress drives some people to eat too much, but it certainly does happen.

One possibility is that the behavior of eating helps to relieve stress by occupying the nervous system with a familiar activity which discharges its nerves without doing any harm, as actual physical fighting might do.

It could also be that eating, or the food eaten, causes the release of soothing substances in the brain. For instance, brain chemical levels change when a high-carbohydrate diet is eaten. The chemical messengers in the brain, called neurotransmitters, are affected by the type of food eaten.

It also seems that certain types of stress cause the production of opiate-like substances in the brain, such as endorphins. The natural brain opiates in the emotion-governing brain regions promote both eating and the reduction of activity. Some proteins, when they are digested, also apparently release peptides which have a hormonal or opiate-type activity. Of course, much more study is needed in this field. But for now, let us say that the person who is subject to this type of behavior—that is, excessive eating during periods of stress—and who may develop obesity because of this, is best advised to find some different type of behavior that will ease the pains of stress, such as exercise, meditation, or starting a hobby.

Overeating during stress, or stress eating, also shows why exercise is important both before and during stress periods. In fact, it may indeed be harmful not to exercise when one is under acute stress. As we mentioned, in the stress response, muscle fuel floods the bloodstream and it needs to be used, or else it will be stored as fat. Emotionally, as well, exercise is good for people who are upset, angry, anxious, depressed, or even too excited or happy to express their feelings through physical actions. Punching pillows, running, lifting weights, dancing, singing, or whatever physical outlet one chooses, releases tensions that would otherwise build up and increase stress.

Exercise during stressful times builds up muscle and bone, promoting the retention of essential nutrients, and also may release pain-killing chemicals which can alleviate a dark mood to some extent, or ease physical pain and/or illness.

NUTRITION WHEN ONE IS RECOVERING FROM STRESS

When the period of great stress is over and the body can recover, a person has the ability to replenish depleted body stores. If weight has been lost, it should be regained by healthful eating and exercise which brings back both lean and fat tissue. If weight has been gained, diet and exercise should be used to remove those excess pounds. People should also learn how better to prepare themselves emotionally for the next stressful situation.

SUCROSE

Sucrose is a complex of two simple sugars, glucose and fructose, and is, therefore, called a disaccharide. Sucrose is used widely in the food industry—in baking, confection making, and soft drink preparation. Consumption has increased considerably since the early part of this century, and many people have been concerned that our high sucrose consumption may be detrimental to our health. The major areas of concern are: dental caries (cavities), obesity, diabetes, and atherosclerosis. (The relation of sucrose to each of these diseases is discussed in the section on that disease.) In general, however, sucrose is a major contributor to dental caries (see DENTAL DECAY), is involved in obesity only to the extent that it supplies calories in a sweet-tasting form, is not involved in the cause of diabetes, and is only important in atherosclerosis in some sensitive individuals. (See also CARBOHYDRATE.)

SULFUR

Sulfur is an important part of all proteins. The harder the protein, the higher the sulfur content, which means that skin, hair, and nails all have a high sulfur content. All protein-rich foods, including meats, fish, wheat germ, beans, peas, and peanuts, contain significant amounts of sulfur, which ensures that, provided your diet contains some protein, it is impossible to become sulfur deficient. It is also not possible to overdose on sulfur from the food you eat. No signs of sulfur overdose or deficiency have been reported in people.

TAURINE

Taurine is an amino acid that is not essential for adults because it can be made from other essential sulfa-containing amino acids. However, taurine is essential for infants of various species probably including humans. The older child or adult has no dietary need for this amino acid and there is no reason to use it as a supplement. (See also AMINO ACIDS.)

TEA

This beverage is prepared from the tender leaves, leaf buds, and tender stalks of different varieties of *Camellia sinensis*. Black tea is perhaps the most popular variety. It is produced by fermenting the leaves before drying them. Of the black teas, orange pekoe is made from the first opened leaf, pekoe from the third leaves, and souchong from the next leaves. Flowering pekoes, another type of black tea, are made from the top leaf buds. Green tea is light in color and higher in tannin than black tea is. This is not fermented but simply steamed and dried. Oolong tea is slightly fermented and is intermediate, between black and green.

The tea made from one tea bag contains .05 milligrams of vitamin B_2, .25 milligrams of nicotinic acid (niacin), and a significant amount of caffeine and caffeine-like substances called theobromides, which are mild stimulants to the brain. (See Dietary Sources of Caffeine (page 77) in CAFFEINE for the caffeine content of teas brewed for various lengths of time.)

As well as supplying nutrients to the diet, tea can detract from the diet. Tannin impairs iron absorption and caffeine increases the rate of excretion of calcium in the urine. (See also CAFFEINE.)

TRYPSIN

Trypsin is an enzyme that is important in the digestion of protein. In the presence of trypsin, the large protein molecules are broken down to smaller molecules and finally to individual amino acids. The individual amino acids are then absorbed from the gastrointestinal tract into the bloodstream. Trypsin has also been used to break down protein in food processing. (See also ENZYMES; PROTEIN.)

TRYPTOPHAN

Tryptophan is an amino acid (building block of protein) that the body cannot make and so it must be supplied by the diet. It is usually found in extremely small amounts in dietary proteins, but as long as 12 to 13 percent of the dietary calories are supplied in the form of good quality protein, sufficient tryptophan will be supplied to satisfy the body's needs.

In recent years tryptophan has been promoted as a therapeutic agent in a number of disorders. It is widely used in sleep clinics as an aid for people who take longer than normal to get to sleep, but it does not help insomnia due to anxiety. It has also been used as a therapeutic agent for people with depression associated with carbohydrate craving. As far as we know, tryptophan in the doses used (usually no more than 3 grams a day) is harmless, but supplementation of this kind should only be done under the advice of a doctor. (See also AMINO ACIDS.)

VEGETARIAN DIETS

Vegetarianism, which is becoming more popular in western society, is already widely practiced in other parts of the world. Therefore, it should not be viewed as a special diet, but rather as an alternative to usual eating patterns. The two major types of vegetarian diets are the ovo-lacto diet, which consists of foods of plant origin along with eggs and dairy products, and the vegan diet, which only includes foods of plant origin. The former is a perfectly acceptable diet and will provide adequate amounts of all the essential nutrients when properly balanced. The latter, if strictly adhered to, must be practiced with some care and should be supplemented with vitamin B_{12}.

OVO-LACTO VEGETARIANS

For various reasons, some people choose to omit foods of animal origin, restricting themselves to plant and milk products. They are called lacto-vegetarians. The inclusion of eggs in an otherwise all-plant diet makes someone an ovo-vegetarian. Vegetarians who consume both are called ovo-lacto vegetarians.

The nutrients which may be scarce in a diet derived from foods of plant orgin are protein, iron, and vitamin B_{12}. If adequate amounts of eggs and milk, cheese, and other milk products are eaten, then these nutrients will be provided in sufficient quantities to meet all requirements. A person should avoid consuming too much saturated fat and cholesterol however, and so should not eat large amounts of egg yolks, whole milk, and certain cheeses. In addition, it should be noted that most cheeses contain large amounts of salt and, hence, should only be eaten in small amounts if salt restriction is desired. This diet is usually rich in protein and will contain adequate amounts of iron and vitamin B_{12}. In addition, the amount of calcium consumed is usually quite high and the relatively low phosphorus intake favors calcium absorption.

Thus, the ovo-lacto vegetarian need not be strictly supervised unless serum cholesterol levels are such as to require dietary fat restrictions. If this is so, then by simply reducing the number of egg yolks to two per week and changing from butter to a soft margarine the problem will be solved. If the person is hypertensive and some salt restriction is desired, then cheeses of most types should be discouraged and natural, rather than processed, vegetables encouraged.

VEGANS

The diet followed by vegans allows

for consumption of nutrients from plant origin only. Thus no meat, poultry, fish, milk or their products are consumed. With the exception of vitamin B_{12} and possibly iron, all of the required nutrients can be obtained from this diet. The most important consideration here is in meeting protein requirements. The proteins present in plants are incomplete. This means that different vegetables must be added to the diet in order to meet the protein needs of the vegan. In general, eating cereals and legumes such as beans and peas in the daily menu is the answer.

PROTEIN

Concern over protein consumption arises from its critical role in the growth and maintenance of body tissue. Proteins, the constituents of muscles, hair, skin, enzymes, and other body tissues, are made up of twenty-two different amino acids. These amino acids are combined in different sequences and numbers, resulting in thousands of proteins with different characteristics. This explains why egg whites and fingernails—both composed of proteins—differ so much in appearance and properties.

Of the twenty-two amino acids, eight of these must be provided in the diet—they are called essential amino acids. The other fourteen amino acids can, with the necessary materials available, be made by the body—they are called nonessential. Without an adequate intake of essential amino acids, protein deficiency will develop.

The proteins found in animal tissues—muscle, eggs, organ meats, milk, and cheese—contain all eight essential amino acids (in addition to some of the other fourteen). They are appropriately called complete proteins. The proteins found in plants do *not* contain all eight essential amino acids and are therefore incomplete proteins. One exception to this is the protein found in soya beans, which is as good as some animal-derived proteins.

It might be assumed from all this that choosing a diet consisting entirely of incomplete plant proteins will result in an inadequate intake of essential amino acids. However, nature has taken care of this possible dilemma. Those essential amino acids that are low or missing in plants such as grains, are abundant in other plants such as legumes. By simply combining different plant foods containing protein at the same meal, all the essential amino acids are present at one time. The resulting combined proteins are then complete. This practice is called "complementing proteins" and is based on the fact that by eating two incomplete proteins in which different essential amino acids are missing, you end up with a complete protein.

Foods most suitable for complementing are grains, a group of plant foods generally low in the amino acid lysine and high in the amino acid methionine, with legumes, a group generally low in methionine and high in lysine. This concept of complementing proteins has been empirically practiced by many civilizations for thousands of years. For example, Latin Americans regularly consume corn tortillas (a grain) and red beans (a legume).

Other amino acids will also match to form a protein of comparable value to that of meats and dairy products. Of course, if a protein of animal origin is added to a meal the total protein value is increased. It is important to remember that the actual consumption of complementary proteins must occur together in order for the individual to receive a complete protein.

Some typical complemented protein meals are described in the Dietary Guidelines. Figure 1 on page 293 illustrates the general rules for selecting specific foods.

One particular concern should be noted in regard to vegetarian diets. With the increased trend toward vegan families, we are seeing more and more small children weaned to diets of pure plant origin. The weaned child is particularly prone to protein deficiency and cases of protein-calorie malnutrition are appearing with alarming frequency. It is very important at this stage of life to encourage the consumption of adequate amounts of complete proteins. This means either continuing the use of soy-based milk or milk products beyond the weaning period, or carefully complementing plant proteins to form a food which the child will eat. To this end, peanut butter can serve a useful purpose. The same effect can be achieved by using soya beans or lentils. The rate of growth of children growing up in a vegan family should be carefully watched so as to make sure the child's growth is not being stunted through a lack of adequate dietary protein. (See PROTEIN-CALORIE MALNUTRITION.)

VITAMIN B$_{12}$

Vitamin B$_{12}$, a vitamin involved in red blood cell production, is available only from animal sources. Thus, a vegan will become deficient in vitamin B$_{12}$. Since symptoms of this deficiency often take a long time to develop, especially when the supply of folacin (a related vitamin) is adequate, it is often overlooked. People consuming a vegan diet must be provided with a source of vitamin B$_{12}$. This can be accomplished in several ways. One usually acceptable source is brewer's yeast, or the soy-fermented product tempeh, and still another is fortified breakfast cereal. Direct vitamin supplementation is also a possibility. (See VITAMIN B$_{12}$.)

IRON

Iron intake can also be a problem for the vegan. The richest sources of iron are those foods of animal origin such as red meats and liver. Another good source is egg yolk. Plant sources only provide a form of iron that may not be easily absorbed, and unless carefully chosen, a deficiency can occur. Ingestion of high amounts of vitamin C or any acidic food (such as tomatoes) will help by promoting iron absorption. Due to the high intake of citrus fruits and many green vegetables, the vegan diet should be relatively high in vitamin C; however, all strict vegetarians must be considered at risk for iron deficiency. There are several ways of approach-ing this problem. One is to make meal choices which bear in mind the iron content of the food. The following table lists the iron content of certain vegetable foods that are relatively good sources of iron. A second approach is to eat iron-enriched foods, such as certain breakfast cereals. Finally, direct iron supplementation of 20 milligrams per day can be used.

During certain periods of life, iron supplementation is mandatory in people consuming strictly vegetarian diets. These times include pregnancy, early childhood, and adolescence. In addition, any major loss of blood, even through voluntary blood donation, should be accompanied with iron supplementation. (See ANEMIAS; IRON.)

IRON CONTENT OF PLANT FOODS

Food	Amount	Grams	Iron (mg)
Enriched white rice (cooked)	1 cup	205	1.8
Brown rice (cooked)	1 cup	195	1.0
Bread (whole wheat & white)	1 sl	23	0.7
Egg (large)	1	57	1.2
Spinach (cooked)	1 cup	190	4.8
Kale (cooked)	1 cup	130	1.3
Tofu	1 piece	120	2.3
Beans (e.g., kidney)	1 cup	255	4.5
Peanut butter	2 tbsp	32	0.6
Bean sprouts (raw)	1 cup	105	1.4
Brewer's yeast	1 tbsp	8	1.4
Torula yeast	1 oz	28	5.5
Fruit (e.g., banana)	1	200	1.0
Dried fruit (e.g., raisins)	1½ oz	42	1.5

CALCIUM

Calcium, although present in the largest amounts in dairy products, is also present in certain foods of plant origin. Figure 2 (below) shows foods rich in calcium. Since most people consuming a vegan diet will be eating relatively small amounts of phosphorus and protein (which tend to impair calcium absorption), absorption of calcium will be very efficient and hence calcium supplementation is unnecessary. During pregnancy and lactation, however, when calcium requirements are very high, supplementation is recommended. This can be most easily accomplished by consuming 500 milligrams of calcium gluconate daily. (See CALCIUM.)

Thus a vegetarian, whether a vegan or an ovo-lacto vegetarian, can consume a healthful and varied diet with only minor adjustments. Such diets have the advantage of being high in fiber and—in the case of strict vegetarians or those consuming only occasional dairy products—low in calories, low in total fat, and low in saturated fat. A vegetarian diet is one way of consuming the so called prudent diet, and hence will offer a certain amount of protection against coronary artery disease. Therefore, we feel there is no reason to discourage vegetarianism.

DIETARY GUIDELINES

As discussed previously, the principal need for the vegetarian is to consume proteins adequate in both quality and quantity. The recommended dietary allowances (1979) for protein are summarized as follows:

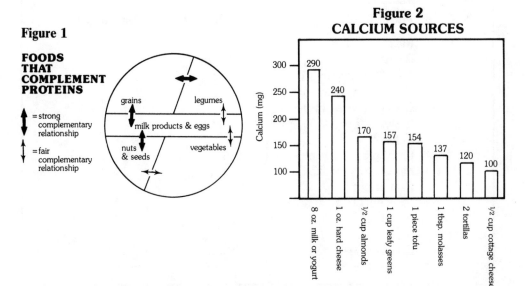

Figure 1

FOODS THAT COMPLEMENT PROTEINS

↕ = strong complementary relationship

↑↓ = fair complementary relationship

grains   legumes
milk products & eggs
nuts & seeds   vegetables

Figure 2
CALCIUM SOURCES

Calcium (mg)

290 — 8 oz. milk or yogurt
240 — 1 oz. hard cheese
170 — ½ cup almonds
157 — 1 cup leafy greens
154 — 1 piece tofu
137 — 1 tbsp. molasses
120 — 2 tortillas
100 — ½ cup cottage cheese

Group	Ages	Protein (g)
Infants	0–1	approx. 13
Children	1–3	approx. 23
	4–6	approx. 30
	7–10	approx. 34
Males	11–14	approx. 45
	15+	approx. 56
Females	11–18	approx. 46
	19+	approx. 44
Pregnant		approx. +30
Lactating		approx. +20

As the following table indicates, it is very easy to consume the recommended amount of protein without eating meat. Since almost all vegetables contain approximately 2 grams of protein per ½ cup cooked serving, these foods add to the total available protein per day.

PROTEIN SOURCES

Food	Amount	Protein (g)
Rice	1 cup	10
Beans	½ cup	10
All milk & yogurt	8 oz	8
Cheese (sandwich-type)	1 oz	7
Cottage cheese (pot-style, or regular)	½ cup	14
Tofu (2″ × 3″)	120	9.4
Leafy green vegetables	1 cup	4–5
Most beans (cooked)	1 cup	14–15
Peanut butter	2 tbsp	8
Most nuts (e.g., almonds)	½ cup	7–12
Bread	1 slice	2–3
Noodles (cooked)	1 cup	7
Brewer's yeast	1 tbsp	3

Pitfalls, as noted earlier, can be avoided by seeking a wide variety of plant foods, thereby ensuring adequate consumption of many nutrients. An ovo-lacto vegetarian should find this diet interesting and certainly as, if not more, economical than a diet with meat.

Breakfasts can be very similar to nonvegetarian meals, minus sausage or other meat additions. If eating at home, boost the protein quality of pancakes, oatmeal, or other home-prepared grain dishes by adding 2 or 3 tablespoons of nonfat dry milk to the batter or pot. Likewise, fortify your fluid milk with a similar proportion of dry milk. Be sure to include fruits and juices.

Lunches for school children can consist of peanut butter, an age-old favorite, or a spread of pot cheese (in place of low-protein cream cheese) on bread. Try plain yogurt, refrigerated and drained overnight in a cheese cloth (save the whey liquid that drips out) for a similar type of cream-cheese spread. These sandwiches can be perked up with sprinkled cinnamon, raisins, or cooking herbs and seasonings. If eaten within three to four hours of preparation, refrigeration is not needed. If possible, however, keep them chilled. Many restaurants now offer yogurt, cottage cheese plates, and salad bars as meatless selections.

Snacks are the key to making sure children and adolescents get enough calories. For everyone, they are a chance to augment light protein meals taken at other times during the day. Finger foods for children can include celery stuffed with cottage cheese or peanut butter, small peanut butter sandwiches, or a candy made of three parts peanut butter, two parts powdered milk, and one part (or less) of honey, all rolled in nut crumbs or graham cracker crumbs and chilled.

The dinner meal can be any version of the following:

Chili sin carne (without meat) with rice
Baked beans and brown bread
Okra, corn, lima, and tomato gumbo
Macaroni and cheese
Zucchini or spinach quiche
Bean sprouts and tofu with rice
Squash stuffed with cottage cheese or tofu

When vegetables and fruits are added these meals are both nutritious and tasty.

Desserts can and should be nutritious complements to all meals. For ovo-lacto vegetarians, flavored yogurt, frozen or fluid, or milk-based puddings are recommended. Egg custards are also protein-rich additions to meals. High protein vegan desserts can consist of sweetened and flavored blends of tofu.

Entertaining is as easy as making minimeals. Items such as stuffed mushrooms, cheese and olives, raw vegetables and yogurt-dill dip, quiche, bean dip and tortilla chips, and mixed dried fruit and nuts are tasty and extraordinary hors d'oeuvres.

Dining out will be different, as the check may be slightly less! Entrees such as eggplant Parmesan, or spaghetti with marinara sauce and Parmesan cheese are good selections at Italian restaurants. Jewish dairy restaurants can be a vegetarian's delight. Steak restaurants may restrict someone more to certain a la carte selections, the soup of the day, or side dishes of vegetables. However, it should be understood that these selections are not necessarily low-calorie or nonfilling. The choice of butter and cream or cheese sauces can significantly alter the calorie and satiety value.

As always, your appetite, personal preferences, and nutritional education are the best guides to the diet suited to you. (See also BREWER'S YEAST; CARBOHYDRATE; FIBER; MACROBIOTIC DIETS; OSTEOPOROSIS.)

VITAMIN(S)

A vitamin is an organic substance the body needs but cannot make and that is therefore an essential component of the diet in very small amounts. The vitamins were discovered, isolated, and synthesized during the early part of this century. Because of their discovery many important diseases known to be caused by a deficiency in one or more vitamins can now be cured by supplying the missing vitamin in pure form or by consuming a diet which is rich in the missing vitamin. The best way for a person to prevent a vitamin deficiency from occurring is to consume a diet which is varied and includes foods from as many groups as possible. In general, vitamins A, D, K, and E (the fat soluble vitamins) are found in a variety of oils from animal and vegetable sources. The B complex vitamins are found in whole grains and some, such as folacin (folic acid), are also found in meat. Vitamin C (ascorbic acid) is found mostly in citrus fruits but certain other foods, such as the potato, contain this vitamin. Vitamin B_{12} is found only in meat or animal products (dairy foods) and hence the pure vegetarian will be deficient in this vitamin.

The vitamins can be divided into two major groups: those which are fat soluble (will dissolve in oils), and those which are water soluble (will dissolve in water).

FAT SOLUBLE VITAMINS

The fat soluble vitamins only dissolve in fat or oil and therefore are found in foods containing these substances. Since they must be transported to the cells of the body via the bloodstream, a water based liquid, they must be carried by special molecules which are soluble in water. Hence, these vitamins are all associated with carrier proteins which act as their vehicles as they go into and come out of the cells in our body.

There are four fat soluble vitamins—A, D, K, and E. They all have certain properties in common, such as their mode of transport in blood, their ability to be stored by the body, and their greater deficiency symptoms in young children. However, each has its own unique purpose in our body's metabolism, and a deficiency of one of these vitamins is accompanied by very specific signs and symptoms.

WATER SOLUBLE VITAMINS

The water soluble vitamins are the B complex vitamins (B_1, B_2, B_3, B_6, folacin and B_{12}) and vitamin C (ascorbic acid). In addition, two other water soluble substances, biotin and pantothenic acid, have recently been shown to be essential and, therefore, are classified as vitamins.

All of these vitamins, with the exception of vitamin B_{12}, are rapidly excreted from the body since the capacity to store them is extremely limited. Thus, they are required on a regular basis or deficiency symptoms will occur. Some of these vitamins (B_1, B_2, B_3, and B_6) are cofactors in certain reactions necessary for the body to utilize its main sources of fuel properly. Hence, when fuel is scarce these vitamins are necessary in smaller amounts and deficiency symptoms may not occur. For this reason, populations suffering from semistarvation may not show signs of specific vitamin deficiencies. Ironically if calories are rapidly supplied without supplementation of these vitamins deficiency symptoms may be induced. (See also entries for specific vitamins.)

VITAMIN A (RETINOL)

There are two dietary forms of vitamin A. Retinol (vitamin A) itself comes from animal sources usually associated with fat; for example, fish liver oils. However, the major source of vitamin A in our diets is B carotene, which comes from plant sources; for example, carrots or other yellow vegetables. The B carotene is broken down and converted to vitamin A within the intestines. The vitamin A is absorbed and transported with the fat in our diets from the intestine to the liver. The liver plays a central role in the body's metabolism of vitamin A. It stores any excess amounts and hence is the main storage site for the release of vitamin A when the body's supply becomes low. The liver also synthesizes a specific protein, retinol binding protein (RBP), which as its name suggests, binds the vitamin A and then transports it via the bloodstream to the tissues of the body.

Not all the actions of vitamin A have been defined. In fact the only function of vitamin A which has been totally worked out is its role in maintaining certain specialized pigment within the retina of the eye. This pigment is necessary for the eye to see when light is dim or absent; hence, a deficiency of vitamin A will result in night blindness. Vitamin A is also important for certain tissues which cover our body (skin) and line our organs (epithelial tissue) to grow and regenerate themselves normally. One such tissue is the cornea of the eye, a transparent membrane covering and protecting the deeper parts of the eye which are more directly concerned with vision. Vitamin A deficiency, particularly in young children, can cause the cornea to lose its transparency. This change, if not treated promptly with vitamin A, can lead to permanent scarring of the eye and blindness. The most common cause of blindness in children the world over is vitamin A deficiency. This form of blindness, which is totally preventable, has affected and is still occurring in millions of children throughout the third world because of widespread vitamin A deficiency. In our own country, such serious vitamin A deficiency rarely occurs. However, milder forms are seen quite commonly. These usually involve roughening and peeling of the skin accompanied by low levels of vitamin A circulating in the blood. One manifestation of chronic low level vitamin A deficiency which has been postulated recently is cancer in certain organs. Because the incidence of certain cancers is higher in populations consuming low amounts of vitamin A or B carotene, it is thought by many scientists that vitamin A in normal amounts may offer some protection against these cancers. Some experiments in animals support these conclusions. There is no evidence, however, that vitamin A itself or B carotene have any effect on any cancer that has already formed.

Too much vitamin A can be extremely toxic, causing headache, nausea, vomiting, blurred vision, and brain damage. Thus, doses above the recommended dietary allowance of 5000 international units should not be consumed. By contrast, B carotene in relatively large amounts does not seem to cause any serious effects except for some yellowing of the skin. However, since no benefits have been described from large doses of B carotene its routine use is not recommended.

Vitamin A is found in dried apricots, green vegetables, cantaloupe, carrots, corn, liver, milk, peaches, sweet potato, pumpkin, squash, and tomato juice.

VITAMIN B₁ (THIAMINE)

Thiamine, or vitamin B_1, is found in large amounts in bran, yeast, and whole grain cereals and in smaller amounts in fresh fruits and vegetables. Thiamine plays a central role in the metabolism of both carbohydrate and protein. In addition, it is essential for proper functioning of the nervous system. In developing countries, particularly among rural populations in southeast Asia, primary thiamine deficiency is common. This is probably due to the fact that these populations subsist on a diet in which the staple food is polished rice. The portion of the rice removed in the "polishing" contains thiamine in substantial quantities but is usually discarded for cultural reasons. In more developed countries, including the United States, secondary thiamine deficiency may be encountered. In alcoholics, especially those in a state of chronic malnutrition, thiamine is poorly absorbed in the intestine; hence, thiamine deficiency may ensue.

Severe thiamine deficiency results in a disease known as beriberi. This disease, still quite common in rural areas of southeast Asia and in other developing countries, may manifest itself in one of three major forms: "wet" beriberi where the person retains fluid which swells the tissue (edema) and develops heart failure; "dry" beriberi which affects peripheral nerves causing weakness of the extremities; and infantile beriberi which affects young infants and is still a leading cause of death in infants between two and five months of age in rice-eating rural areas.

In the United States, both the "wet" and "dry" forms of beriberi are seen in alcoholics, particularly those who are on a poor diet as well. Thus it is often seen in the poorer segments of society in individuals who have been consuming large amounts of alcohol for long periods of time. Because alcohol interferes with the absorption of other nutrients, pure thiamine deficiency (beriberi) is rare. More commonly it is mixed with other forms of malnutrition. (See FOLACIN; VITAMIN B_2; VITAMIN B_6; ZINC.)

There is a specific nervous disorder which is seen mainly in alcoholics and is due to thiamine deficiency. It is called the Wernicke-Korsakoff syndrome. If this disease is not treated promptly with generous amounts of thiamine severe irreversible brain damage may ensue.

The present recommended dietary allowance for vitamin B_1 is about 1.5 milligrams per day. There is no evidence that large doses of this vitamin has any health benefits except for the treatment of beriberi and then only for a short time.

Some sources of vitamin B₁ are: asparagus, beans, meat, cereals, green vegetables, dairy products, and oranges.

VITAMIN B₂ (RIBOFLAVIN)

Riboflavin is a yellow-green fluorescent compound which is needed by the tissues to utilize oxygen for burning fuel. The best sources of riboflavin are liver, milk, dairy products, poultry, fish, eggs, and green vegetables. It differs from the other B vitamins in that it is present in relatively large amounts in dairy products but only in small amounts in cereal products. Riboflavin is also found in beer.

Considering its importance in the body's metabolism it is surprising that deficiency of this vitamin is not more common. Severe deficiency may affect the mouth, tongue, and eyes. While these symptoms have been rarely seen in connection with riboflavin deficiency in the United States, surveys have shown that large numbers of people, particularly among poorer segments of our population, have low blood levels of riboflavin and are, therefore, potentially deficient.

There are no known benefits of riboflavin in large doses, and therefore, even though toxic symptoms are not common, the use of these large doses of vitamin B₂ is not recommended.

VITAMIN B₃ (NIACIN)

Niacin is necessary for tissues to burn carbohydrate and protein efficiently in order to produce energy. A deficiency of this vitamin occurs most often among poor peasants who subsist mainly on corn. Until the 1950s, severe niacin deficiency, known as pellagra, was quite common in the southern part of the United States. Pellagra is a very debilitating disease which is accompanied by weight loss, a characteristic rash in areas exposed to the sun, diarrhea, swollen tongue, and severe mental changes. Vitamin B_2 requirements are expressed in niacin equivalents. Milk and eggs have high niacin equivalents. In fact, niacin itself is widely distributed in plant and animal foods, but in relatively small amounts. Meat (especially organ meat), fish, whole grain cereals, asparagus, peas, potatoes, peaches, nuts, and pulses are good sources of niacin. As a result of this widespread distribution even a moderately good diet should easily supply the 6.6 milligrams per 1000 calories of niacin equivalents that constitute the recommended daily allowance. Hence, niacin rarely needs to be supplemented.

Niacin in high doses can produce certain side effects, such as flushing and palpitations, and should therefore never be taken in so called megadoses (ten to one hundred times the RDA) without a physician's supervision.

VITAMIN B₆ (PYRIDOXINE)

Vitamin B_6 is essential for a number of important reactions concerned with protein metabolism. Primary deficiency is rare because vitamin B_6 is widely distributed in both animal and plant tissues. It is found in large amounts in meat, fish, nuts, bananas, potatoes, dairy products, and bran. Most human diets provide 1 to 2 milligrams a day which is quite sufficient for most people. Several cases of primary pyridoxine deficiency occurred in the 1950s when one of the infant formulas then on the market failed to add vitamin B_6. Severe neurological consequences including convulsions occurred in a number of infants before the cause was discovered and the problem corrected. Secondary pyridoxine deficiency is more common. Certain drugs, including oral contraceptives and isoniazid (a drug commonly used for the prevention and treatment of tuberculosis), interfere with vitamin B_6 metabolism. Thus, people taking these drugs should consume a vitamin B_6 supplement. In those people who are deficient in pyridoxine because of an interfering drug that they are taking, larger doses of the vitamin than are normally needed may be necessary to reverse the deficiency (ten to twenty times the RDA). Symptoms of vitamin B_6 deficiency may include depression and for that reason some people have recommended the use of this vitamin in very large doses (one thousand times the RDA) for the treatment of depression. Vitamin B_6 will help only a depression caused by a deficiency. Most depressions have nothing to do with pyridoxine deficiency and hence will not respond to administration of vitamin B_6 in any amount.

VITAMIN B₁₂ (CYANOCOBALAMIN)

The only clearly defined action of vitamin B_{12} is to make active folacin (folic acid) available for certain essential metabolic reactions. Thus, the major manifestations of vitamin B_{12} deficiency are identical to those of folacin deficiency; a profound anemia with abnormal red cells. These manifestations can be reversed with folacin as well as with vitamin B_{12}. However, there is another serious manifestation of vitamin B_{12} deficiency which is not present in folacin deficiency; severe irreversible brain and spinal cord damage. Thus, it is essential that any person with the characteristic anemia of either folacin or B_{12} deficiency be carefully studied so the specific cause of the anemia can be determined. If it is due to vitamin B_{12} deficiency this vitamin and only this vitamin will cure the anemia and prevent the neurological disease that might follow.

Vitamin B_{12} is found only in foods of animal origin and hence strict vegetarians are at risk for developing a deficiency. Some types of yeast and other nontraditional foods acceptable to vegetarians, such as tempeh, contain vitamin B_{12}. If these foods are not consumed, strict vegetarians should either use foods fortified with vitamin B_{12} or take a supplement. In general, primary vitamin B_{12} deficiency due to poor dietary intake is quite rare since the requirement is very low (3 milligrams per day) and almost all foods of animal origin, including all dairy products and eggs, contain generous amounts of vitamin B_{12}. (See VEGETARIAN DIETS.)

However, in order to be absorbed through the small intestines, vitamin B_{12} must form a complex with a substance secreted in the stomach known as intrinsic factor. If this substance is missing, as might be the case in people who have diseases involving the stomach or who have had their stomachs removed, vitamin B_{12} deficiency may occur. Under these conditions the vitamin may have to be given by injection in order to be effective.

Vitamin B_{12} is the only water soluble vitamin that is stored by the body in any appreciable amounts. Hence, a deficiency of this vitamin may take several years to develop. There is a rare genetic form of vitamin B_{12} deficiency in infants who cannot utilize the vitamin completely. Such infants may require high doses of this vitamin for the rest of their lives. Other than for the treatment of this extremely rare condition there is no known health benefit from high doses of vitamin B_{12} and, therefore, supplementation at higher amounts than the RDA is not recommended. (See also ANEMIAS.)

VITAMIN C (ASCORBIC ACID)

At the end of the eighteenth century Dr. James Lind discovered that there was a factor in the juice of limes which protected against scurvy, a disease which was common in England during that period and which plagued the seamen of the British navy. British warships began to carry limes among their supplies, scurvy rarely occurred thereafter and the British sailors came to be known as "limeys," a name which has persisted in some circles until today. Thus the classical deficiency disease caused by an insufficient supply of vitamin C in the diet was able to be cured before its cause was actually known. Only in the 1930s were Glen King and Albert Szent-Gyorgi independently able to isolate and synthesize vitamin C and show that it was the missing agent in experimentally induced scurvy.

Vitamin C is essential in maintaining the integrity of connective tissue. Since the walls of small blood vessels are made up largely of connective tissue, bleeding is the most common manifestation of vitamin C deficiency. In scurvy, the bleeding commonly occurs in the gums, and if the disease lasts long enough the teeth loosen and fall out. Bleeding may also occur in the skin and into the space surrounding some of the long bones. When such bleeding occurs it can be extremely painful and debilitating. Since wounds heal primarily through the growth of new connective tissue, vitamin C is important in wound healing and patients who are deficient in this vitamin may heal poorly after trauma involving cuts or fractures and after surgery. Only a few mammals (humans, higher apes, guinea pigs, and bats) require vitamin C. The majority of mammals can synthesize ascorbic acid from other compounds.

Vitamin C is found in fruits, especially citrus fruits and vegetables, including the potato. The normal requirement for vitamin C has become a very controversial subject. Certainly 40 milligrams per day, the present recommended daily allowance, is more than enough to cure scurvy and prevent any of its symptoms from recurring. At this intake blood levels of vitamin C are normal and tissues appear saturated with this vitamin. Some recent data suggests that blood levels of vitamin C are lower in heavy smokers and that their requirements may be somewhat higher. The controversy, however, is whether very high doses of vitamin C (ten to one hundred times the RDA) can protect us against certain diseases; the two most important being the common cold and cancer. The data with the common cold is unclear. One large study showed that 500 milligrams daily of vitamin C taken for a year reduced the severity of the common cold. People taking this supplement had as many colds but their symptoms were fewer and they missed fewer days of work. A second study, however, was unable to show any differences between people taking the supplement and those who did not.

As for cancer, there is data which suggests that populations who consume large amounts of citrus fruits have a lower incidence of certain cancers. However, there is no data to support the claim that huge doses of vitamin C can protect us from getting cancer. Some people have claimed that very high doses of vitamin C can cure certain forms of cancer. So far, all the studies trying to confirm this hypothesis have failed. Although vitamin C even in large doses over long periods of time is relatively safe, some side effects have been noted. High doses of vitamin C will cause an increased excretion of this vitamin in the urine and can also cause diarrhea, urate stones, and interference with glucose testing. Since very little vitamin C is stored in the body the urine will become more acidic than usual (since vitamin C is acid). We do not know if prolonged periods of acidic urine are dangerous.

Recently, another side effect of prolonged high doses of ascorbic acid has been reported in pregnant guinea pigs and is suspected in pregnant women. Guinea pigs exposed to high doses of vitamin C during pregnancy give birth to pups who develop scurvy more rapidly when reared without additional vitamin C. This occurs because vitamin C is broken down more rapidly in these pups and, hence, reserves are used up faster. Thus a sort of vitamin C dependency has occurred which disappears with time if small amounts of vitamin C are consumed. This dependency has been seen in people who have consumed large doses for a long time and then cut back to the usual intake. Their blood levels of vitamin C drop below normal and then over time regain their original level.

Clearly there are no definitive answers about consuming large doses of ascorbic acid. Certainly Americans should increase their intake of citrus fruits. Over and above this there is little evidence that very high doses of vitamin C offer any specific health benefits.

Good sources of vitamin C are: citrus fruit, green vegetables, cantaloupe, green peppers, and berries.

VITAMIN D

Vitamin D is found in certain fish oils and can be made in our skin when exposed to the ultraviolet rays of the sun. This vitamin is unique in the sense that it can be made by the body when exposed to sunlight, and in addition, has its own "backup system" in its presence in the foods we eat. In general, in those areas where sunlight is scarce (polar regions) the inhabitants can get all the vitamin D they need from the fish which make up a significant portion of their diet.

Deficiency of vitamin D, like deficiencies of other fat-soluble vitamins, manifests itself most frequently in young children. It may occur during the first year of life, and has even been diagnosed in utero by examining X rays of fetuses of women who are vitamin D deficient.

During the early part of this century, rickets, the classic vitamin D deficiency disease, was extremely common in this country and in Europe. However, with the addition of vitamin D to milk, primary rickets has been almost eliminated in most developed countries. In developing countries, however, it remains one of the major cripplers of children.

The earliest changes produced by rickets can be detected by X rays. In a small child rachitic changes are seen in the developing bones of the wrists. As growth progresses and weight bearing begins, the tibias become soft and bow due to poor calcification. At the junctions of the ribs and the sternum (breastbone), faulty calcification results in a series of beadlike projections, known as the rachitic rosary. Thus, the child with active rickets is short, deformed, and has extremely painful and tender bone ends.

The disease responds dramatically to small doses of vitamin D and can be prevented by adequate exposure to sunlight or by eating foods containing vitamin D, such as oily fish and enriched foods.

In more advanced countries, secondary rickets—also called vitamin D–resistant rickets because it could not be satisfactorily treated even with massive doses of vitamin D—has remained a problem. In the last few years, several research breakthroughs have improved our understanding of the metabolism of this vitamin and, for the first time, have made specific therapy for certain forms of vitamin D–resistant rickets possible. These recent investigations into the biochemical mechanisms for the action of vitamin D demonstrate, perhaps better than in any other area of nutrition, how fundamental research can have a direct and immediate influence on the treatment of disease.

Strictly speaking, the vitamin D found in the diet or converted in our skin is not a vitamin since it is in an inactive form. In order to become active it must undergo a two-step chemical transformation. The first step occurs in the liver and the final product is made in the kidney. Only the kidney is capable of making this active form of the vitamin (dihydroxy-vitamin D). Thus, in certain disease states where this function of the kidney is destroyed, rickets will develop even though dietary vitamin D is adequate. The active form of vitamin D can now be made in the laboratory and is available for use in certain types of kidney disease. Thus, in order to function, the vitamin D we take in our diet or convert in our skin must first reach the liver. In that organ the first chemical transformation occurs and the resulting product is transported through the blood to the kidney. In the kidney the final transformation occurs and the active form is created. This active form of vitamin D is really a hormone because it acts on two distant systems; the gastrointestinal tract and the bones. In the gastrointestinal tract, the active hormone of vitamin D (dihydroxy-vitamin D) stimulates the absorption of calcium into the bloodstream. In the bones it stimulates the deposition of that calcium into the bony structure. Thus, the vitamin D hormone pulls calcium into the body and causes its deposition into bone. If this hormone is present in inadequate amounts a deficiency of calcium will ensue and this deficiency will be partially made up by calcium leaving the bones to supply the other tissues. It is this loss of calcium from bone or the failure of calcium to deposit in newly forming bone which results in rickets and the deformed and painful bones described above.

Although vitamin D is found naturally in fish oils (cod-liver oil used to be our major source) our main source today is fortified milk and dairy products. The recommended dietary allowance for vitamin D is 400 international units. This amount is present in 1 quart of milk. Thus, the average person who consumes dairy products and who is moderately exposed to sunlight has no need for vitamin D supplementation.

Vitamin D in large quantities can be extremely toxic causing calcium to deposit in tissues other than bone. The margin of safety between the recommended dietary allowance (RDA) for vitamin D and the level which is toxic in some people is very small; the smallest for any vitamin. Some people develop toxic symptoms at three to four times the RDA. Thus the practice of supplementation with this vitamin should be discouraged.

VITAMIN E (TOCOPHEROL)

Vitamin E is actually a series of compounds known as tocopherols. They are found both in vegetable and animal oils and are associated with polyunsaturated fatty acids. The most potent of these tocopherols is alpha-tocopherol and hence the requirements for vitamin E is in units of tocopherol. The recommended dietary allowance (RDA) for vitamin E is between 10 and 20 international units (IU) per day. The exact action (or actions) or vitamin E is not well understood. It is important in maintaining the structure of cell membranes, and in the adult, long standing vitamin E deficiency when experimentally induced resulted in red blood cells which were more fragile than normal. Under normal conditions, dietary vitamin E deficiency in the adult does not occur. In the newborn infant, particularly the premature infant, vitamin E deficiency can and does occur. Perhaps this is because the premature infant has so little body fat, where vitamin E is normally stored. The deficiency syndrome in premature infants is a severe anemia (caused by the breaking up of the fragile red cells). If not diagnosed and treated with vitamin E this anemia can be very serious even leading to death.

Considering the very low prevalence of vitamin E deficiency it is surprising that this vitamin has received the attention that it gets. It has been hailed by some as a potential panacea. Exaggerated claims are being made including suggestions that it increases libido and sexual potency in both males and females. To be sure, vitamin E, even in very high doses, does not seem to be toxic. However, the stories we hear that high doses of vitamin E can prevent aging, reduce the risk of cancer, cure skin diseases, prevent habitual miscarriage, heart disease, and menopausal symptoms, and cure infertility, peptic ulcer, burns, and certain neuromuscular disorders are without foundation. Vitamin E in large doses has even been marketed for curing sexual dysfunction in both sexes. Again, there is no basis for such claims.

The lack of toxicity of vitamin E has prompted some people to argue that "It doesn't hurt and since it may do some good why not use it?" This is a very dangerous argument. We do not know that very high doses of vitamin E taken for very long periods of time are not toxic. Recently one of the B vitamins has been shown to be severely toxic in very high doses in certain people. (See VITAMIN B$_6$.) The same could be true with vitamin

E. In addition, this vitamin is stored in the body, in our fat tissue, and therefore the potential for serious toxicity from a cumulative effect of long-term administration is always there.

Certain chemical properties of vitamin E make it an attractive candidate for preventing certain types of damage to the body. Among these is the damage produced in the lung by certain environmental pollutants. There is a large amount of research currently being conducted on this subject. As yet the best we can say is that it works in some animals exposed to large amounts of certain pollutants. The data is not yet strong enough to warrant the use of high doses of vitamin E in the general public.

One rather specific and quite rare condition may respond to high doses of vitamin E in some people. This condition is known as intermittent claudication. It is manifested by a hardening of the arteries of the legs causing reduced circulation and severe pain in walking. Some people suffering from this condition have had the severity and frequency of attacks lessened by large doses of vitamin E (ten to one hundred times the RDA). Since this condition should always be under the care of a physician these doses of vitamin E should not be used without his or her advice.

Vitamin E is found in vegetable oil, nuts, and fish-liver oils.

VITAMIN K

Vitamin K is found in green leafy vegetables (e.g., broccoli, lettuce, cabbage, spinach) and red meat, particularly beef liver. Vitamin K is absorbed from the small intestines together with the fat in our diet and is transported to the liver where it is stored and when needed released into the bloodstream. Vitamin K has one known physiological function. It serves as a cofactor in synthesizing the various proteins needed for blood clotting, the most important being prothrombin.

Since many of the bacteria normally carried in our gastrointestinal tract can synthesize vitamin K, dietary deficiency almost never occurs in the adult. However, under certain circumstances in which bacterial growth is impaired, for example under specific antibiotic treatment, vitamin K deficiency can be induced unless adequate quantities are consumed in the diet. In young infants (particularly during the newborn period), before the bacterial flora of the gastrointestinal tract has become estab-lished, vitamin K deficiency can occur. Its main manifestation is bleeding, and if the bleeding occurs in vital organs it can be extremely dangerous. For this reason in many hospitals vitamin K is routinely given at delivery by injection.

There are certain times when a physician may deliberately want to reduce the ability for blood to clot. Under these circumstances an anticoagulant may be used. One class of these drugs, the coumarins, of which dicumarol is the most common, blocks the action of vitamin K and thereby reduces blood clotting. If a patient is taking one of these drugs and begins to bleed, vitamin K is the specific antidote.

High doses of vitamin K should never be used except under careful medical supervision. There are no known benefits of high doses of this vitamin and because of the effect such doses might have on blood clotting, taking vitamin K in large amounts is potentially very dangerous.

WOMEN

In the United States, within the adult population, nutrient deficiencies occur almost exclusively in women. While both men and women consume too many calories, too much fat, and too much salt, deficiencies of such nutrients as calories, iron, calcium, and folacin (folic acid) are primarily problems in children of both sexes and in adult women.

The near obsession with thinness in our society has led many women to a life of constant calorie restriction. In some young women, this concern with thinness can distort their body image and lead to the perception that they are obese even when they are below ideal weight. Weight loss is then carried to extremes and a condition known as anorexia nervosa develops. (See ANOREXIA NERVOSA.) In most women, however, restriction of calories in itself may not be a problem, but by restricting calories, they are limiting the amount of food consumed. Reduced intake of food, in turn, will result in a reduction in the intake of certain nutrients which are present only in limited amounts in our food supply. For example, it is very difficult to meet the body's requirement for iron when consuming only 1200 calories per day.

In addition to restricting the amount of food they eat, women require more of certain nutrients during particular periods of their life cycles. For example, during pregnancy and lactation, there is an increased requirement for all vitamins and minerals and particularly for iron, calcium, zinc, and folacin. Because of menstruation, women are constantly losing iron, which must be replaced from their food supply. Also, the new life-styles contribute to certain nutrient deficiencies in women. Oral contraceptives interfere with the metabolism of folacin, vitamin B_{12}, and vitamin B_6, and hence the requirement for these nutrients increases. Liberal consumption of alcohol will also interfere with the metabolism of these same nutrients, placing the woman who is on the Pill and who drinks in double jeopardy.

Finally, with one nutrient, calcium, a combination of factors is involved in making women more prone to deficiency. While both men and women go into negative calcium balance in adult life (they lose more calcium than they retain), women do so before men, usually in the third decade. In addition, women require enormous amounts of calcium during pregnancy and lactation. Moreover, when women reach menopause, they lose calcium at an even faster rate. Finally, women live longer than men and hence are in negative balance for that extra period of time. This combination of factors makes osteoporosis (brittle bones) a much more common and severe problem in older women than in older men.

IRON

It is estimated that up to 30 percent of American women have reduced iron stores in their bodies. About 10 percent are anemic due to iron deficiency. Women whose menstrual periods are heavy are more at risk than women who bleed lightly. Likewise, women who have had several pregnancies are more at risk. For these reasons, all women should consume a diet rich in iron.

We recommend that all women take an iron supplement during pregnancy (30 to 60 milligrams per day). (See IRON.)

CALCIUM

Calcium stores must be built up in the bones, and this must be done early in life—during childhood, adolescence, and young adulthood. This is particularly important for women, as we have pointed out. The amount of calcium which ultimately gets into the bones depends not only on the amount in the diet but also on the amount of protein and phosphorus

consumed together with the dietary calcium. The more protein and phosphorus there is, the less calcium is absorbed. Thus, children and young women must consume foods rich in calcium, dairy products and certain green leafy vegetables.

In addition, since protein and phosphorus consumed at the same time will decrease calcium absorption, women of all ages should limit the amount of meat (which is rich in both protein and phosphorus) consumed at the same meal as calcium. During pregnancy and lactation, the amount of calcium which is absorbed increases. However, unless care is taken to consume calcium-rich foods, the increased absorption may not be enough and supplementation may be desirable. After menopause, it is particularly important to get enough calcium, not because calcium can cure osteoporosis (it can't), but because calcium deficiency may further aggravate the state of calcium loss and make osteoporosis worse. (See CALCIUM.)

FOLACIN

Folacin deficiency is the most common vitamin deficiency in the United States and is found most often in women. The American diet is marginal in its content of this vitamin, and therefore women consuming limited numbers of calories are at risk for deficiency. Requirements for folacin increase during pregnancy because it is needed for making new red blood cells and for the fetus to grow properly. For this reason, we recommend that all pregnant women be supplemented.

If a woman is taking oral contraceptives she is more prone to folacin deficiency due to the known interference by the Pill with the metabolism of this vitamin. If she drinks moderately to heavily, she is also at greater risk for deficiency since alcohol blocks the absorption of folacin. Obviously, if she is on the Pill and consumes large quantities of alcohol, she is at even greater risk. (See FOLACIN.)

ZINC

Zinc has been known for many years to be an essential trace mineral. Only recently have we come to realize that its deficiency is fairly common. Children of both sexes, particularly adolescents, and women, especially pregnant women, are at risk. Severe deficiency does not occur in the United States. It has been described in adolescents in several Middle Eastern countries, where it results in dwarfism and poor sexual development, and is due not only to a low zinc diet but to the presence of a specific substance called phytate in certain locally grown grains. The phytate binds zinc in the intestinal tract and makes it unavailable to the body.

In the United States, milder forms of zinc deficiency have been reported in children. Such children may fail to grow properly and may exhibit a variety of skin rashes. Recently we have become concerned about zinc deficiency during pregnancy. Animal experiments have demonstrated that a diet devoid of zinc throughout pregnancy will result in severe congenital malformations in the offspring. In addition, even moderate zinc deficiency during pregnancy results in a slowing of the rate of cell division in all fetal organs, including the brain.

Finally, behavioral abnormalities have been described in the offspring of zinc-deficient pregnant rats. In humans, several reports have demonstrated an association between low levels of zinc in maternal blood and congenital malformations in the fetus. One report showed a high incidence of malformations in fetuses in which the amniotic fluid had low zinc levels. The new research strongly supports the position that women during pregnancy should consider the zinc content of food when making their selections.

Zinc is present in large amounts in many of the foods which are rich in iron. If those foods are included in the diet, there is no need for zinc supplementation. (See ZINC.)

If we were to recommend a diet specifically for American women, it would be a diet rich in iron, Calcium, folacin, and zinc. (See also BREAST-FEEDING; OSTEOPOROSIS; PREGNANCY.)

WORKPLACE

Each day, over ninety million Americans go to their places of work. The fact that so many people are assembled in such diverse locations as plants, shops, offices, or classrooms gives rise to three significant questions about the ecology of nutrition and the workplace. The first question is what are the reciprocal effects of nutrition and work performance, and conversely, in what ways do work demands influence nutritional status? The second question asks whether or not eating habits at the workplace affect workers' performance. Can a worker's sense of well-being be enhanced rather than impaired by foods eaten at the office? And finally, how can the workplace be a site for intervening in the nutrition-related killer diseases, like cardiovascular diseases (heart attack, stroke, high blood pressure), cancer, diabetes, and cirrhosis of the liver? While many of the answers to these questions are complex, there remain areas in which one can offer clear-cut recommendations.

NUTRITION AND THE WORKPLACE

Work performance relates to the ability of an individual to perform a task within normal expectations. In most industries work performance is assessed qualitatively (attitude) and quantitatively (output). In almost all cases, the more healthy a person is, the better his or her performance will be. One of the most important elements involved in maintaining good health is sound nutritional status. Hence, the link can definitely be made between nutritional status and work performance.

Consider fatigue, which is probably the most common excuse given for poor work performance. Nutritional deficiencies are just as responsible for fatigue as the more apparent factors, such as inadequate rest or an excessive work load. The table on page 321 summarizes the possible role of nutrition and fatigue. Overall, poor general nutritional status diminishes a person's abilities and can lead to exhaustion, apathy, poor concentration, and reduced strength.

Theories abound regarding the potential of various components of the diet to aid in work performance. Most are either untrue or unproven. What is consistently shown in performance studies is that supernutrition—the taking of large doses of nutrients—does not increase the capacity of already healthy people. In special cases, where there may be a nutritional compromise such as anemia, food intolerances, or nutrition depleting medications, special supplementation is necessary. The discussion which follows explores how the principal elements of diet affect work performance.

ENERGY

In general terms, energy means the capacity to do work. Energy is also used to describe the fuels involved in getting the work done. Determining human energy potential is a matter of balancing the energy taken in (fuel) with the energy going out (activity). The basic human energy-requiring activities are such functions as respiration and digestion. Increased amounts of energy are needed for the physical demands of movement. The critical point to remember concerning energy and work performance is that inadequate fuel (calories) will diminish a worker's energy level and, consequently, performance potential. Futhermore, on low or reduced calorie diets (as seen with weight control plans) the concentration of the intrinsic nutrients may fall to inadequate levels. Therefore, it is important to make sure workers receive adequate, nutrient-rich calories for the tasks to be performed.

It stands to reason that a job which requires a great deal of physical labor requires a larger amount of calories. However, studies done with people of average weight, employed in heavy labor, have revealed curious variances in their energy intake and energy output levels. Based on these findings, one would expect to see significant gains or losses in body weight, but neither occurred. Other surveys have shown that in most jobs, sitting accounts for approximately one-third of the total energy required in a workday—even for those workers who spend a considerable part of the day in moderately heavy to heavy activities. In fact, for most people, energy output in nonwork and nonsleep activities exceeds the energy expended at the workplace.

In the United States, the recommended dietary allowances for energy (calorie) intakes for a 150 pound man and a 130 pound woman in light industry occupations are 2700 (range of 2300 to 3100) and 2000 (range of 1600 to 2400) calories, respectively. However, the 1977–1978 National Food Consumption Survey found the adult males consumed an average of 2182 to 3100 calories and adult females consumed an average of 1530 to 1607 calories—up to 25 percent less than recommended levels.

This raises a question of whether or not there is a real or potential energy crisis at the workplace. It may be that the high prevalence of obesity (upward of 30 percent in adults) in the US is due in part to the fact that close to 25 percent of the life of the labor force is spent in sedentary activities, hence incurring a low energy output. Therefore, a moderate or occasionally high energy intake would seem to predispose many workers to obesity.

A reciprocal consequence is that many people may consume fewer calories in order to maintain their weight and therefore consume a diet with an inadequate nutrient density. One way to prevent this possible problem is to encourage workers to engage in some regular activity to better enable them to maintain a calorie intake at a level commensurate with an adequate nutrient intake.

CARBOHYDRATES

The theories about the relationship between carbohydrates and work performance can probably be credited to the alleged ability of sugars to fire a quick energy boost or to relieve fatigue. Actually, sugars and starches are equally effective at accomplishing an immediate rise in blood sugar level. However, there is no evidence that giving a carbohydrate supplement (e.g., a soft drink) improves performance. In fact, occasional rest periods seem to be the best refreshers. On the other hand, workers who experience reactive hypoglycemia (a rise in blood sugar level followed by a rapid drop to below fasting level, usually in reaction to a high-carbohydrate, low-protein meal)

may benefit from a light snack. For suggestions on managing this problem, see the Dietary Guidelines at the end of this section.

Carbohydrate is a very efficient fuel for muscle work. It is best if dietary carbohydrate contributes 55 percent of the day's total calories. Low-carbohydrate diets (20 to 25 percent of all calories) have been shown to produce symptoms of fatigue and reduced muscle strength. It is quite clear then that a low-carbohydrate diet would indeed compromise work performance. (See CARBOHYDRATE.)

FAT

At a level of 30 percent of total calories, fat provides sufficient energy for activities. As long as total calories and protein are adequate, lower fat intakes (as low as 10 percent of calories) will not compromise performance and may impart long-range health benefits. In very cold environments, a high-fat diet (50 to 60 percent of total calories) seems to aid in body temperature control.

PROTEIN

Contrary to popular belief, additional dietary protein has no metabolic advantage in improving work performance at any level of activity. The recommended protein levels of 56 and 46 grams per day for men and women, respectively, are sufficient to meet physical demands. Muscle building requires additional calories, more than additional protein. As the volume of food is increased to meet the extra calorie needs, the protein level will likewise rise. Extra protein is used by the body for energy. Furthermore, a diet which derives a significant percentage of calories from protein sources imposes a heavy nitrogen load on the kidneys. This could prove hazardous in individuals with kidney problems.

Borderline or low protein intakes—levels which could lead to protein deficiency states—may increase the danger of liver damage in workers exposed to hepatotoxic agents such as chloroform.

VITAMINS AND MINERALS

In well-nourished workers not exposed to agents which affect their vitamin metabolism, supplementation with vitamins A, D, and B-complex has not been shown to improve muscular ability, resistance to fatigue, or recovery from exertion.

On a global basis, iron deficiency anemia is the condition most responsible for fatigue and low performance. Fortunately, detection and treatment are relatively simple, and the overall improvement in health brought about by correct treatment is reflected by improved work productivity. (See ANEMIAS; IRON.)

EMPLOYMENT CONDITIONS

Now, let us turn our attention to how conditions of employment exert a significant influence on the health and nutritional status of the worker.

Very cold temperatures induce an increased need for energy (for the extra effort involved in locomotion in protective clothing and for thermal regulation), and for vitamin C. Very high temperatures, which cause sweating, produce an increased need for water and sodium. Water needs are particularly critical in overweight workers. For control of body temperature it is necessary to replace water above the level dictated by thirst. When individual variations are considered, the amount of water needed is approximately 8 to 16 ounces per hour. For most people involved in sweat-producing tasks, replacement of sodium is not necessary if dietary intake includes convenience foods or salted condiments. Glucose and electrolytic beverages have no advantage over water in controlling thirst and body temperature.

No matter what the source is, most people who do work experience stress. Stress may manifest itself in gastrointestinal disturbances (e.g., ulcers), respiratory allergies, cardiovascular problems, or in emotional terms. Methods, as well as products, are currently being promoted to aid the body's ability to tolerate stress. No clinical evidence exists to support the use of B-complex vitamins. But, because their toxicity is unlikely there has not been any need for a campaign to discourage their consumption. It is hypothesized that the vitamin C found in the adrenal gland is utilized at a significantly higher rate when adrenaline is released in response to stress. However, there is no definitive evidence at this time to advocate increased intakes of vitamin C—a vitamin which is potentially toxic in high doses—to aid in stress tolerance. (See STRESS.)

Preliminary data exists on the influence of nutritional status on pollutant toxicity. It seems that workers exposed to environmental pollutants, carcinogens, and even excess noise may derive some protection from these damaging effects through administration of large doses of various vitamins. However, until the risk-benefit issues are resolved, recommendations on dose levels will not be released.

HEALTH PROMOTION AT THE WORKPLACE

Each year, poor health and accidents cost industry millions of dollars in medical expenses, disability compensation, absenteeism, and low productivity rates. Likewise, the workers and their families suffer from a restriction in their ability to participate in active life-styles. Clearly, there is a great deal of concern about preventing the loss of human resources.

Strict safety standards issued by the Occupational Safety and Health Administration (OSHA) of the US Department of Labor are intended

---

FATIGUE—A PRIMARY CAUSE OF IMPAIRED PERFORMANCE POSSIBLE CAUSES & NUTRIENTS INVOLVED

Possible Causes	Nutrients Involved
Anemia	iron, vitamin C, folacin, vitamin B_{12}, protein
Undernutrition	total calories, all nutrients at inadequate levels
Obesity	excess calories, some nutrients at inadequate levels
Reactive hypoglycemia	excess sugars, low protein at meals
Vitamin toxicity	excess vitamin A
Dehydration	water (and sodium)

to protect workers on the job from hazards that may cause, or are likely to cause, death or injury. But a gap still exists in ensuring optimal health of workers. The growing field of industrial medicine is expanding the knowledge and application of pro-grams to control the synergistic effects of life-style and occupational health. Within the field, nutritional monitoring has been found to be a valuable means of detecting, treating, and preventing those health problems for which nutrition is a

---

NUTRITION-RELATED HEALTH PROBLEMS*
Impact on Worker-Workplace & Dietary Factors Involved

Health Problem	Magnitude of Influence	Dietary Factors
Alcoholism	$2,000,000,000/year lost	alcohol
Allergies	approx. 16 million people are allergic to foodstuffs	gluten, milk, fruits, nuts, others
Anemia	(not estimated)	iron, protein, vitamin C
Cancer	over 320,000 deaths	fat, vitamin C, fiber, smoking, others
Cardiovascular disease	over 1 million deaths/year	sodium, cholesterol, fat, fiber, total calories, smoking
Dental health	$6.5 billion spent on dental services	carbohydrates, calcium, fluoride, vitamin C
Diabetes	35,000 deaths/year	carbohydrates, fat, total calories
Digestive disorders	8,495,000 workdays lost, $4.2 billion in annual costs	allergies, fat, several other factors
Malnutrition	324.5 million workdays lost, 51.8 million people needing medical attention and/or restricted activity	total calories, protein, fat, carbohydrates, vitamins, minerals
Obesity	30–40% of adults in population	total calories, exercise

*Adapted from US, Congress, Senate, Select Committee on Nutrition and Human Needs, "Table 1, Magnitude of Benefits from Nutrition Research," in *Dietary Goals for the United States*, 2nd ed., December, 1977.

major component. The table opposite summarizes the impact on the worker and the workplace from the major nutrition-related health problems. From this evidence, it seems clear that the integration of sound practices within the sphere of industrial medicine should have enormous potential for diminishing the morbidity and mortality caused by these problems.

Recently, many companies have begun to implement various nutrition strategies to help with these problems. Some of the more elaborate programs have been funded through the National Institutes of Health or by private foundations. Other companies have simply instituted improvements within their own structures to achieve the desired outcome. The features that almost all health promotion programs have in common are: voluntary participation by employees, identified risk classifications, behavioral objectives, and evaluation components.

For example, several health promotion–integration programs have been developed around reducing the employee's risk of developing heart disease. Using a four-phase format such as the one given below, employers have a tool to launch an effective occupational health program.

Phase I: Setting Objectives. In the first phase, overall objectives are identified. Take for example:

1. cessation of smoking
2. reduction of serum cholesterol
3. reduction of blood pressure level
4. reduction of body weight
5. improved fitness

The success level of each objective is determined (e.g., achieving a reduction of 10 milligrams per 100 milliliters in serum cholesterol level). The success level should be in a unit which is easy to quantify.

Phase II: Screening. In the second phase the company establishes who among the employees needs to modify their risk for heart disease. The use of questionnaires makes it possible to learn of employees' family histories of heart disease, dietary practices, regular exercise levels, and smoking. Modified physical exams have been performed to acquire information on pulse recovery rates, blood pressures, weights, heights, and cholesterol levels.

Phase III: Intervention. The extent of Phase III depends on the characteristics of the participants. All participants may not necessarily be at risk for the health problems which are identified in the objectives; many seemingly healthy or risk-free workers have gotten involved in the program. The kinds of services which have been offered include workshops, diet counseling, access to recreational facilities, modifying food service selections, and referrals to outside agencies. In-house and outside experts have been used. Self-monitoring and behavior modification techniques are stressed to maximize motivation among participants. Employee incentives have included financial bonuses, subsidized membership in outside facilities, or release-from-work time for participation in such programs.

Phase IV: Follow-up and Evaluation. In Phase IV, such tools as telephone calls, rescreening, and self-evaluation have aided in determining the effectiveness of the programs and in maintaining levels of success among participants.

Because of the labor intensity of a four-phase health promotion approach, many companies have sought simpler approaches. These have included such innovations as:

- nutrition education articles in company periodicals.
- nutrition education materials in lounges.
- supplying vending machines, coffee wagons, canteens, etc., with nutritious, low-salt, low-fat items (see the table on page 327).

One particular effort concerned with healthful eating at the workplace is the New York Heart Association's "Lighten Up" program. Quantity recipe cards based on the American Heart Association's dietary recommendations have been designed for use in company cafeterias or coffee shops. Now the salad platter need not be the only offering open to those wanting a healthful lunch. (The recipe cards are available through local affiliates of the AHA.)

DIETARY GUIDELINES: EATING ON AND FOR THE JOB

No matter what your functions are on your job, the day goes more smoothly if you are feeling up to it. Aside from issues of personal satisfaction, your sense of motivation is directly related to your feelings of well-being.

Eating right for the task at hand begins with good food choices. Several guides have been designed to instruct consumers on selecting the amounts and kinds of foods necessary to be well-nourished. More recently, the issues of excess fat, salt, and alcohol have been reflected in the dietary goals for Americans. The quantities eaten should be proportional to the amounts represented. The total amount to be included in a person's normal intake is usually determined by the age and activity level. It is important to remember that the energy demands on the job are usually less than for the remainder of the day; keep the amount of food eaten at the level on which you can maintain a desirable weight. There seems to be some truth to the idea that what you eat will affect your mood and performance. This is related to certain mechanisms in the body, such as those which regulate appetite, fluid and electrolytic balance, and neurotransmitter levels in the brain.

The best way to start the day is with a good breakfast. Actually, bacon, fried eggs, buttered toast, and coffee are not the ideal foods to choose. The high-fat diet offers no advantage in starting the day. A good breakfast should average from 300 to 400 calories. The sample breakfasts shown further on in this section are examples of how to distribute the calories in a nourishing and appealing way. Of the total calories, carbohydrate should contribute approximately 50 percent, protein 15 to 20 percent, fat 30 to 35 percent. It has been shown that by consuming more than 25 percent of the day's calories in the morning meal incorrectly, reduced efficiency may result. Making allowances for individual variances in tolerance to food in the morning, the first meal can be somewhat smaller or larger and the foods eaten can be substituted. Hot cereal, the stick-to-the-ribs favorite of breakfast advocates, can be appropriately substituted with a bowl of hot soup or leftovers from the night before. In doing this the importance of the meal need not be dismissed because the traditional breakfast foods are either unavailable or unpopular. Even if the meal is eaten after leaving home, try to get to it at the first possible opportunity. Even from a vending machine or newsstand, a can of vegetable juice, a bag of peanuts (preferably unsalted), a package of raisins with hot chocolate makes for a good picniclike breakfast. One thing not to do, however, is to toss a raw egg in with other ingredients to make a shake. The raw egg white contains a substance, avidin, which will bind to the vitamin biotin and make it unavailable for use. Cooking the egg will render the avidin harmless. If you like shakes for breakfast, add one or two tablespoons of nonfat dry milk to milk, yogurt, or fruit nectar and blend until frothy.

Another good companion beverage could be water or a caffeine-free drink. Because of the stimulating effects of caffeine, sensations of irritability and jitters may plague you at your job. Higher levels, in excess of eight cups per day, have been shown to increase the likelihood of breast cysts, low grade fevers, and other unpleasant side effects.

A morning meal of coffee and a pastry may result in a late morning slump. To prevent this phenomenon, it is helpful to have more than a token amount of protein at the first meal.

Other meals at the workplace should aim to satisfy hunger without creating a sluggish feeling by adding

SAMPLE BREAKFASTS

	Calories	Protein	Carbohydrate	Fat
1 whole grapefruit	82	0.5	10.8	0.1
1 English muffin	138	5.3	28.3	1.4
2 tsp margarine	72	–	–	8.0
1 medium egg	78	6.2	0.4	5.5
	370	12.0	39.5	15.0
1 medium orange	71	1.1	18.1	0.3
6 oz 1% fat milk	77	6.0	9.0	2.0
1 cup puffed rice	54	0.9	12.6	0.1
1 sl whole wheat toast	70	2.5	15.0	–
1 tbsp peanut butter	86	3.9	3.2	7.2
	358	14.4	57.9	9.6

excess calories. The prohibition of alcohol in many jobs is obviously related to its ability to impair judgment and generally compromise efficiency. Following breakfast, there does not seem to be an exact, ideal spacing or frequency of meals; as long as the daily needs are met, individual preference seems to be the rule. If hypoglycemia is experienced, then a three-hour spacing of smaller meals has been shown to help some people.

Water is an often omitted, but very important, element in a good diet. To break into the water habit, begin by substituting a glass of water for one of your usual cups of another daily beverage (whether it is coffee, tea, or a soft drink). Aim for a level of three glasses of water per day in addition to other beverages normally consumed.

THE COFFEE BREAK

The nutritional practice at the workplace most in need of amending is the ever-popular coffee break. In fact, it is the pause—not the food—that refreshes the worker. But, workers are drawn to that coffeepot and it is as ingrained in the workday as chicken soup is for a cold. The following table describes the usual items eaten at the coffee break and proposes some alternatives. By using this guide, one can develop better habits in making selections, in a variety of similar situations.

Keep in mind that even nutritious foods can be overeaten. And there is no rule that says you have to eat just because it's break time. If you need more stimulation, indulge in some stretching or jumping

REVISING THE REFRESHMENT BREAK

Item	Reason for Omitting	Alternative
Coffee & tea	caffeine causes gastric distress, high in caffeine & sugar	caffeine-free coffee or tea, herb teas, fruit juices
Sugar & saccharin	low nutrient density, linked to cancer	cinnamon
Cream & coffee lighteners	high in saturated fat	skimmed, evaporated milk
Lemon juice	—	—
Whole milk	high in saturated fat	low-fat milk
Cocoa	high in sugar	low-sugar varieties
Pastries	high in sugar & saturated fat	low-fat muffins, raisin bread
Candy bars	high in sugar & saturated fat	fresh or dried fruit

in place instead of a food or beverage.

Just as each worker brings to the job her or his own style of working and eating, the best nutritional improvement campaign at the workplace is one which the worker will carry home for the benefit of all those in the family.

ZINC

Zinc is required by many enzymes in the body including those concerned with growth and the degradation of protein and carbohydrate. The recommended dietary allowance (RDA) for zinc is 15 milligrams, which can be obtained from foods such as beef, clams, lamb, liver, oysters, popcorn, brown rice, whole wheat products, wheat germ, corn, fish, and egg yolks. A poor intake of this nutrient results in poor wound healing, ulcers, dermatitis of the face and limbs, and a loss of appetite associated with a loss of taste. A zinc deficiency during pregnancy can result in fetal growth retardation and is the most likely time that a deficiency will occur as requirements increase at this time to 20 milligrams daily. Growth retardation and delayed sexual maturation in children has also been reported, especially in countries where dietary intake is low and dietary fiber high. Both fiber and calcium impair zinc absorption.

A toxic dose of zinc would be 500 milligrams. Such an overdose causes nausea, vomiting, and diarrhea. To achieve a toxic intake could necessitate megadose supplements, although acidic foods and drinks can leach enough zinc from galvanized containers to cause an overdose and so should not be stored in such containers. Zinc impairs the absorption of both copper and iron and can cause a deficiency in either.

TABLE 4
ZINC CONTENT OF FOODS IN MILLIGRAMS (mg) PER SERVING

.2 to .5 mg/serving	.5 to 1 mg/serving	1 to 1.5 mg/serving
egg . . . . .1 med.	puffed wheat . . . . .1 oz	clams . . . . .3 oz
gefilte fish . . . . .3½ oz	cheddar cheese . . . . .1 oz	brown rice . . . . .1 cup
mango .½ med.	tuna . . . . .3 oz	whole wheat bread . . . . .2 slices
applesauce . . . . .1 cup	white rice . . . . .1 cup	popcorn .2 cups
pineapple juice . . . . .8 oz	white bread . . . . .2 slices	wheat germ . . . . .1 tblsp
tomato . . . . .1 med.	cranberry-apple drink . . . . .8 oz	bran (cooked, dryed) . . . . .¾ cup
potato, cooked . . . . .1 med.	chicken breast . . . . .3 oz	
	milk (whole or skim) . . . . .8 oz	

4 to 5 mg/serving	Other
beef (lean only) . . . . .3½ oz	9.4 mg · Pacific oysters (raw) . . . . .3½ oz
pork (lean only) . . . . .3½ oz	74.7 mg · Atlantic oysters (raw) . . . . .3½ oz
lamb (lean only) . . . . .3½ oz	
liver (beef and calf) . . . . .3 oz	

APPENDIX

FOOD AND NUTRITION BOARD, NATIONAL ACADEMY OF SCIENCES–NATIONAL RESEARCH COUNCIL
RECOMMENDED DAILY DIETARY ALLOWANCES,[a] Revised 1980
Designed for the maintenance of good nutrition of practically all healthy people in the U.S.A.

	Age (years)	Weight (kg)	Weight (lb)	Height (cm)	Height (in)	Protein (g)	Fat-Soluble Vitamins			Water-Soluble Vitamins							Minerals					
							Vitamin A (µg RE)[b]	Vitamin D (µg)[c]	Vitamin E (mg α-TE)[d]	Vitamin C (mg)	Thiamin (mg)	Riboflavin (mg)	Niacin (mg NE)[e]	Vitamin B-6 (mg)	Folacin (µg)[f]	Vitamin B-12 (µg)	Calcium (mg)	Phosphorus (mg)	Magnesium (mg)	Iron (mg)	Zinc (mg)	Iodine (µg)
Infants	0.0–0.5	6	13	60	24	kg × 2.2	420	10	3	35	0.3	0.4	6	0.3	30	0.5[g]	360	240	50	10	3	40
	0.5–1.0	9	20	71	28	kg × 2.0	400	10	4	35	0.5	0.6	8	0.6	45	1.5	540	360	70	15	5	50
Children	1–3	13	29	90	35	23	400	10	5	45	0.7	0.8	9	0.9	100	2.0	800	800	150	15	10	70
	4–6	20	44	112	44	30	500	10	6	45	0.9	1.0	11	1.3	200	2.5	800	800	200	10	10	90
	7–10	28	62	132	52	34	700	10	7	45	1.2	1.4	16	1.6	300	3.0	800	800	250	10	10	120
Males	11–14	45	99	157	62	45	1000	10	8	50	1.4	1.6	18	1.8	400	3.0	1200	1200	350	18	15	150
	15–18	66	145	176	69	56	1000	10	10	60	1.4	1.7	18	2.0	400	3.0	1200	1200	400	18	15	150
	19–22	70	154	177	70	56	1000	7.5	10	60	1.5	1.7	19	2.2	400	3.0	800	800	350	10	15	150
	23–50	70	154	178	70	56	1000	5	10	60	1.4	1.6	18	2.2	400	3.0	800	800	350	10	15	150
	51+	70	154	178	70	56	1000	5	10	60	1.2	1.4	16	2.2	400	3.0	800	800	350	10	15	150
Females	11–14	46	101	157	62	46	800	10	8	50	1.1	1.3	15	1.8	400	3.0	1200	1200	300	18	15	150
	15–18	55	120	163	64	46	800	10	8	60	1.1	1.3	14	2.0	400	3.0	1200	1200	300	18	15	150
	19–22	55	120	163	64	44	800	7.5	8	60	1.1	1.3	14	2.0	400	3.0	800	800	300	18	15	150
	23–50	55	120	163	64	44	800	5	8	60	1.0	1.2	13	2.0	400	3.0	800	800	300	18	15	150
	51+	55	120	163	64	44	800	5	8	60	1.0	1.2	13	2.0	400	3.0	800	800	300	10	15	150
Pregnant						+30	+200	+5	+2	+20	+0.4	+0.3	+2	+0.6	+400	+1.0	+400	+400	+150	h	+5	+25
Lactating						+20	+400	+5	+3	+40	+0.5	+0.5	+5	+0.5	+100	+1.0	+400	+400	+150	h	+10	+50

[a] The allowances are intended to provide for individual variations among most normal persons as they live in the United States under usual environmental stresses. Diets should be based on a variety of common foods in order to provide other nutrients for which human requirements have been less well defined. See text for detailed discussion of allowances and of nutrients not tabulated. See Table 1 (p. 20) for weights and heights by individual year of age. See Table 3 (p. 23) for suggested average energy intakes.

[b] Retinol equivalents. 1 retinol equivalent = 1 µg retinol or 6 µg β carotene. See text for calculation of vitamin A activity of diets as retinol equivalents.

[c] As cholecalciferol. 10 µg cholecalciferol = 400 IU of vitamin D.

[d] α-tocopherol equivalents. 1 mg d-α tocopherol = 1 α-TE. See text for variation in allowances and calculation of vitamin E activity of the diet as α-tocopherol equivalents.

[e] 1 NE (niacin equivalent) is equal to 1 mg of niacin or 60 mg of dietary tryptophan.

[f] The folacin allowances refer to dietary sources as determined by *Lactobacillus casei* assay after treatment with enzymes (conjugases) to make polyglutamyl forms of the vitamin available to the test organism.

[g] The recommended dietary allowance for vitamin B-12 in infants is based on average concentration of the vitamin in human milk. The allowances after weaning are based on energy intake (as recommended by the American Academy of Pediatrics) and consideration of other factors, such as intestinal absorption; see text.

[h] The increased requirement during pregnancy cannot be met by the iron content of habitual American diets nor by the existing iron stores of many women; therefore the use of 30–60 mg of supplemental iron is recommended. Iron needs during lactation are not substantially different from those of nonpregnant women, but continued supplementation of the mother for 2–3 months after parturition is advisable in order to replenish stores depleted by pregnancy.

INDEX

Abortion, spontaneous, 16, 78, 79
Acetaldehyde, 29
Acetylcholine, 215
Acetylsalicilic acid, *see* Aspirin
Acid-base balance, 99
Additives, 11–13
  antioxidants as, 49
  cancer and, 83, 88
Adipocytes, 228
Adolescents, 14–20
  alcohol abuse by, 18–19
  anorexia nervosa in, 44, 45
  athletic, 20
  bone growth in, 239, 241–42
  caffeine use by, 78
  energy and protein needs of, 14–15
  high-fiber diet for, 150
  normal growth of, 14
  obese, 228, 230–31
  pregnant, 16–18, 261
  vegetarian, 19–20
  vitamins and minerals for, 15–16
  zinc deficiency among, 315
Adrenocortical hormones, 238, 239
Aflatoxin, 88
African Bushmen, 274
Aging, 21–26
  alcohol and, 31
  bee pollen and, 64
  drug-nutrient interactions and, 127–29
  fiber and, 148–50
  hydrochloric acid production and, 175

hypertension and, 178
immune system and, 193, 194, 200
Alcohol, 27–32
  adolescent abuse of, 18–19
  cancer and, 78
  folacin deficiency and, 39, 154
  gastritis and, 166
  heartburn and, 165
  immune system and, 199, 200
  indigestion and, 165
  low blood sugar and, 186, 187
  magnesium deficiency and, 218, 219
  moderate consumption of, 30–32, 126
  obesity and, 231
  oral contraceptives and, 313, 315
  pantothenic acid and, 246
  during pregnancy, 259–60
  thiamine deficiency and, 301
  zinc deficiency and, 40
Allergies, 33–34
  bee pollen and, 64
  cytotoxic testing for, 110
  in infants, 93
Aluminum, 35
  in antacids, 129
  phosphorus and, 249
Alzheimer's disease, 35
  lecithin for, 215
Amenorrhea, 44, 45
American Dental Association Council on Dental Therapeutics, 113
American Heart Association, 106, 123, 324

American Indians, 274

American Medical Association, 106

American Psychological Association, 75

Amino acids, 36
  in aspartame, 62, 63
  in infant formula, 190
  iron and, 211
  in vegetarian diet, 290–91
  See also specific amino acids

Amphetamines, 233

Anemia, 37–43
  in adolescents, 16
  alcohol-induced, 27
  in athletes, 224
  in celiac disease, 201
  folacin deficiency, 38–40, 154
  immune system and, 196
  iron deficiency, 37–38, 209
  vitamin B$_{12}$ deficiency, 41–42, 305
  work performance and, 320
  zinc deficiency, 40–41

Angel dust, 18

Angina pectoris, 100
  alcohol and, 31
  hypertension and, 177

Animal studies
  of hypertension, 180–81
  of immune system, 196
  of pregnancy, 252, 259

Anorexia, drug-induced, 130

Anorexia nervosa, 44–47, 313
  bulimia and, 75
  calcium deficiency and, 242

Antacids, 129, 175
  for heartburn, 165
  for peptic ulcer, 167

Antibiotics
  bee pollen as, 64
  calcium and, 80
  as contaminants, 91–92

Antibodies, 33, 193, 196

Anticarcinogens, 48

Anticoagulants, 130, 312

Antidiuretic hormone, 32

Antigens, 33

Antioxidants, 49

Appetite depressants, 233

Appetite regulation, 50–53
  drugs affecting, 130
  environmental factors in, 50–51
  metabolic factors in, 51
  regulation of body weight and, 52–53
  satiation and, 51–52

Applesauce gingerbread, 207

Arginine, 53

Arteriosclerosis, 22, 54–57, 99
  alcohol and, 30–31
  cholesterol and, 100–101
  in diabetes, 116, 119
  EPA and, 131
  gout and, 29
  hypertension and, 177, 179
  prevention of, 106, 107
  sucrose and, 286

Arthritis, aspirin for, 127

Artificial sweeteners, 11

Ascites, 29

Ascorbic acid, *see* Vitamin C

Aspartame, 62, 63, 248

Aspartic acid, 62, 63

Aspirin, 127–28, 173
  gastritis caused by, 166
  ulcers and, 167

Asthma, bee pollen and, 64

Athletics, 20
  bee pollen and, 64
  nutrition and, 223–25
  See also Exercise

Atkins diet, 234, 235, 269–70

Atropine, 222

Australian Aborigines, 274

B cells, 192–96
B-complex vitamins, 297, 298
  for adolescents, 15
  aging and, 25
  in brewer's yeast, 74
  in high-fiber foods, 148
  immune system and, 196
  for nursing mothers, 72
  stress and, 284, 321
  work performance and, 320
  See also specific vitamins
Baby food, 158–59, 180, 189, 276
Bacteria
  drug-resistant, 92
  in plaque, 111, 112
Balanced diet, 155
  reducing, 271–73
Banana and Milk Diet, 269
Bee pollen, 64
Behavior modification therapy
  for anorexia nervosa, 46
  for obesity, 232
Belching, 167
Belladonna, 222
Beriberi, 301, 302
Beta carotene, 48, 299, 300
BHA, 49
BHT, 49
Bile, 148
Bioflavonoids, 65
Biological amplification, 90, 91
Biotin, 65, 298
Blacks
  hypertension among, 178, 181, 275, 276
  obesity among, 226
Bladder cancer, 11
Blanching, 156
Bland diet, 166, 167
Blindness, vitamin A deficiency and, 299
Blood cells, folacin and, 153–54

Blood clotting, 312
Blood pressure, high, *see* Hypertension
Body image, disturbance of, 44
Body weight
  "ideal," maintenance of, 125
  regulation of, 52–53
Bone marrow, 192, 193
  iron storage in, 209
Bonemeal, 82
Brain
  aluminum deposits in, 35
  effect of alcohol on, 19, 29
  fat in, 104
  folacin and, 154
  glucose and, 145
  prenatal growth of, 17
  tumors of, 164
Bran, 147
Breakfast, 325–26
Breast cancer, 69, 83–84
  polyunsaturated fat and, 195
Breast-feeding, 66–73, 93, 189
  advantages for infant of, 66–68
  advantages for mother of, 68–69
  calcium and, 241, 242
  iron and, 38
  mother-child interactions during, 69–70
  mother's diet during, 70–73
  postpartum weight loss and, 231, 259
  practical tips for, 70
  supplemented with formula, 190
  weight gain during pregnancy and, 252, 253
Brewer's yeast, 74, 291, 305
  chromium in, 108
Brittle bones, *see* Osteoporosis
Bromelain, 74
Bruch, Hilda, 45
Bulimia, 44, 47, 74–75
Butter, 76

Cadmium, 90
  copper and, 109
  hair analysis for, 172
  immune system and, 198
Caffeine, 76–79, 325
  heartburn and, 165
  indigestion and, 165
  during pregnancy, 260
  in tea, 287
  ulcers and, 167
Calcitonin, 238
Calcium, 80–82
  in adolescence, 15, 18
  aging and, 21, 22, 24–25
  aluminum and, 35
  in butter, 76
  diuretics and, 129
  drug interactions with, 130
  factors affecting absorption of, 42
  fluoride and, 153
  hypertension and, 181–82
  immune system and, 198
  in kidney stones, 214
  in macrobiotic diet, 218
  magnesium and, 218
  in milk, 221
  for nursing mothers, 70, 71
  osteoporosis and, 237–39, 241–45
  phosphorus and, 249
  during pregnancy, 254, 261
  stress and, 282–84
  tea and, 287
  tooth formation and, 113
  in vegetarian diet, 289, 293
  vitamin D and, 309
  for women, 313, 314
Calories
  for adolescents, 14–15
  aging and, 23
  in alcohol, 19, 27, 28, 126
  for athletes, 20, 223
  in balanced diet, 155

  in butter, 76
  in carbohydrates, 24, 87
  in diabetic diet, 117, 121
  expended in different activities, 136
  from fats, 56, 57
  fiber and, 147, 148
  in junk food, 212
  in milk, 221
  for nursing mothers, 71
  osteoporosis and, 242–43
  during pregnancy, 17, 18, 252, 254,
      256–57, 261
  in processed foods, 158
  reduced efficiency in utilization of,
      267
  weight reduction and, 231–36
  work performance and, 318–19
Cameron, Ewan, 197
Cancer, 83–85, 317
  additives and, 11, 12
  alcohol and, 27, 30
  antioxidants and, 49
  bladder, 11
  breast, *see* Breast cancer
  caffeine and, 77, 78
  colon, *see* Colon cancer
  copper and, 109
  cruciferous vegetables and, 279
  death rate from, 100
  diet and, 123
  fluoride and, 114
  folacin needs and, 154
  glutathione peroxidase and, 171
  immune system and, 193–95
  of ovary, 85
  of prostate, 85
  protection from, 48
  selenium and, 278
  of stomach, 85, 88
  vitamin A and, 299–300
  vitamin C and, 197, 307
  See also Carcinogens

Carbohydrates, 86–87
  in adolescent diet, 15
  aging and, 24
  for athletes, 20, 223–25
  in diabetic diet, 116, 118, 119
  in enteral nutrition, 131
  exercise and, 133–35, 138, 142–44
  gas and, 168
  hypoglycemia and, 187
  increased consumption of, 124
  in infant formula, 190
  in milk, 221
  neurotransmitters and, 285
  niacin and, 303
  in parenteral nutrition, 247
  in reducing diets, 267–70
  stress and, 282
  thiamine and, 301
  in weight-loss diets, 234–35
  work performance and, 319
  See also Fiber
Carcinogens, 84–85
  in food, 88
Cardiac sphincter, 164
Cardiovascular disease, *see*
        Arteriosclerosis; Heart disease
Carnitine, 89
Casein, 36, 190
Cavities, 111
Celiac disease, 201–2
Cellulase, 89
Cellulose, 86, 147
Cerebrovascular accident, *see* Stroke
Ceruloplasmin, 108
Cesarean sections among teenage
        mothers, 16
Chemical contaminants, 90–92
Chemical fertilizers, 13
Chemical preservation of foods, 158
Children, 93–94
  anemia in, 37
  arginine for, 53
  bone growth in, 239
  caffeine and, 77–78
  celiac disease in, 201–2
  diabetic, 115, 117, 119
  gastrointestinal disorders in, 164
  histidine for, 174
  hyperactivity in, 11–13
  iodine deficiency in, 208
  lactose intolerance in, 203–4
  lead poisoning in, 214
  on macrobiotic diet, 218
  malnutrition in, 265–66
  obese, 158, 226, 227, 229, 230, 232
  selenium deficiency in, 277
  on vegetarian diets, 291, 295
  zinc deficiency in, 41, 315
Chloride, 99
Chlorinated hydrocarbons, 91
Cholecystokinin (CCK), 52
Cholesterol, 23, 99–107, 176, 179
  arteriosclerosis and, 54–56
  blood levels of, 101–2
  in breast milk, 67, 190
  in butter, 76
  in diabetic diet, 116, 119
  exercise and, 137, 179
  in fad diets, 235
  fiber and, 87, 149
  immune system and, 195
  lecithin and, 215
  in ovo-lacto vegetarian diet, 289
  protein and, 104–5
  reduced consumption of, 106–7, 124
  saturated and unsaturated fats and,
        102–4
Choline, 215
Chromium, 108
  immune system and, 198
Cigarette smoking, 176
  alcohol and, 30
  arteriosclerosis and, 54, 56
  cardiovascular disease and, 100

Cigarette smoking (*cont.*)
  exercise and, 137
  heartburn and, 165
  immune system and, 199, 200
  oral contraceptives and, 105
  during pregnancy, 260
  ulcers and, 167
  vitamin C and, 306
Cimetidine, 167
Cirrhosis, 27–29, 126, 317
Cobalt, immune system and, 198
Cocaine, 18
Coeliac disease, 202
Coenzyme A, 246
Coffee breaks, 326–27
Colitis, 122
Colon cancer, 22, 23, 84–85, 149
  polyunsaturated fat and, 195
  vitamin C and, 197
Coloring dyes, 11, 12
Colostrum, 66
Common cold
  bioflavonoids and, 65
  vitamin C for, 197, 307
Complementary proteins, 290–91
Congenital malformations
  caffeine and, 78–79
  folacin deficiency and, 40
  zinc deficiency and, 41
Congestive heart failure, 164, 177
Congress, U.S., 12
Constipation, 128, 169
  fiber and, 148, 150
  during pregnancy, 257
Contamination
  additives to prevent, 11
  cancer and, 83, 88
  chemical, 90–92
  heavy metal, 82
Copper, 42, 108–9
  immune system and, 198
  iron and, 211

molybdenum and, 222
Coronary artery disease, 23
  diet and, 123
Cortisone, 239
Coumarins, 312
Cow milk, 189, 191, 221
  in infant formula, 190
Crenshaw, Mary Ann, 269
Cruciferous vegetables, 279
  anticarcinogenic properties of,
    48
Cucurbocitrin, 173
Cyanocobalamin, *see* Vitamin B$_{12}$
Cysteine, 36, 110
Cytotoxic testing, 110

DDT, 88, 91
Delaney Clause (1958), 12, 88
Dental decay, 111–14
  sucrose and, 286
Depression
  among bulimics, 75
  pyridoxine deficiency as cause of,
    304
  tryptophan for, 288
Diabetes mellitus, 115–22, 317
  arteriosclerosis and, 54
  aspartame and, 62
  carbohydrates and, 124
  cardiovascular disease and, 100
  chromium supplements for, 108
  complications of, 116
  eating behavior in, 51
  fiber and, 149
  low blood sugar in, 186, 187
  obesity and, 226
  pregnancy and, 261–62
  sucrose and, 286
Dialysis, 213
Diarrhea, 164, 168–69
  in celiac disease, 201–2

from fat and carbohydrate
 malabsorption, 268
in kwashiorkor, 266
in lactose intolerance, 203, 204
magnesium deficiency and, 219
in marasmus, 265
potassium loss in, 250
stress-induced, 284
Dicumarol, 312
Diet
 additive-free, 12
 bland, 166, 167
 bone mass and, 239, 241–45
 for breast-feeding, 70–73
 calcium sources in, 80
 cancer and, 83
 cholesterol and, 101–3, 106–7
 to control obesity, 232–36
 diabetic, 116–22
 for elderly, 25, 26
 elimination, 33–34, 205
 exercise and, 134–35, 139–44
 high-fiber, 148–52
 macrobiotic, 218, 269
 milk-free, 206
 during pregnancy, 18, 255–57
 recommendations for, 123–26
 sodium-restricted, 182–85, 275–76
 vegetarian, *see* Vegetarian diets
 weight-loss, *see* Reducing diets
 wheat-free, 206
Dietary Goals for the United States,
 The, 123, 324
Dimethyl nitrosamine, 30
Disaccharides, 286
Diuretics, 129
 herbal, 173–74
 magnesium deficiency and, 219
 potassium loss from, 250
 during pregnancy, 262
 sodium excretion and, 275
Diverticulitis, 149, 170

Diverticulosis, 22, 87, 149, 150, 164,
 169–70
Dolomite, 81–82
Drug abuse, adolescent, 18–19
Drugs
 alcohol and, 29, 32
 caffeine in, 77
 low blood sugar and, 186, 187
 nutrient interactions with, 127–30
 during pregnancy, 261
 ulcers and, 167
 for weight reduction, 233
Drying of foods, 157
Dual Center theory of feeding
 behavior, 50
Duodenal ulcer, 167
Dyes, 11, 12
Dynamic exercise, 138
Dysentery, 92
Dysmenorrhea, alcohol for, 32

Eclampsia, 16
Edema
 in beriberi, 301
 in heart disease, 129
 in kwashiorkor, 265–66
 during pregnancy, 16, 262
EDTA, 49
Eicosapentinoic acid (EPA), 131
Elderly, *see* Aging
Elimination diet, 33–34, 205
Enamel hypoplasia, 113
Endorphins, 285
Enteral nutrition, 131
Enzymes, 132
 copper and, 109
 digestive, reduced availability of, 170
 inactivation of, in food processing,
  156
 phosphorus in, 249
 See also specific enzymes

Esophagus, 164–65, 222
Essential fatty acid (EFA), 216
Essential hypertension, 177
Estrogen, 238, 239, 243
  high-density lipoprotein and, 105
Exchange lists, 119–21
Exercise, 133–44
  for adolescents, 15
  aging and, 23
  by anorexics, 45
  arteriosclerosis and, 56
  bone mass and, 239–41
  cholesterol and, 105, 107
  constipation relieved by, 169
  diet and, 134–35, 139–44
  fuels utilized during, 133–34
  hypertension and, 179
  nutrition and, 138–44, 223–25
  reducing diets and, 268
  starting program of, 135–37
  stress and, 283, 285
  weight reduction and, 232

Fad diets, 233–35
  calcium deficient, 243
  protein-calorie malnutrition on, 265
  for weight loss, 268
Family therapy for anorexia nervosa,
    46
Fast foods, 212
  obesity and, 231
Fasting, 145, 269
  protein-supplemented, 269–71
  stress and, 284
Fat soluble vitamins, 297
  See also Vitamin A; Vitamin D;
    Vitamin E; Vitamin K
Fatigue, 317, 320
Fats, 58–61, 146
  in adolescent diet, 14
  aging and, 23

  alcohol and, 29
  for athletes, 223, 224
  in butter, 76
  calories in, 155
  cancer and, 84, 85
  cholesterol and, 55, 56
  in diabetic diet, 116, 117, 119
  in enteral nutrition, 131
  exercise and, 138, 144
  heartburn and, 164
  high-fiber diet and, 148, 149
  in human milk, 66, 67
  immune system and, 195
  indigestion and, 165
  in infant formula, 190
  in junk food, 212
  in milk, 221
  in parenteral nutrition, 247
  reduced consumption of, 123–24
  in reducing diets, 234–35, 267–70
  stress and, 282
  work performance and, 319
Fatty acids, 216
Feingold, Benjamin, 12
Fermentation, 157–58
Fertilizers, chemical, 13, 91
Fetal alcohol syndrome, 259–60
Fiber, 24, 86–87, 147–52, 169, 170
  aging and, 22
  cholesterol and, 105
  colon cancer and, 85
  in diabetic diet, 116, 118
  high nutrient density and, 148
  hypoglycemia and, 187
  increased consumption of, 124, 150–
    52
  iron and, 211
  in reducing diets, 267
  specific benefits of, 148–49
  in vegetarian diets, 293
Fish oil, 131
Fitness, *see* Exercise

Fluoride, 113–14, 153
for infants, 68, 153
Fluorosis, 114
Folacin (folic acid), 153–54, 297, 305
for adolescents, 15
alcohol and, 19, 27
aspirin and, 127–28
deficiency of, 37–40, 129–30
factor affecting absorption of, 42
in high-fiber foods, 148
immune system and, 196, 199, 200
lost in food processing, 156
in milk, 221
during pregnancy, 254
for women, 313–15
Food additives, *see* Additives
Food and Agricultural Organization/World Health Organization, 81
Food balancing, 155
Food and Drug Administration (FDA), 88, 90
Food poisoning, 166
Food processing, 156–59
Formula feeding, 189–91
marasmus and, 265
Fraenkel, G., 89
Free radicals, 48, 171, 210, 278
Freezing, 157
Fructose, 86, 286

Galactose, 86
Gall bladder disease, 122
Galton, L., 179
Gas, 21, 167–68
Gastrointestinal system
abnormalities of, low blood sugar due to, 187
aging and, 21–22
alcohol and, 27–28, 31
defense against infection in, 192

in diabetes, 122
diseases of, 164–70
See also specific diseases
enzymes in, 132
fiber in, 147–50
folacin in, 153
Gastric ulcer, 167
Gastritis, 165–67
General adaptation syndrome, 280
Genetic factors
in cirrhosis, 28
in hypertension, 178, 181
in obesity, 228–30
Gingerbread, applesauce, 207
Glaucoma, 222
Glucose, 86, 87, 286
chromium and, 108
in diabetes, 115–17
exercise and, 133, 224
fasting and, 145
stress and, 282
Glucose tolerance factor (GTF), 108
Glucostatic hypothesis of appetite regulation, 51
Glutamic acid, 171
Glutathione peroxidase, 171
Gluten intolerance, 201–2, 206
Glycine, 172
Glycogen, 133–35
exercise and, 224–25
fasting and, 145
stress and, 282
Goitrogens, 208
Gonorrhea, 92
Gout, 29
Granulocytes, 192, 193
Greenland Eskimos, 274
Growth, 93–94
arginine and, 53
charts, 95–98
effect of alcohol on, 19

Growth (*cont.*)
iron and, 38
normal, 14
prenatal, 17
vitamins and minerals and, 15, 16
Growth hormone, 239

Hair analysis, 108, 172
Heart disease, 316
alcohol and, 27
calcium and, 81
diabetes and, 122
diet and, 124
diuretics for, 129
EPA and, 131
exercise and, 137
high blood pressure and, 176, 177
obesity and, 226
risk ratings for, 106
selenium deficiency and, 277
workplace intervention to prevent, 323–24
See also Arteriosclerosis
Heartburn, 21, 164–65, 175
during pregnancy, 257
Heat processing, 156–57
Heavy metal contamination, 82, 90
Hemicellulose, 86, 147
Hemoglobin, 209
Herbal medicines, 173–74
Herpes, lysine for, 217
Hesperidin, 65
High blood pressure, *see* Hypertension
High-density lipoproteins (HDLs), 31, 55, 104–5
EPA and, 131
High nutrient density, 148
in balanced diets, 155
Histamine, 174
Histidine, 174
Hormones

alcohol and, 30, 32
bone loss and, 237–40
breast-feeding and, 69
cancer and, 84
carcinogenic, 88
in stress response, 280, 282
for weight reduction, 233
Human Chorionic Gonadotropin (HCG) diet, 269
Hunger, 50
perception of, 45
Hydrochloric acid, 175
Hydroxyapetite, 80, 153, 237
Hyperactivity, 11–13
caffeine and, 77–78
Hyperlipidemia, 226
Hyperplastic obesity, 228, 230, 232
Hypertension (high blood pressure), 11, 100, 107, 176–85, 317
alcohol and, 27
arteriosclerosis and, 54
calcium and, 80, 181–82
diet for, 182–85
diuretics for, 129
exercise and, 137, 179
herbal diuretics and, 173–74
obesity and, 178–79, 226
during pregnancy, 16, 262
role of nutrition in, 178
sodium and, 124, 158–59, 179–81, 274–76, 279
Hyperthyroidism, 213
Hypertrophic obesity, 228
postpartum, 259
Hypocupremia, 109
Hypoglycemia, 186–87, 319, 326
exercise and, 133, 135
Hypothalamus, 50

Immune system, 188, 192–93
aging and, 193, 194, 200

dietary fat and, 195
minerals and, 198–200
nutrition and, 193–94, 198–99
obesity and, 188, 194, 199
protein and, 194–95
vitamins and, 195–97, 199–200
Indigestion, 164, 165
See also Nausea; Vomiting
Industrial medicine, 322
Infants, 93
arginine for, 53
bone growth in, 239, 241
copper deficiency in, 109
feeding, *see* Baby food; Breast-feeding; Formula feeding
histidine for, 174
immune system of, 193, 194
iron requirements of, 38
linoleic acid for, 216
low-birthweight, 17
malnutrition in, 265–66
obesity in, 228, 229
removal of sugar and salt from foods
for, 158–59
taurine for, 287
vitamin B$_{12}$ deficiency in, 305
vitamin E deficiency in, 310
vitamin K deficiency in, 312
Infection, 192–200
body surface defenses against, 192
resistance to, 188
Insomnia, tryptophan for, 288
Insulin, 108, 115–19, 121
Intermittent claudication, 311
Intestinal bypass, 233
Intolerance, 201–7
Intrinsic factor, 167, 305
Iodine, 208, 277
immune system and, 198
in kelp, 213
Iron, 209–11
in adolescence, 15, 16, 18

aging and, 25
aspirin and, 127
for athletes, 224
in breast milk, 67–68
in brewer's yeast, 74
in butter, 76
copper and, 108–9
deficiency of, 37–38
drug interactions with, 130
exercise and, 139
factors affecting absorption of, 42
in high-fiber foods, 148
immune system and, 198, 200
for infants, 93, 191
in junk food, 212
in macrobiotic diet, 218
manganese and, 219
in milk, 221
for nursing mothers, 70, 71
pica and, 214
during pregnancy, 254, 261
tea and, 287
in vegetarian diet, 289, 290, 292
for women, 313, 314
work performance and, 320
Irritable bowel syndrome, 170
Isoleucine, 36
Isoniazid, 306

Jews, hypertension among, 275
Jolliffe, Norman, 56
Junk food, 212

Kelp, 213, 277
Keshan disease, 277–78
Ketones, 145, 235, 269, 270
Kidney disease, 164, 213
diabetes and, 122
hypertension and, 177
magnesium deficiency in, 219

Kidney disease (*cont.*)
  potassium loss in, 250
  vitamin D in, 309
Kidney stones, 214
King, Glen, 306
Kwashiorkor, 265–66

Labor, U.S. Department of, 321
Lactic acid, accumulation in muscles,
    224
Lactose, 86
  gas and, 168
  in human milk, 66, 67
  in infant formula, 190
Lactose intolerance, 21, 27, 201, 203–
    4, 206
Last Chance diet, 269, 271
Laxatives, 128–29
Lead, 90, 214–15
  hair analysis for, 172
  immune system and, 198
Lecithin, 215
Let down reflex, 66
Leucine, 36, 216
Leukemia, 109
Lind, Dr., 306
Linoleic acid, 104, 195, 216
Lipoproteins, 55, 104–5
  alcohol and, 31
Liver disease
  alcoholic, 19, 27–30
  in diabetes, 122
Low blood sugar, *see* Hypoglycemia
Low-calorie diets, *see* Reducing diets
Low-density lipoproteins (LDLs), 31,
    55, 104–5
  EPA and, 131
Lungs, lining of, 192
Lymph nodes, 192
Lymphocytes, 192
Lysine, 36, 217, 220, 291

Macrobiotic diet, 218, 269
Macrophages, 192
Magnesium, 218–19
  calcium and, 80, 82
  immune system and, 198
  phosphorus and, 249
Maillard Reaction, 157
Malignant hypertension, 177
Malnutrition, 265–66
Maltose, 86
Manganese, 219
  immune system and, 198
Marasmus, 265, 266
Marijuana, 18
  during pregnancy, 261
Mayer, Jean, 51
Mayo Clinic, 197
Mayo Clinic diet, 269
Measles, 266
Megaloblastic anemia, 154
Memory, lecithin and, 215
Menarche, 17
Menopause
  calcium loss in, 313
  cholesterol levels and, 105
  osteoporosis and, 21, 238–39
Menstruation
  anemia and, 37, 39
  in anorexia nervosa, 44
  in athletes, 224
  bulimia and, 75
  iron needs and, 16, 313, 314
  painful, 32
Mental development, protein-calorie
    malnutrition and, 266
Mercury, 90, 220
  immune system and, 198
Metabolic stimulants, 233
Methionine, 36, 110, 220–21, 291
Metropolitan Life Insurance Company
    Tables, 262
Milk, 221

Milk-free diet, 206
Milk intolerance, 201, 203–4, 206
Minerals
    for adolescents, 15–16, 18
    in breast milk, 67
    diuretics and, 129
    in enteral nutrition, 131
    exercise and, 139
    hair analysis for, 172
    in high-fiber foods, 148, 150, 152
    immune system and, 188, 198–200
    in infant formula, 191
    lost in food processing, 156
    in parenteral nutrition, 247
    during pregnancy, 260–61
    stress and, 284
    work performance and, 320
    See also specific minerals
Molybdenum, 222
    copper and, 109
Monocytes, 192, 193
Monosodium glutamate (MSG), 279
Monounsaturated fats, 55, 103
Mucus, 192
Muscle mass
    aging and, 23
    iron and, 16
Myocardial infarction, 109

Narcotics, 18
    during pregnancy, 261
National Academy of Sciences, 24, 249
    Food and Nutrition Board of, 106,
        109, 123, 124, 210
National Cancer Institute, 114
National Food Consumption Survey,
    318
National Institutes of Health, 323
Nausea, 164, 170
    in gastritis, 166, 167
    during pregnancy, 257

NDGA, 49
Neuroses, gastrointestinal symptoms
    in, 164
Neurotransmitters, 171, 174, 215, 285
New York City Department of Health,
    56
New York Heart Association, 324
Niacin (B$_3$), 303
    in adolescence, 15
    in high-fiber foods, 148
    in milk, 221
    in tea, 287
Nightshades, 222
Nitrites, 83
Nitroglycerin, 31

Obesity, 226–36, 318–19
    in adolescence, 14–15
    aging and, 23
    arteriosclerosis and, 54, 56
    aspartame and, 62
    cardiovascular disease and, 100
    childhood, 158
    definition of, 226–28
    diabetes and, 115
    diagnosis of, 229–30
    etiology of, 228–29
    exercise and, 137
    heartburn and, 165
    high-density lipoproteins and, 105
    hypertension and, 178–79, 274
    immune system and, 188, 194, 199
    osteoporosis and, 243
    postpartum, 259
    prevention of, 230–31
    as public health problem, 226
    risk factors for, 230–31
    saccharin and, 11–12
    stress eating and, 285
    sucrose and, 286
    treatment of, 231–36

Occupational Safety and Health
  Administration (OSHA), 321
Oral contraceptives, 129–30, 313, 315
  folacin deficiency and, 39–40, 154
  hypertension and, 178
  immune system and, 200
  pyridoxine deficiency caused by, 304
  risk of heart disease and, 105
Osteoclasts, 238
Osteoporosis, 21, 22, 80, 237–45, 314
  aluminum and, 35
  dietary guidelines for preventing,
    241–45
  laxatives and, 128
  nature of, 237–41
  phosphorus and, 249
  risk factors for, 240
Ovary, cancer of, 85
Ovo-lacto vegetarianism, 289
Oxylate in kidney stones, 214

Pancreas
  cancer of, 78
  in diabetes, 115
  hypoglycemia and, 187
Pancreatitis, 27–28
Pantothenic acid, 246, 298
  immune system and, 196
Papain, 246
Parathyroid hormone, 237, 238
Parenteral nutrition, 247
Pasteurization, 157
Pauling, Linus, 196–97
PCP, 18
Pectin, 86
  cholesterol and, 105
Pellagra, 303
Penicillin, 173
Peptic ulcer, 122, 164, 165, 167
Perfluoracetyl bromide, 268
Periodontal disease, 22

Peritonitis, 167
Pesticides, 88, 90–91
Phenylalanine, 36, 62, 248
Phenylketonuria, 62, 248
Phospholipids, 215
Phosphorus, 15, 22, 24, 219
  breast-feeding and, 71
  in butter, 76
  calcium and, 80
  deficiency of, 35
  drugs causing loss of, 128, 129
  fluoride and, 153
  in milk, 221
  osteoporosis and, 237, 244
  tooth formation and, 113
Physical fitness, *see* Exercise
Phytate, 209, 315
Pica, 214
  during pregnancy, 257
Pituitary gland, 239
Plaque, 111, 112
Pneumonia, 92, 164
Polynesians, 274
Polyunsaturated fats, 55, 56, 58–61,
    103–4
  immune system and, 195
Postpartum obesity, 259
Potassium, 250–51
  in brewer's yeast, 74
  in butter, 76
  diuretics and, 129
  exercise and, 134
  fasting and, 145
  sodium and, 279
  stress and, 282, 284
Preeclampsia, 16
Pregnancy, 252–63, 313
  adolescent, 16–18, 261
  alcohol consumption during, 30
  bone growth during, 239, 241
  caffeine consumption during, 77–79
  calcium needs during, 81, 113, 314

diabetes mellitus and, 261–62
folacin during, 40, 153
iodine deficiency during, 208
iron needs during, 38, 209, 314
ketosis during, 235
lead contamination during, 215
macrobiotic diet during, 218
nutrition prior to, 262–63
pantothenic acid during, 246
proper diet during, 255–57
specific nutrient requirements dur-
    ing, 254–55
specific nutritional problems of,
    257–59
substances to avoid during, 259–61
toxemia of, 262
vegetarian diet during, 293
vitamin C during, 307
vitamin depletion during, 200
weight gain during, 252–53
zinc deficiency during, 40, 315
Premature births, 16
    alcohol as preventive of, 32
Premature infants
    amino acid requirements of, 36
    cysteine for, 110
Preservatives, 11, 13
Pritikin diet, 269, 270
Processing of food, 156–59
Progesterone, 238, 239
Prostate cancer, 85
    polyunsaturated fat and, 195
Protein, 36, 264
    for adolescents, 14–15, 17, 18
    aging and, 23
    alcohol and, 29
    for athletes, 223
    in bee pollen, 64
    in breast milk, 66, 67
    in brewer's yeast, 74
    calcium and, 24–25, 244–45
    cholesterol and, 104–5

in diabetic diet, 116, 117, 119
in enteral nutrition, 131
exercise and, 134, 138, 141, 144
fasting supplemented with, 269–71
growth and, 94
heartburn and, 164–65
hypoglycemia and, 187
immune system and, 194–95
in infant formula, 190
kidney disease and, 213
lost in food processing, 156, 157
in macrobiotic diet, 218
in milk, 221
neurotransmitters and, 285
niacin and, 303
for nursing mothers, 71
in parenteral nutrition, 247
during pregnancy, 17, 18, 254,
    261
pyridoxine and, 304
in reducing diets, 234–35, 267–70
stress and, 282–84
sulfur in, 286
thiamine and, 301
in vegetarian diet, 19–20, 289–91,
    293–94
work performance and, 319–20
zinc and, 16
Protein-calorie malnutrition (PCM),
    265–66
Prothrombin, 312
Prudent Diet, The, 123
Psychoses, gastrointestinal symptoms
    in, 164
Psychotherapy for anorexia nervosa,
    46
Puberty, 14
Pyridoxine (B_6), 130, 304
    in adolescence, 15
    in high-fiber foods, 148
    immune system and, 196, 200
    during pregnancy, 254

Ranitidine hydrochloride, 167
Reactive hypoglycemia, 187, 319
Recommended dietary allowances (RDAs)
  for calcium, 81
  for copper, 109
  for folacin, 153
  for iron, 210
  for magnesium, 219
  for niacin, 303
  for protein, 293–94
  for Vitamin C, 306
  for Vitamin D, 245, 309
  for Vitamin E, 310
  for zinc, 328
Red dye II, 12, 83
Reducing diets, 267–73
  balanced, 271–73
  folacin deficiency and, 39
  high-fiber, 150
  impaired absorption in, 267–68
  reduced efficiency of utilization in, 267
  unbalanced, 268–70
  zinc deficiency in, 40–41
Refrigeration, 157
Respiratory infections, vitamin C for, 197
Retinol, *see* Vitamin A
Rheumatoid arthritis, copper and, 109
Riboflavin (B₂), 302
  in adolescence, 15
  in butter, 76
  in high-fiber foods, 148
  immune system and, 196
  in milk, 221
  oral contraceptives and, 130
  in tea, 287
Rickets, 308, 309
Royal College of Physicians, 114

Saccharin, 11–12, 62, 83, 88
Salmonella, 92
Salt, 11, 274–76
  in baby food, 158
  chloride in, 99
  depletion of, during exercise, 134
  in diabetic diet, 121–22
  diet low in, 275–76
  hypertension and, 179–81
  in junk food, 212
  during pregnancy, 262
  See also Sodium
Samburu tribesmen, 274–75
Satiation, 51–52
Saturated fats, 55, 56, 102–3
  in fad diets, 235
  immune system and, 195
  reduced consumption of, 123–24
Scarsdale diet, 234, 269, 270
Scurvy, 306, 307
Seaweed, 277
Selenium, 277–78
  as anticarcinogen, 48
  as antioxidant, 49
  glutathione peroxidase and, 171
  immune system and, 198
Senate Select Committee on Nutrition and Human Needs, 123
Senility, hypertension and, 177
Senses, effect of aging on, 22
Serotonin, 36
Set-point theory, 52–53
Skin, defense against infection in, 192
Skin-fold calipers, 229
Smoking, *see* Cigarette smoking
Sodium, 279
  calcium and, 245
  diet low in, 182–85
  diuretics and, 129
  fasting and, 145
  potassium and, 250
  reduced intake of, 124

stress and, 282, 284
Soft drinks, caffeine in, 77
Spirulina, 277
Spleen, 192
  iron storage in, 209
Spoilage, additives to prevent, 11
Spontaneous abortion, 16
  caffeine and, 78, 79
Sprouts, 279
Sprue, 109
Starches, 24, 86
Sterilization, 157
Stillman diet, 234, 269, 270
Stomach cancer, 85, 88
Stress, 280–85
  body reserves used during times of,
    282
  effects of, 280–82
  gastrointestinal disorders due to,
    166–68
  nutrition and, 282–85
  overeating during times of, 284–85
  in workplace, 320–21
Stroke, 100–101, 317
  hypertension and, 176, 177
  obesity and, 226
Sucrose, 286
  dental decay and, 112
Sucrose polyester, 267–68
Sugars, 24, 86
  in baby food, 158
  dental decay and, 111–12
  in processed foods, 158
  See also specific sugars
Sulfur, 286
Szent-Gyorgi, Albert, 306

T cells, 192–96
Tagamet, 167
Taurine, 287
Tea, 287

Tempeh, 19, 291, 305
Testosterone, alcohol and, 30
Tetracycline, 80–81, 113, 130
Thiamine (B$_1$), 301
  in adolescence, 15
  alcohol and, 27
  in high-fiber foods, 148
  immune system and, 199
  in milk, 221
Threonine, 36
Thymus, 192, 193
Thyroid gland, 208, 213, 238
Thyroid hormone, 239
Tobacco, *see* Cigarette smoking
Tobacco pyrolyzate, 30
Tocopherol, *see* Vitamin E
Tooth decay, *see* Dental decay
Toward Healthful Diets, 123
Toxemia, 262
Toxicity of antioxidants, 49
Triglycerides, 195
Trypsin, 288
Tryptophan, 36, 288
Tryptophan pyrolyzate, 30
Tuberculosis, 164
Tumors
  brain, 164
  intestinal, 170
Type A personality, 100–101
Tyrosine, 248

Ulcer, *see* Peptic ulcer

Valine, 36
Vegans, 289–90
Vegetarian diets, 155, 289–96
  in adolescence, 19–20
  aging and, 25
  breast-feeding and, 71
  brewer's yeast and, 74

Vegetarian diets (*cont.*)
  calcium in, 293
  guidelines for, 293–96
  iron in, 292
  macrobiotic, 218
  osteoporosis, 245
  ovo-lacto, 289
  during pregnancy, 257–58
  protein in, 290–91
  vegan, 289–90
  vitamin B_{12} and, 41–43, 291, 305
  zinc and, 16
Vitamin A, 297, 299–300
  in adolescence, 15
  alcohol and, 19
  as anticarcinogen, 48
  in butter, 76
  immune system and, 195–96
  laxatives and, 129
  lost in food processing, 157
  in milk, 221
  during pregnancy, 260
  work performance and, 320
Vitamin B_1, *see* Thiamine
Vitamin B_2, *see* Riboflavin
Vitamin B_3, *see* Niacin
Vitamin B_6, *see* Pyridoxine
Vitamin B_{12}, 37, 297, 305
  in adolescence, 15
  aging and, 25
  alcohol and, 19
  in gastritis, 166–67
  immune system and, 196, 200
  macrobiotic diet and, 218
  potassium and, 251
  vegetarian diets and, 19, 289–91
Vitamin C, 297, 306–7
  in adolescence, 15
  as anticarcinogen, 48
  as antioxidant, 49
  aspirin and, 128
  in high-fiber foods, 148

  immune system and, 196–97, 199
  iron and, 16, 210, 211, 292
  lost in food processing, 157
  in milk, 221
  for nursing mothers, 72
  oral contraceptives and, 130
  during pregnancy, 260
  stress and, 284, 321
Vitamin D, 297, 308–9
  in adolescence, 15
  in breast milk, 68
  calcium and, 80, 81, 237–38, 242, 245
  laxatives and, 128, 129
  in milk, 221
  during pregnancy, 260
  tooth formation and, 113
  work performance and, 320
Vitamin E, 42, 297, 310–11
  in adolescence, 15
  as anticarcinogen, 48
  as antioxidant, 49
  immune system and, 196
  selenium and, 278
Vitamin K, 130, 297, 312
  laxatives and, 129
Vitamin P, 65
Vitamins, 297–98
  for adolescents, 15–16, 18
  aging and, 25
  in breast milk, 67
  in enteral nutrition, 131
  exercise and, 139
  fat soluble, 297
  hair analysis for, 172
  in high-fiber foods, 148, 150, 152
  immune system and, 188, 195–97, 199–200
  in infant formula, 191
  in junk food, 212
  lost in food processing, 156
  for nursing mothers, 70, 72

in parenteral nutrition, 247
during pregnancy, 260–61
stress and, 284
water soluble, 297–98
work performance and, 320
See also specific vitamins
Vomiting, 164, 170
in bulimia, 75
in gastritis, 167
during pregnancy, 257
stress-induced, 284

Water, 326
conservation of, in stress response,
282, 284
exercise and, 20, 139, 225
fluoridated, 153
potassium and, 250
retention of, 180
working conditions and, 320
Water soluble vitamins, 297–98
See also specific vitamins
Weight loss
in adolescence, 14–15
in anorexia nervosa, 44
breast-feeding and, 67–68, 72
diabetes and, 115
exercise and, 133
through fasting, 145
saccharin and, 11
See also Reducing diets

Weight Watchers, 232
Wernicke-Korsakoff syndrome, 301
Wheat-free diet, 206
White muscle disease, 277
Williams, Roger, 246
Women, 313–16
See also Breast-feeding; Menstrua-
tion; Pregnancy
Workplace, 317–27
conditions in, 320–21
health promotion at, 321–24
nutrition and, 317–20
World Health Organization (WHO),
81, 92

Xanthine oxidase, 222

Zantac, 167
Zinc, 37, 40–41, 328
in adolescence, 15, 16
alcohol and, 19
as antioxidant, 49
in brewer's yeast, 74
copper and, 109
factors affecting absorption of, 42
immune system and, 198
in junk food, 212
in milk, 221
during pregnancy, 254
for women, 313, 315